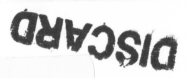

AGING

The Health Care Challenge

Third Edition

An Interdisciplinary Approach
to Assessment and Rehabilitative
Management of the Elderly

AGING

The Health Care Challenge

Third Edition

An Interdisciplinary Approach
to Assessment and Rehabilitative
Management of the Elderly

**CAROLE BERNSTEIN LEWIS,
PT, GCS, MSG, MPA, PhD**

President, Physical Therapy Services of Washington, DC, Inc.

Associate Professor of Clinical Medicine
George Washington University College of Medicine
Washington, DC

 F. A. DAVIS COMPANY • Philadelphia

F. A. Davis Company
1915 Arch Street
Philadelphia, PA 19103

Printed in the United States of America

Last digit indicates print number: 10 9 8 7 6 5 4 3 2 1

Publisher: Jean-François Vilain
Developmental Editor: Ralph Zickgraf
Production Editor: Jessica Howie Martin
Cover Designer: Louis J. Forgione

As new scientific information becomes available through basic and clinical research, recommended treatments and drug therapies undergo changes. The author and publisher have done everything possible to make this book accurate, up to date, and in accord with accepted standards at the time of publication. The author, editors, and publisher are not responsible for errors or omissions or for consequences from application of the book, and make no warranty, expressed or implied, in regard to the contents of the book. Any practice described in this book should be applied by the reader in accordance with professional standards of care used in regard to the unique circumstances that may apply in each situation. The reader is advised always to check product information (package inserts) for changes and new information regarding dose and contraindications before administering any drug. Caution is especially urged when using new or infrequently ordered drugs.

Library of Congress Cataloging-in-Publication Data

Aging, the health care challenge : an interdisciplinary approach to assessment and rehabilitative management of the elderly / [edited by] Carole Bernstein Lewis. — 3rd ed.
   p. cm.
Includes bibliographical references and index.
ISBN 0-8036-0042-9 (hardcover : alk. paper)
  1. Aged—Diseases. 2. Aged—Rehabiliation. 3. Aged—Medical care. I. Lewis, Carole Bernstein.
RC952.5.A48 1995
362.1'9897—dc20
                                     95-460
                                     CIP

Dedication

The editor and contributors to *Aging: The Health Care Challenge* dedicate this third edition to our most memorable older patients, mentors, and role models, especially:

Susan Mellette, MD, long-time colleague and friend

Mary Alexandria Di Michele

Margaret Langdon and *Cornelius Vanderbilt Roosevelt,* memorable patients and wonderful souls

Anna Addicks

George Mackechnie, role model, mentor, and friend

Vernon and *Lorene Irwin*

James R. Bohannon, Jr., who encouraged me to write and taught me to work

Anne Laffey, my most special older patient

James C. Laflin, my twice-widowed 77-year-old father, who recently experienced an intellectual, emotional, spiritual, and physical awakening through his marriage to a younger woman (she's 75)

Sara Williams, who refuses to grow old

Clarissa Marie deVillers Gruppo

Helen Foley, in memory of my mom

Henry and *Florence Yee,* who helped support me in my academic career

Sui Wah Young Yee and *Leong Yun Lai,* whose lives gave me the inspiration to pursue a career in gerontology

Gerald Canter, PhD

Sam Chernoff, my father

Malcolm Muggeridge and *Jacques Ellul,* men of wisdom, men of God

Alice Ajamiam, age 92, who shared her life with me

Jim Tout, my first and most dignified guide through dying and death

Preface

The title of this book, *Aging: The Health Care Challenge, An Interdisciplinary Approach to Assessment and Rehabilitation Management of the Elderly*, Third Edition, accurately sums up the contents of this comprehensive textbook for the rehabilitation professional, written to meet the needs of practitioners and students working in the field of geriatric rehabilitation. The first edition was the first text of its kind; now, there are several textbooks on the topic, but this remains one of the few written for the entire allied health team.

Clinicians will appreciate this book because of the clinical emphasis in each chapter. Each author provides fundamental concepts and explanations followed by assessment and treatment modifications for the older patient. The student will appreciate the clear explanations of treatment techniques and evaluation tools. Background information is provided to help students develop a strong foundation for working with older patients.

This book covers a wide variety of topics directly applicable to clinical practice, as well as those that are peripheral. All topics covered have an important impact on the health care management of the older person. The topics are divided into three sections describing internal variables, physical aspects, and external variables. Each chapter can stand by itself as a specific course unit or be used as a specific study tool for the practicing clinician. Behavioral objectives for each area of clinical study provide the reader with a list of what follows in each chapter. All chapters describe normal and pathologic changes, and evaluation and treatment strategies commonly seen in geriatric rehabilitation practices. Each author is nationally recognized for his or her expertise and has provided a clear, concise chapter.

The third edition has been expanded to include more information in the areas of treating patients with Alzheimer's disease and frail patients as well as new chapters on documentation and health care systems and assessment for the elderly. Also included are clear outlines so that the reader can get a sense of each chapter at a glance.

To get the most from the textbook, readers should have a basic understanding of rehabilitation and current rehabilitation procedures. Each chapter focuses on how these basic procedures can be modified for use with older persons. Thus, students using this book should have some background in rehabilitation procedures. For clinicians currently practicing in rehabilitation, this book should be easy to understand and should expand their current knowledge base.

By the end of Section One, Theories and Psychosocial Aspects of Aging, the reader will have a grasp of classical theories of aging and knowledge of the most recent developments in these theories. This section also includes a chapter on psychosocial changes and other nonorganic aging complications commonly seen in rehabilitation settings.

Section Two, Physical Aspects of Aging, is a review of the body systems with which rehabilitation professionals work directly, including the musculoskeletal, cardiopulmonary, neurologic, and sensory systems. In addition, several chapters deal with important elements of life that are affected by the physical aspects of aging. Each author cites normal and pathological changes, as well as detailed treatment strategies for the practicing clinician and student.

Section Three, External Aspects of Aging: The Current Status, is an investigation of important issues in geriatric rehabilitation. The topics of health promotion, stress, nutrition, sexuality, dying, research, and drugs are all discussed in terms of the older population. The contributors have covered the clinical implications of all these topics in detail and provided comprehensive summaries of current programs and bibliographies.

When one enters the realm of geriatric rehabilitation, the treatment strategy changes; this book provides a strong foundation for clinical expertise in this area, as well as information for further study. The topic of geriatrics can confuse students because so much information must be extrapolated to the needs of the older person.

The editor has selected experts, not generalists, as contributors for this text, so that the level of information available to the reader is high. Specific treatment protocols encompassing current theories in the various areas of rehabilitation are discussed in depth.

To be a good clinician in the geriatric field, it is important to know every aspect of treatment. This book has taught me a great deal, and it is my hope that the reader will feel the sense of challenge, excitement, and rewards to be gained from working with older people that is felt by its contributors.

C.B.L.

Acknowledgments

I would like to extend my deepest appreciation to those who helped make this book possible. The task was made easier by the outstanding contributors, who have been patient and understanding. My thanks to those contributors who have updated their chapters and to those who are new to this edition for providing a strong foundation for use in geriatric rehabilitation.

My thanks as well to Jean-François Vilain, Publisher, Allied Health, F. A. Davis Company, for his support in producing this third edition. I would also like to acknowledge the staff at Physical Therapy Services of Washington, DC, Inc. Special thanks to Theresa Slabe and Tina Conway for their help, to Mai Nguyen for typing and organizing the manuscript, and to my son Gerald Wagner for being such a good baby, thus allowing me the time to meet the tight deadlines.

Contributors

Mary Ferguson Livingstone Belmont, EdD, RN
President
Belmont Healthcare Management, Inc.
New York, New York
Clinical Nurse Specialist for Pain Management
Long Island College Hospital
New York, New York
Adjunct Associate Professor
Columbia University, Teachers College
and New York University
New York, New York
Major, Army Nurse Corps
United States Army Reserve
Visiting Professor
Epsom and Kingston College of Nursing and Midwifery
Surrey, England

Richard W. Bohannon, EdD, PT, NCS
Professor
School of Allied Health
University of Connecticut
Storrs, Connecticut
Coordinator for Clinical Research
Department of Rehabilitation
Hartford Hospital
Hartford, Connecticut

Linda C. Campanelli, PhD
Director and Associate Professor
Graduate Health Professions
Trinity College
Washington, DC

Leora Reiff Cherney, PhD, CCC/SLP
Assistant Professor
Physical Medicine and Rehabilitation
Northwestern University Medical School
Chicago, Illinois
Clinical Researcher, Communicative Disorders
Rehabilitation Institute of Chicago
Chicago, Illinois

Ronni Chernoff, PhD, RD
Associate Director
Geriatric Research Education and Clinical Center
John L. McClellan Memorial Veterans Hospital
Professor, Nutrition and Dietetics
College of Health Related Professions
University of Arkansas for Medical Sciences
Little Rock, Arkansas

Carol M. Davis, EdD, PT
Associate Professor
University of Miami School of Medicine
Department of Orthopaedics and Rehabilitation
Division of Physical Therapy
Coral Gables, Florida

Stephen A. Gudas, PT, PhD
Assistant Professor
Department of Physical Medicine and Rehabilitation
Physical Therapist
Cancer Rehabilitation Program
Medical College of Virginia
Richmond, Virginia

Alona Harris, EdD, RN
Professor
Epsom and Kingston College of Nursing and Midwifery
Surrey, England
Associate Professor
University of Maine at Fort Kent
Fort Kent, Maine
Clinical Nurse Specialist for Complementary Medicine
Belmont Healthcare Management, Inc.
New York, New York

Z. Annette Iglarsh, PT, PhD
Vice President, Eastern Operations
Theraphysics Corporation
Adjunct Associate Professor
University of Delaware
School of Life and Health Sciences
Department of Physical Therapy
Newark, Delaware

Scot C. Irwin, MS, PT, CCS
Director
Department of Physical Therapy and Rehabilitation
Clayton General Hospital
Riverdale, Georgia

Kathleen Kline, PhD, PT, GCS
Assistant Professor of Physical Therapy
Beaver College
Glenside, Pennsylvania

Kristin N. Koehler, MA, RN
Assistant Director of Nursing
Mary Manning Walsh Home
New York, New York
Clinical Nurse Specialist for Elder Care
Belmont Healthcare Management, Inc.
New York, New York

Molly Laflin, PhD
Associate Professor
Bowling Green State University
Bowling Green, Ohio

Carole Bernstein Lewis, PT, GCS, MSG, MPA, PhD
President
Physical Therapy Services of Washington, DC, Inc.
Associate Professor of Clinical Medicine
George Washington University College of Medicine
Washington, DC

Gail Hills Maguire, PhD, OTR/L, FAOTA
Professor, Occupational Therapy
Florida International University
Miami, Florida

Lynn M. Phillippi, MS, PT
Vice President of Career Development
MJ Care, Inc.
Racine, Wisconsin

Jerome F. Singleton, PhD, CTRS
Professor
Leisure Studies Division
School of Recreation, Physical and Health Education
Dalhousie University
Halifax, Nova Scotia, Canada

Betty J. Williams, PhD
Professor of Pharmacology
Associate Dean of Graduate School of Biomedical Sciences
University of Texas Medical Branch
Galveston, Texas

Barbara W. K. Yee, PhD
Associate Professor
Department of Health Promotion and Gerontology
University of Texas Medical Branch
Galveston, Texas

Cynthia Coffin Zadai, MS, PT, CCS
Director
Chest Physical Therapy
Beth Israel Hospital
Boston, Massachusetts

Contents

SECTION TWO: Physical Aspects of Aging

Chapter 3: Activities of Daily Living

Gail Hills Maguire, PhD, OTR/L, FAOTA

Chapter 4: The Effects of Aging on Communication

Leora Reiff Cherney, PhD, CCC/SLP

Chapter 5: Leisure Skills

Jerome F. Singleton, PhD, CTRS

Chapter 9: Cardiopulmonary Rehabilitation of the Geriatric Patient

Cynthia Coffin Zadai, MS, PT, CCS, and
Scot C. Irwin, MS, PT, CCS

Chapter 10: Implications of Oncology in the Aged

Stephen A. Gudas, PT, PhD

Chapter 11: Health Promotion for the Elderly

Mary Ferguson Livingstone Belmont, EdD, RN;
Kristin N. Koehler, MA, RN; and Alona Harris, EdD, RN

SECTION THREE: External Aspects of Aging: The Current Status   277

Chapter 12: Stress and Aging   279
Z. Annette Iglarsh, PT, PhD

Chapter 13: Nutritional Rehabilitation and the Elderly   305
Ronni Chernoff, PhD, RD

Chapter 14: Medication Management and Appropriate Substance Use for the Elderly   325
Barbara W.K. Yee, PhD, and Betty J. Williams, PhD

Chapter 15: Sexuality and the Elderly
364

Molly Laflin, PhD

Chapter 16: Working with the Dying Older Patient
392

Linda C. Campanelli, PhD

Introduction

Carole Bernstein Lewis, PT, GCS, MSG, MPA, PhD

One of the questions most frequently asked by rehabilitation professionals is "What's so different about treating the older person? A hip is a hip." My response is contained in the pages of this book. Although it is true that a hip is a hip, if you can expand your focus and look at the whole picture— the person and his or her support system, living environment, and history— you will have a much better idea of the needs of that particular hip.

When I lecture, I often tell the following story. A friend returned from the mountains with a beautiful photograph of a mountain goat, and in the far left corner was the earnest, excited face of her kid. I told my friend that I loved the picture and wanted a copy. He said, "Sure, I'll crop out the extra features and center the goat." I was aghast. He was going to cut out the kid. For me, the little kid's expression was the essence of the picture.

This experience taught me the importance of guiding others to see the whole picture. Focus on the wholeness of events is crucial to the rehabilitation of the elderly, and it is the approach taken in this text. The various sections do not deal solely with the physiologic systems, but explore the other aspects of the older person as well.

This text focuses on rehabilitation strategies. It is meant to be an introductory text, but even seasoned clinicians will find new insights into common challenges. As rehabilitation professionals are becoming more and more aware of the comprehensive clinically oriented health care programs for the elderly, their concerns lead to a need for more information on the subject. This book fills that need and responds to the increased need for improved health care of the elderly.

Statistics on aging are startling. For example, in the late 1800s, 3 percent of the population was aged 65 or older; today it is approximately 11 percent.[1] In the year 2020, as much as 30 percent of the population could be over 65. In addition, health care needs of the elderly make the older person a major consumer of the various forms of health care. Elderly persons have twice as many hospital stays as their younger counterparts, and the stays last twice as long. In addition, people over age 65 visit the doctor 43 percent more often than those under age 65. The variety of health care settings currently required for the elderly is also much greater than for other segments of the population. Elderly people use hospitals, long-term care settings, rehabilitation facilities, outpatient clinics, respite centers, home care, hospices, and day care centers on a regular basis.[1]

Rehabilitation professionals are concerned about how to provide the best services for each setting. In order to provide appropriate services, however, one must be acutely aware of the statistics on the elderly and the need for improved health care. Some of the innovative health care techniques for managing the increasing health care needs of the elderly are presented here. In addition, suggestions for optimizing care in multiple settings are discussed.

The importance of achieving and maintaining independence for the elderly is emphasized. This concept, along with the concern for improving and optimizing the older person's quality of life, is discussed. The focus on a functional approach emphasizes quality of life and independence through understanding. This understanding is achieved by integrating all facets of the elderly patient's existence into the treatment approach.

Each contributor to this text uses a simple writing style. The emphasis is threefold: (1) to provide the most information in the simplest way; (2) to encourage the reader to use the information in the daily clinical setting, and to think about and share this information with patients; and (3) to serve as a framework for establishing communication among therapists, patients, and support groups.

The text is presented so that even someone with very little experience with elderly patients can develop a useful treatment strategy. Not only clinical skill modifications but also excellent baseline level information on the elderly are provided.

When describing the uniqueness of the elderly, I often refer to the multiplicity of problems that can be seen in this population. For example, as most geriatric practitioners know, a common finding on the chart of newly admitted elderly patients is a list of diagnoses ranging from diabetes to depression. Often the primary diagnosis is only the tip of the iceberg and may not address the real problem, for example, "difficulty with walking because of improper foot care."

To be a top-notch rehabilitation professional in the field of aging, strong investigative skills and the ability to recognize potential problems are required. A statement that is relevant to the treatment of the elderly patients is "the eyes cannot see what the mind does not know." This text is designed to provide the mind with the necessary information to improve the eyes' ability to clinically see rehabilitation problems in a clearer light.

The unique aspect of the elderly is the wide variation that exists within this group. Even though this text describes an average for changes that occur with age, the reader is encouraged to see the extremes that can exist in younger people and understand that with age these variations result in clinical symptoms and responses specific to each individual.

This concept of variation is also useful in encouraging the reader to use carefully considered labels. A label can be useful in some contexts and harmful in others. The authors here are careful to provide useful information on how to avoid using labeling that may preclude proper care for older persons.

Initially, the text provides general information on values, theories, and psychological aspects of aging that are intangible parameters of approaching the elderly patient; the various aspects of function and independent living are explored in terms of activities of daily living, communication, and leisure skills, all crucial aspects for designing a rehabilitation program that focuses on improving the quality of life.

The approach of the middle section of the text is one of review; the areas of the senses, muscles, bones, nervous system, cardiopulmonary system, and the field of oncology are explored. For each of these areas, specific changes with age, ways of integrating information, and avenues of future investigation are explored.

The final section discusses additional aspects of care for elderly persons and treats the aging patient in a holistic fashion. Some controversial yet crucial areas of rehabilitation are explained in detail. The concept of stress is defined and discussed. Implications for creative programming are given.

Drugs as variables to patient outcome are described along with the complications and importance of understanding how drugs can affect the patient's independent functioning.

Aspects of sexuality other than sexual intercourse—a touch, a wink, or a smile—are explored. The focus is on understanding sexuality and learning to enhance and maintain it.

It is hoped that the chapter on research will provide impetus for further study of the health care needs of the elderly. Research on aging can be different from research on other age groups.

In this section, one chapter deals with dying. As Elizabeth Kübler-Ross has said, "Death is a final stage of growth."[2] What therapists must teach is how to plan for and accept death, and how to help patients and families with this stage of life.

Two new chapters have been added to the third edition, one on Medicare documentation and one on treating the frail elderly. These two areas of caring for the aged are constantly changing, yet important to today's practicing clinician.

It was my hope in planning this book to bring together the best clinicians, educators, and writers to create a text that would be comprehensive in the area of rehabilitation and aging. It is meant to provide the clinician with information on how to investigate multiple clinical areas, how to integrate ideas, and how to teach others.

Rehabilitation professionals are now realizing the importance of a multifaceted approach to patient care. This book uses that ideology in the presentation of its material.

One final hope that I have for this book is that it will answer the question "What's so different about treating the older person? A hip is a hip." If those who need this book are able to develop new thoughts on improving health care for the elderly and devising new and more challenging areas of exploration for health professionals working with the elderly, it will have been a success.

REFERENCES

1. American Association of Retired Persons. A Profile of Older Americans. AARP, Long Beach, CA 1992.
2. Kübler-Ross, E. Death: The Final Stage of Growth. Prentice Hall, Englewood Cliffs, NJ 1975.

SECTION ONE

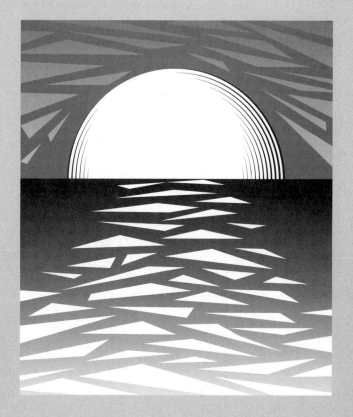

Theories and
Psychosocial Aspects
of Aging

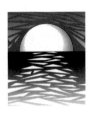

CHAPTER 1

Theories of Aging

Linda C. Campanelli, PhD

BEHAVIORAL OBJECTIVES

Upon completion of this chapter, the reader will be able to:

1 List at least four principal theories of aging.
2 Describe two differences and similarities in the four theories of aging.
3 Identify a factor in each principal theory of aging that may affect rehabilitation.
4 Differentiate between genetic and nongenetic theories.
5 Discuss the reasons why there is no universal theory of aging.
6 Summarize the concept of aging as a developmental process and not a sudden occurrence.

BASIC ASSUMPTIONS

The search for the cure for that nemesis called "old age" has led many scientists to the laboratory. Although several theories of aging have been proposed, only the principal ones will be reviewed here. In theoretic gerontology there are several underlying assumptions that form an important basis for acquiring further knowledge.

1. **Aging is developmental:** This concept is simple but easily forgotten. We do not suddenly age. Our aging time capsules do not go off at 65! We develop into more mature adults and grow older developmentally, not chronologically. This is why later life is unique among all developmental stages. Someone who is 70 years old chronologically may have the physiologic age of a 50-year-old person. Or a 50-year-old may have enough chronic diseases to parallel the physiologic decline of a 90-year-old person.

2. **Old age is a gift of 20th-century science and technology:** Gerontologist James Birren makes the point that our current extended life expectancy is really a gift of modern medicine and modern technology. We are blessed with longer lives because of the discovery of insulin, vaccinations, a decline in infant mortality, and the development of modern surgical techniques and advanced treatment modes for formerly fatal diseases. Also, we are staying older *longer.* The whole phenomenon is new.

3. **Normal aging must be differentiated from pathologic aging:** Often we assume that a functional decline is due to aging. But pathology may often cause functional decline, which is not a normal aging process. For example, if one has adult-onset diabetes, then the probability of cardiovascular disease increases, owing to the effect of the diabetes. However, it is not "normal" to get diabetes; it is a function of lifestyle and heredity in North America. But anyone who lives long enough will develop cataracts, the progressive opacity of the lens of the eye. Cataracts are an example of normal age changes.

4. **There is no universally accepted theory of aging:** Although aging is a universal phenomenon, no one really knows what causes it or why we age at different rates.

Aging theories can be divided into two major categories: genetic and nongenetic. Genetic theories focus on the mechanisms for aging located in the nucleus of the cell. Nongenetic theories focus on areas located elsewhere, such as organs, tissues, or systems. In order to understand the theories, a basic understanding of the three somatic cell types is necessary.

Not all somatic cells age at the same rate; nor do they have similar aging characteristics. Somatic cells are divided into three major categories: continuously proliferating cells, reverting postmitotic cells, and fixed postmitotic cells.[1]

Continuously proliferating cells never cease to replicate themselves, and injury done to these cells is healed through regeneration. Such cells include superficial skin cells, red blood cells, cells of the lining of the intestine, and bone marrow cells. Reverting postmitotic cells have a slower rate of division than continuously proliferating cells, but when there is injury, the rate of division is speeded up and regeneration is possible. Examples of these are kidney and liver cells. Fixed postmitotic cells never replicate once they reach maturity.[1, 2] Muscle cells and nerve cells are primary examples of fixed postmitotic cells. In our adult life, therefore, nerve and muscle cells repair themselves only if the nucleus is intact. Because the postmitotic cell does not replicate itself, no new vital cells are produced. Therefore, the need for residual fixed somatic cells to remain vital is crucial to the well-being and life expectancy of the individual.

GENETIC THEORIES

The study of cellular aging has been somewhat retarded by a historic event in biologic science. Beginning in 1912, Carrel and Ebeling conducted a series of experiments using normal chick embryo fibroblasts cultured in vitro. (In vitro experiments are conducted in an artificial environment, such as a test tube, as opposed to in vivo experiments, which are conducted within the body.)

Based on Carrel's series of experiments, it was thought that fibroblasts could replicate indefinitely and remain virtually immortal. It was not until much later that others, replicating Carrel's studies, found they did not get the same results. Scientists later discovered that the method of preparation of the chick embryo extract was continuously contaminated with fresh embryonic cells. The result was erratic miotic activity coinciding with the periodic addition of chick embryo extract.[2] In other words, these cells lived forever because young embryo cells were mixed with the older prepared culture. Recently, one of Carrel's laboratory assistants, now in her nineties, admitted this.

Hayflick Limit Theory

In 1961, a landmark study by two then-unknown cell biologists, Hayflick and Moorehead,[3] turned the study of senescence of cultured cells completely around. They concluded from their in vitro studies of fetal fibroblast cells (lung, skin, muscle, heart) that human fibroblasts have a limited life span in culture. Fries and Crapo[1] describe their experiment, illustrated in Figure 1–1, as follows:

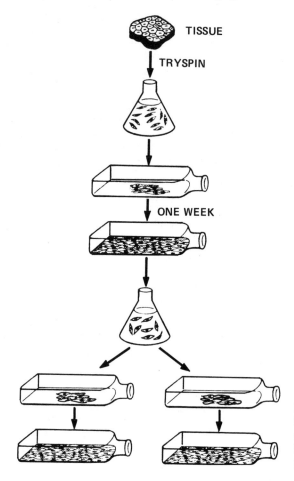

FIGURE 1–1. A schematic drawing of the Hayflick-Moorehead serial cultures of human fibroblasts. (From Fries and Crapo,[1] p. 48, with permission.)

Placed in a flask with liquid tissue culture medium, the cells were grown until they formed a layer across the bottom of the flask. After formation of this primary culture, the enzyme trypsin was added to break the attachments between the cells, which were then divided in half and cultured again to confluence in two new flasks. This subcultivation produces a population doubling, since just enough cells to cover the bottom of one flask become just enough to cover the bottom of two flasks. And the process can be repeated until the cells no longer proliferate. (p. 47)

The Hayflick-Moorehead experiment launched the study of cellular biology and aging and remains a classic to this day.

Repeated studies by Hayflick and others show that the number of cell population doublings ranges from 40 to 60, the average doubling being 50. The developmental senescence process of cultured cells is graphically described in Figure 1–2. Does this mean that the Hayflick limit is intrinsic for embryo cells or that we are mortal because studies in vitro are applicable to humans in vivo? Probably not.

Hayflick noted alterations and degeneration within the cells before they reached their growth limit.[4] These alterations were evident in cell organelles, membranes, and genetic material. What Hayflick may have shown in these studies is that functional changes within cells are responsible for aging and that the cumulative effect of improper functioning of cells and eventual loss of cells in organs and tissues is responsible for the aging phenomenon.

Hayflick's limit has served as a model to others who have shown that population doubling potential is a function of donor age; that is, an inverse correlation exists between donor age and the population doubling potential.[5,6] Evidence of the Hayflick limit has also been seen in cultures taken from individuals with progeria (Hutchinson-Guilford syndrome and Werner's syndrome). Inasmuch as progeria is a premature aging syndrome, the decreased life span of the donors' cells shows a lower Hayflick limit, as expected.[1] Finally, although not as reliable as originally thought, the length of the longest life span for different species and the number of population doublings are correlated. For example, the Galapagos tortoise has a maximum life span of 175 years, with a maximum doubling number of 125, whereas the human maximum life span is 110 years, with a maximum doubling number of 60.[7]

Error Theory

The error theory, also known as the error catastrophe theory, was first presented by Orgel in 1963. The theory specifies that "any accident or error

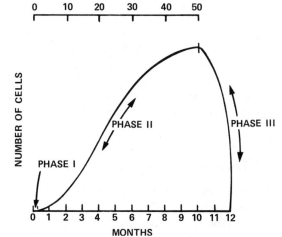

FIGURE 1–2. Growth characteristcs of human embryo fibroblast cultures in vitro. Notice the rapid cell proliferation in phase II and the final cessation of division in phase III. Note that this entire schema represents one individual's entire lifetime. (From Fries and Crapo,[1] p. 49, with permission.)

in either the machinery or the process of making proteins would cascade into multiple effects."[8] A decrease in the fidelity or accuracy of protein synthesis was specifically hypothesized to be caused by errors in proper initiation of the pairing of messenger RNA codon with an anticodon of transfer RNA. However, Hayflick[9] notes that it may not be possible to tell the difference between contributions to cellular aging caused by mistakes in protein synthesis and mistakes due to an accumulation of somatic mutations. Is inaccurate protein synthesis distinguishable from inaccurate DNA synthesis? Is the accuracy of both processes dependent on the fidelity of the other? Are intracellular and extracellular mechanisms of aging coupled, inasmuch as inaccurate protein synthesis affects extracellular events? The interdependence and cumulative effects of errors remain deeply intertwined and somewhat indistinguishable.

Recent experiments contradict Orgel and no longer lend support to the error theory. Experiments have shown that not all aged cells accumulate misspecified molecules and that aging is not necessarily accelerated when misspecified molecules are purposely introduced.[9] However, from a historical viewpoint, it was important to test these hypotheses in order to move toward a more plausible theory.

Redundant DNA Theory

Medvedev[10] has devised a theory that may be coupled to the error theory. He believes that biologic age changes are a result of errors accumulating in functioning genes; but as these errors accumulate, reserve genetic sequences with identical information take over until the system's redundancy is exhausted. This theory is known as the redundant message theory. Medvedev believes that different species' life spans may be a function of the degree of *repeated* genetic sequences. If error occurred in a nonrepeated gene sequence, the chance of preserving intact a final gene product during evolution or a long life span would be lessened.

Redundancy seems to protect mammals from losing vital genetic information during the life span. The major criticism of this theory is that it fails to explain other possible aging factors, such as radiation-induced aging and quantitative aspects of normal aging.

Transcription Theory

Other scientists have developed theories focused specifically on stages of genetic processing. One of these processes, transcription, is the first stage in the transfer of information from DNA to protein synthesis. It entails the formation of messenger RNA, so it contains, in the linear sequence of its nucleotides, the genetic information located in the DNA gene from which mRNA is transcribed.

This theory, according to Hayflick,[9] maintains that:

1. With increasing age, deleterious changes occur in the metabolism of differentiated posmitotic cells.
2. The alterations are the results of primary events occurring within the nuclear chromatin.
3. There exists in the nuclear chromatin complex a control mechanism responsible for the appearance and the sequence of the primary aging events.
4. This control mechanism involves the regulation of transcription, although other regulated events may occur.

There appears to have been insufficient experimentation regarding this hypothesis, but, as Hayflick suggests, this should not imply that the hypothesis is wrong.

When contemplating these theories thus far, one must ask why some cells, such as germ cells and some cancer cells (HeLa and other strains), never age or die. Hayflick[9] suggests that in order to maintain immortality, genetic information is exchanged between these cells, much like the reshuffling of genetic cards when egg and sperm fuse. The reshuffling of a fused sperm and egg cell leads to a fixed life span. As with all species, there appears to be a specific time for decrement and eventual death. Hayflick and others refer to this as "mean time to failure." Perhaps species-related genetic apparatus runs out of correctly programmed material and some species-related repair systems are better than others because they have a longer life span. If so, does that mean we are programmed to age as nature intended it? Is there a programmed theory of aging per se?

NONGENETIC THEORIES

Cross-Linkage Theory

In 1942, Johan Bjorksten[11,12] first related the concept of cross-linkage to developmental aging. Prior to the 1940s, cross-linking was used as a method to stabilize macromolecules for individual purposes, such as vulcanizing rubber. Basically, Bjorksten looked at large reactive protein molecules within the body—such as collagen, elastin, and DNA molecules—and regarded their cross-linkage as responsible for secondary and tertiary causes of aging. According to Bjorksten,[11]

> Crosslinking reactions result in the union of at least two large molecules. A bridge or link between these is usually formed by a crosslinking agent: a small, motile molecule or free radical with a reactive hook or some other

mechanism at both ends, capable of reacting with at least two large molecules. It is also possible for two large molecules to become crosslinked by the action of their own side chains or reactive groups present on one or both of them, or pathologically formed by ionizing radiation. (p. 66)

Figure 1–3 shows the conceptual cross-linkage of DNA.

The implications of cross-linking are enormous. Bjorksten[12] implies that it is the primary cause of sclerosis, failure of the immune system, and loss of elasticity. Aging of the skin is perhaps the most obvious example of cross-linking. Because the tanning process is a form of cross-linkage, exposure to solar radiation promotes cross-linkage. Tanning is the same process used by Native Americans to toughen hides for clothing and shelter. The long-term effect of chronic sun exposure without the use of a sunscreen accelerates aging and promotes significant loss of elasticity of the dermal superficial and deeper layers.

It was once thought that the inflexibility of the body with age was primarily due to the cross-linking of tendon, bone, and muscle tissue. It has since been noted that more active individuals remain more flexible despite constant exposure to cross-linking agents. A combination of exercise and proper diet seems to help inhibit the cross-linking process.

The popularity of the theory stems from the fact that potential cross-linking agents are ubiquitous. Unsaturated fats, polyvalent metal ions (Al, Mg, Zn), and exposure to radiation are a few. The prophylactic use of vitamin E as an antioxidant has been recommended,[13] as well as dietary and drug restrictions of compounds containing cross-linking agents. Such agents are contained in antacids, baking powder, and coagulants, all of which contain aluminum. There is considerable controversy about vitamin E supplements, especially dosage and possible adverse side effects. Selenium and

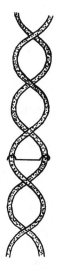 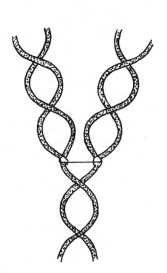

FIGURE 1–3. Representation of cross-linkage splitting a protein molecule. (From Bjorksten,[11] p. 66, with permission of the publisher.)

lecithin have also proven to be effective cross-linking inhibitors (antioxidants); however, the extent of their effectiveness in vivo is not certain.[11]

Free-Radical Theory

Basically, free radicals are highly charged ions whose outer orbits contain an unpaired electron. Free radicals have been shown to damage cell membranes, lysosomes, mitochondria, and nuclear membranes through a chemical reaction called lipid peroxidation. Both membrane damage and the cross-linking of biomolecules result from free-radical chain reactions.[14] The net result of free-radical reactions, as summarized by Leibovitz and Siegel,[15] is a decline in cellular integrity caused by reduced enzyme activities, error-prone nucleic acid metabolism, damaged membrane functions, and accumulation of aging pigments (lipofuscin) in lysosomes.

The accumulation of age pigments does not refer to the dark brown spots on one's hands. Age pigments (lipofuscin) are seen at microscopic levels in self-selected tissues of the body, such as nerve and muscle tissue. The rate of accumulation of age pigments is a good index of chronologic age and perhaps one of the few aging phenomena universally demonstrated in mammals. Age pigments as an entity are examples of degenerative change. When accumulated in tissue, they choke off oxygen and nutrient supplies to surrounding areas, causing further degeneration and eventual death of tissue.

The free-radical theory of aging is attributed to Harmon,[16] whose studies have a history of almost 30 years. There is much support for free-radical reactions and their implications in the aging process as well as their probable pathologic effects as a hypothesized cancer-causing and atherosclerosis-causing agent.

Extensive research has been done regarding the use of antioxidants with free radicals. Vitamin E, vitamin C, selenium, glutathione peroxidase, and superoxide dismutase have been used as free-radical and lipid peroxidase inhibitors.[15] The implication is that there appear to be effective free-radical inhibitors that may prevent further cellular degeneration, such as reduced accumulation of age pigments.

Autoimmune Theory

There have been several theories regarding the phenomenon of autoimmunity. According to these theories, the regulatory machinery of the immune system allows cells reactive against non-self-antigens to flourish by suppressing immune cells reactive against non-self-antigens. In other words, the immune system no longer recognizes some of its own members and becomes self-destructive by literally reacting against itself.

Autoimmune diseases include those affecting the young (for example, lupus erythematosus and scleroderma) and those affecting the old (for example, adult-onset diabetes and senile amyloidosis).[16] Hayflick[9] points out that this hypothesis may not be universally applicable since age changes occur in animals that lack an immune system (invertebrates). What we see, therefore, is a possible genetic explanation as the basis for a nongenetic theory.

Hormonal Theory

D. Donner Denckla, an endocrinologist turned gerontologist, believes that the seat of aging is located in the brain.[17] His theory is based on past studies of hypothyroidism, a disease that mimics mature aging. Hypothyroidism can be fatal if untreated with thyroxine, inasmuch as all the manifestations of aging are evidenced, such as a depressed immune system, wrinkling of the skin, gray hair, and a slowed metabolic rate.

The pituitary gland controls the thyroid gland, and thus the secretion of thyroxine. Thyroxine is the master rate-controlling hormone within the body. However, it is not the release of thyroxine upon which Denckla focuses. Rather, it is the proposed ability of the pituitary to release a hormone labeled decreasing oxygen consumption (DECO), which blocks the cell membrane from taking up thyroxine. Denckla has not isolated the antiaging serum, but he has given us an alternative point of view in theoretic gerontology: the in vivo versus the in vitro controversy. Denckla believes that the aging process in vitro is an artifact and unrelated in any meaningful way to true aging.

Other theories have been proposed with regard to functional decline of various organs and systems. As Hayflick[9] notes, they may simply be the result of more fundamental causes, or the organ system in question may not be universally present in all aging animals.

Data attempting to relate endocrine function to aging do not lend satisfactory evidence to substantiate a significant contribution of endocrine gland function to the process of aging.[18, 19] For example, in response to stress and trophic hormones, the adrenal cortex and thyroid gland remain intact. In women, menopause is a hormone-mediated event that chronicles but does not regulate aging. The ovary is the sole endocrine gland whose functional capacity predictably declines with normal aging. On the other hand, in men, androgen production by the testes is not as predictable because there are individual differences.

Energy-Restriction Theory

Roy Walford[20] is a highly respected research physician and gerontologist at UCLA Medical School and a staunch proponent of a diet based on calorie restriction, also known as energy restriction (ER).

As a result of years of in vivo animal experimentation and research on longevity and life-span potential, Walford has developed a high-nutrient, low-calorie diet that appears to retard the functional, if not the chronological, aging process. Walford has committed himself to a lifestyle based on his own high-low diet, coupled with moderate vitamin and mineral supplementation and regular exercise.

The ER program requires that an individual gradually lose weight over several years until a point of maximum metabolic efficiency is reached for maximum health and maximum life span. Despite more recent reports associating being a little overweight as "healthier" than being underweight, most recent results from the National Institutes of Health Nutrition Committee and the Centers for Disease Control have concluded that "the weights associated with the greatest longevity are below average weights of the population," as long as such weights are not associated with illness.

The high-low diet influences both aging rate and disease susceptibility. Implicit in this dietary practice is abstinence from smoking, limited or no alcohol intake, and control of stress produced by anxiety or frustration, as opposed to stress induced by hard work. Before embarking upon his program, however, Walford recommends that individuals who wish to adopt his dietary regimen have their aging biomarkers evaluated. These include testing for vital capacity, autoantibody levels in the blood, creatinine clearance, glucose tolerance, and serum cholesterol with a determination of levels of high-density lipoproteins (HDL) and low-density lipoproteins (LDL).

Once one has taken the proper evaluation steps, such as engaging the permanent services of a physician to follow one through these lifestyle changes and the initial testing of biomarkers, one is ready to begin losing weight. The high-quality nature of the diet allows individuals to lose weight gradually, over a period of not less than 4 to 6 years, until one is 10 to 25 percent below one's set point for body weight, or 50 percent below whatever is recommended for body fat. "Set point" is defined as one's weight after a considerable period of not overeating or undereating. Walford recommends using the set point for greater accuracy. However, if you are an average-size person with a medium build, targeting a weight 10 to 25 percent below the standard tables used by life insurance companies for your height and body frame will amount to the same degree of loss. Walford cautions, however, that rapid weight loss is counterproductive and that his regimen (usually 1500 to 2000 calories per day, progressing to less than 1500 per day) is not to be used as a crash diet.

ER and Dietary Supplementation

To supplement or not to supplement? That is the question Walford has often addressed, with rather controversial responses. Once a proponent of large-dose supplementation, Walford[20] presently holds the following position:

1. To avoid borderline deficiencies of minerals and vitamins, individuals on the high-low diet should take small amounts of the necessary vitamins and minerals.
2. Supplementing more than the recommended daily allowance (but not in megadose amounts), will, within reasonable probability, enhance average survival prospects.

Walford recommendations and believes that ER, with adequate supplementation, will eventually bring about the desired results.

ER and Exercise

Walford's[20] personal exercise program is "aimed at balancing the positive effects of physical fitness on disease susceptibility against the potentially negative effects of exercise and increased energy turnover on the generation of free radicals" (p. 183). He follows a cross-training approach, which includes weight lifting, swimming, bicycling, jogging, and walking. Emphasizing cardiovascular fitness, Walford recommends exercising three or four times a week for 15 or 20 minutes in order to achieve a target heart-rate range of 70 to 85 percent of one's maximum heart-rate level. A consistent regimen will enable one to increase HDL levels, decrease cardiovascular risk, increase flexibility and strength, and enhance self-perception. It is important to note that this regimen follows the guidelines of the American College of Sports Medicine as well as those of the American Heart Association.

How ER Affects Life Extension Capacity

It has been said that the immune system is the pacemaker of aging.[18] ER has been shown to affect the immune system. For example, it slows down the immune system's decline and inhibits the increased autoimmune reaction.[21] Further, pilot studies in mice point toward evidence that ER may also slow the decline in DNA repair capacity,[22] as well as affect the generation or persistence of free radicals.[23] Recent studies regarding the latter show that lipid peroxidation is lower and that catalase reactions are higher in ER mice than in controls.[24]

Relationship of ER to Other Aging Theories

ER influences widely diverse phenomena, particularly those whose mechanistic possibilities include effects on the immune system, cell basal state and proliferation potential, metabolic rate, DNA repair, levels of free-radical scavengers, chromatin structure, and protein synthesis and turnover.

As can be seen by other theories discussed in this chapter, aging may be caused by a single factor or by many. Thus, the ER model might be useful in analyzing single-factor theories of aging; it might also clarify the significance of physiologic aging markers that correlate with differences in maximum life spans between species.[25]

THEORETICAL IMPLICATIONS OF THE AGING PROCESS FOR PERSONAL HEALTH

Gerontologists and physiologists alike have increased their efforts to convince the public to adopt healthy ways and to learn more about the interrelation of health and aging. Terms such as *biointervention, sarcopenia,* and *set point* have been introduced into the vocabulary. Never before have laboratory and clinical research data been wielded in such a vigorous effort to educate and motivate the public to change unhealthy and age-accelerating behaviors.

Two recently published books address preventive health practices and the aging process. *Biomarkers: The Ten Determinants of Aging You Can Control*[26] and *The Anti-Aging Plan*[27] illustrate the new determination of scientists to educate the general public regarding preventive intervention and personal lifestyle. The authors of these two books speak of assessing one's functional age by using biomarkers, most of which have some predictive value. Walford's list of biomarkers includes forced vital capacity, autoantibodies, static balance, fasting blood sugars, and white blood cell count. He duly notes that after 6 months inside Biosphere 2 there were significant changes in biomarkers and other health-status indicators in the eight people who followed his nutrient-rich antiaging diet.[27]

Evans and Rosenberg emphasize exercise, particularly strength training, as a necessary complement to any aerobic training. They use data from clinical research studies on older adults to support their concept of an individual's "health span," which can be extended by the proper balance of such exercises.[26] These authors, too, cite biomarkers, including muscle mass, strength, basal metabolic rate, percent body fat, blood-sugar tolerance, cholesterol/HDL ratio, blood pressure, bone density, and the body's ability to regulate internal temperature. According to Evans and Rosenberg, the first four markers are closely related and highly indicative of success in preventing sarcopenia.

Although Walford's suggested biointerventions differ from those of Evans and Rosenberg, it is safe to infer that the combination of proper exercise (including aerobic exercise and strength and flexibility training) and proper diet (high in fiber, low in saturated fat and cholesterol) will yield the best possible antiaging results.

SUMMARY

Theories of aging may be divided into genetic and nongenetic. Differences of opinion exist regarding the use of in vitro methods (continued experiments under glass) and in vivo methods (within-the-body observations).

Although Hayflick's limit is the greatest contribution to the history of cellular biology within the past 30 years, Harmon and Tappel's work regarding free-radical theory and Bjorksten's work regarding cross-linking theory also have contributed plausible mechanisms for the implications of their theories. For example, the accumulation of lipofuscin and destruction to cell membranes and organelles may result from free radicals. And cross-linking may play a role in the development of arteriosclerosis and the eventual sclerotic processes seen in scleroderma and progeria patients.

Gerontology has evolved into a more sophisticated science in that we are now able to distinguish between logical, plausible explanations and idealistic searches for the fountain of eternal youth. But the question remains: What causes us to age?

Frolkis, a Soviet gerontologist, was quoted as saying, "the number of hypotheses is generally inversely proportional to the clarity of the problem."[17] This brief overview of theories should confirm the complicated nature of theoretic gerontology. Although there is no universal aging theory, there does exist a universal aging phenomenon of which we are a part, and one day we, too, shall be old.

REFERENCES

1. Fries, I and Crapo, L: Vitality and Aging. WH Freeman, San Francisco, 1981.
2. Hayflick, L: Senescence and cultured cells. In Shock, N (ed): Perspectives in Experimental Gerontology. Charles C Thomas, Springfield, IL, 1966.
3. Hayflick, L and Moorhead, PS: The serial cultivation of human diploid all strains. Exp Cell Res 25:585, 1961.
4. Hayflick, L: The cellular basis for biological aging. In Finch, C and Hayflick, L (eds): The Handbook of the Biology of Aging. Van Nostrand Reinhold, New York, 1977.
5. Martin, GM, Sprague, CA, and Epstein, CJ: Replicative lifespan of cultivated human cells. Lab Invest 23:26, 1970.
6. Schneider, EL and Mitsui, Y: The relationship between *in vitro* cellular aging and *in vivo* human age. Proceedings of the National Academy of Sciences 73:3584, 1976.
7. Stanley, JF, Pye, D, and MacGregor, A: Comparison of doubling numbers attained by cultural animal cells with life span of species. Nature 255:158, 1975.
8. Sonneborn, T: The origin, evolution, nature and causes of aging. In Behnke, J, Fince, C, and Moment, G (eds): The Biology of Aging. Plenum Press, New York, 1979, p 341.
9. Hayflick, L: Theories of aging. In Cape, R, Coe, R, and Rodstein, M (eds): Fundamentals of Geriatric Medicine. Raven Press, New York, 1983.
10. Medvedev, Z: Possible role of repeated nucleotide sequences in DNA in the evolution of life spans of differential cells. Nature 237:453, 1972.
11. Bjorksten, J: The crosslinkage theory of aging: Clinical implications. Compr Ther II:65, 1976.
12. Bjorksten J: Crosslinkage and the aging process. In Rockstein, M (ed): Theoretical Aspects of Aging. Academic Press, New York, 1974, p 43.
13. Bjorksten, J: The place of vitamin E in the quest of longevity. Rejuvenation 3:37, 1975.
14. Tappel, AL: Lipid peroxidation damage to cell components. Fed Proc 32:1870, 1973.
15. Leibovitz, BE and Siegel, B: Aspects of free radical reactions of biological systems: Aging. J Gerontol, 35(1):45, 1980.

16. Harmon, D: Prolongation of life: Roles of free radical reactions in aging. J Am Geriatr Soc 17:721, 1969.
17. Walford, RL: The immunologic theory of aging: Current status. Fed Proc 33:2020, 1974.
18. Rosenfeld, A: Are we programmed to die? Saturday Review 10(2):10, 1976.
19. Davis, PJ: Endocrinology and aging. In Behnke, A, Finch, C, and Moment, G (eds): The Biology of Aging. Plenum Press, New York, 1979, p 273.
20. Walford, RL: The 120-Year Diet. Pocket Books, New York, 1986.
21. Walford, RL: The Immunologic Theory of Aging. Munksgaard, Copenhagen, 1969.
22. Weindruch, R, Chia, D, Barnett, EV, and Walford, RL: Dietary restriction in mice beginning at 1 year of age: Effects in serum immune complex levels. Age 5:111–112, 1982.
23. Harman, D: Free radical theory of aging: Role of free radicals in the origination and evaluation of life, aging, and disease processes. In Johnson, JE, Walford, RL, Harmon, D, and Miguel, J (eds): Free Radicals, Aging, and Degenerative Diseases. Liss, New York, 1986, pp 3–50.
24. Koizumi, A, Weindruch, R, and Walford, RL: Influence of dietary restriction and age on liver enzyme activities and lipid peroxidation in mice. J Nutr 117:361–367, 1987.
25. Walford, RL, Harris, S, and Weindruch, R: Dietary restriction and aging: Historical phases, mechanisms and current directions. J Nutr 117:1650–1654, 1987.
26. Evans, W and Rosenberg, I: Biomarkers. Simon & Schuster, New York, 1991.
27. Walford, RL and Walford, L: The Anti-Aging Plan. Four Walls and Eight Windows, New York, 1994.

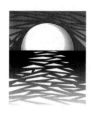

CHAPTER 2

Psychosocial Aspects of Aging

Carol M. Davis, EdD, PT

BEHAVIORAL OBJECTIVES

Upon completion of this chapter, the reader will be able to:

1 List the three challenges of aging in all human beings.
2 Discuss the normal psychologic processes undergone by all aging people, such as emotional development and maturity, changes in motivation, changes in relating to the body as it ages, and minimal change in learning capacity.
3 Differentiate between acute and chronic brain syndromes and between depression and dementia.
4 Contrast the major sociologic theories of aging.
5 Describe psychoneuroimmunology and its impact on the aging process.
6 Identify ways in which the family plays a central role in caring for the elderly person.

Growing older can be one of the richest of life's stages. All too often, the process of aging is associated with lack and limitation, decline and helplessness. This chapter presents some current psychologic and sociologic perspectives in geriatrics that emphasize aging as a positive developmental process. Theories of both normal and abnormal psychologic and sociologic aging are reviewed.

Relevant theories of normal psychologic development will be discussed. Although much has been written on the development of personality, Erik Erikson's work serves as a general model of normal psychologic development. The dialectic between the needs of the body and the intentions of the self, and between cognitive development and learning capacity, are reviewed. Finally, the concept of motivation is examined, with special emphasis on the expectations of the elderly person.

Traditionally, we think of rehabilitation as appropriate solely for those who are ill or injured, but this chapter takes a look at the rehabilitation needs of those who are aging psychologically in a normal way. In this instance, the concept of *rehabilitation* includes activities designed to maintain optimal functioning and prevent age-related changes in the neuromusculoskeletal and cardiopulmonary systems.

The focus of the chapter shifts to a consideration of common psychopathology in the elderly person. Hypochondriasis, depression, and dementia will be discussed, followed by rehabilitation concerns for all three conditions.

Attention will then shift from the individual to the group, and common theories of normal sociologic aging will be reviewed. Spiritual considerations of elderly people are briefly reviewed, along with the importance of the family in the care of elderly people. Group rehabilitation focuses on the various approaches that group therapy offers, especially in the presence of pathology. The chapter concludes with a look at the prevalence of burnout among those involved in the rehabilitation of elderly people, with suggestions for its early identification and prevention.

THE ROLE OF REHABILITATION WITH ALL ELDERLY PEOPLE

Berg and Gadow[1] offer the following:

For many, growing old is an enriching, deepening experience; it is distinctly not degenerative or even "business as usual"—that is, trying to remain young or "nearly normal." It is a time of slowing down, of rejecting the physical, material world as ideal, of turning in, distilling experiences for their essences, of becoming clearer, or in some cases, less certain of knowing it all, and, finally, of determining the personal significance of death. (pp. 88,89)

Whitehead[2] suggests three universal challenges that are central to each person's experiencing of aging:

1. Establishing a basis for self-worth less dependent upon economic productivity or social role
2. Interpreting the significance of one's own life
3. Coming to terms with the changes and losses of aging

Whether one finds oneself among the well, the worried well (those with chronic illness) or the ill aging, these challenges prevail. Illness complicates this unfolding process, wherein all attention is focused on day-to-day survival and a return to independent function. Rehabilitation can play a key role in maintaining the highest and deepest quality of life possible. It is important for us, as rehabilitation specialists, to assume that if people could, they would grow old gracefully, with great dignity, peace, and independence in functioning. Many factors can interfere with that goal, however.

NORMAL PSYCHOLOGIC AGING

Erikson's Model of Development

Psychology is the study of the mind. As people age, they undergo changes in the way they view the world and respond to the challenges before them. Many authors have researched normal psychology and personality development, among them Erik Erikson, who is well known for his description of the natural growth process of the personality.[3] Table 2–1 outlines the eight stages of ego development that Erikson predicts each person goes through on the path to mature adulthood. At each stage, life offers challenges to the maturing psyche; the task of the growing person is to overcome the restrictive forces at each stage, and to emerge with a healthy feeling of power and accomplishment. According to Erikson's theory, the family and society exert a major influence on the developing personality. The growing child struggles with opposing forces at each stage, but out of that struggle emerge mature personality traits. For example, in examining the impact of the very first set of forces that challenge the infant (trust versus mistrust) on the final stages of growth (integrity versus despair), Erikson offered this in an interview with E. Hall:[4]

Erikson: A basic sense of trust means both that the child has learned to rely on his (or her) caregivers to be there when they are needed, and to consider himself trustworthy. But just imagine what somebody would be like who had no mistrust at all.

Hall: Gullible, to say the least. We'd probably think such a person wasn't very bright.

Erikson: Out of the conflict between trust and mistrust, the infant develops hope, which is the earliest form of what gradually becomes faith in adults. If you say that an adult has hope, I'd say, "Well, I

Table 2–1. **Erikson's Eight Stages of Development**

Period in Life	Erikson Stage	Description of Major Dialectic Forces at Work
0–12 months	Trust vs. mistrust	Self-confidence and comfort vs. autistic isolation and fear
2–4 years	Autonomy vs. shame	Asserting self through activity— feeding, toileting vs. (if over controlled) shame and self-doubt
4–5 years	Initiative vs. guilt	Expansive imaginative activity and curisioty vs. feelings of guilt and inhibition with evolving of conscience
6–11 years	Industry vs. inferiority	Competition and achievement leads to self-worth vs. doubt about worth due to parents' status, race, or lack of money
12–18 years	Identity vs identity confusion	Striving to be oneself and share with significant other; break from parents vs. hopeless fear that demands of adulthood are too great
Young adulthood	Intimacy vs. isolation	Trust and intimacy while retaining identity vs. fear and distancing from others who threaten identity
Adulthood	Generativity vs. stagnation	Guiding the next generation by parenting, mentoring vs. anger, hurt, and self-absorption
Maturity and late life	Integrity vs. despair	Acceptance of one's self and one's life as "the best I could do"; ego integrity vs. overwhelmed with tragedies, disappointments, and hurts, thus consumed with anger, despair, and fear of impending death; contemptuous displeasure with self and others

Source: From Erikson,[3] with permission.

hope so," but if you say that a baby has faith, I'd say, "That's quite a baby." Real faith is a very mature attitude.

Hall: So the various strengths take different forms in old age, because they're all tempered by the strength of old age, which is "wisdom."

Erikson: Yes, old age is when a certain wisdom is possible and even necessary, as long as you don't make it too darn wizard-like.

Hall: Perhaps . . . changing what you can change and not changing what you can't hope to change, but wise enough to know the difference.

Erikson: Absolutely, although one hesitates to make it all too simple. (p. 25)

Erikson weaves together the challenge of the very first stages of growth with the challenges of the last stages of growth, on a continuum that can, inevitably, foster the development of wisdom. Wisdom, however, is a characteristic reserved for the later stages of life. In *Identity: Youth and Crisis*, Erikson defines wisdom as the detached and yet active concern with life in the face of death, maintaining and conveying the integrity of experience despite the decline of bodily and mental functions.

Erikson,[4] who died recently but lived well into his eighties, stresses the point that the struggle with the opposing forces is necessary for growth to take place.

> Sometimes what we call the "dystonic tendency" can have positive aspects. For example, during old age the life crisis involves the conflict between integrity and despair. How could anybody have integrity and not also despair about certain things in his own life, about the human condition? Even if your own life was absolutely beautiful and wonderful, the fact that so many people were exploited or ignored must make you feel some despair. (p. 29)

Thus, to grow old in a healthy way on a normal developmental path is to respond to both positive and negative forces but to make choices that increase one's sense of self-esteem and result in feelings of personal power and accomplishment. The ability to do this depends in large part on one's ability to overcome negative, destructive beliefs about one's incompleteness and lack of perfection and the ability to take responsibility for one's life. Those who fail to age in a healthy way often suffer from feelings of low self-esteem and tend to blame the forces of the universe for their problems, failing to take personal responsibility for significant moments in their lives.

Carol Gilligan[5] of Harvard University and Jean Baker Miller[6] of the Stone Center at Wellesley College have criticized Erikson's theory for being incomplete in describing mature personality development. Women psychologists suggest that the independence and autonomy held up by men to be the ideal goals are not only unrealistic but unattainable in a world where no one can exist happily and be totally alone. Instead they suggest that the psychology of personality development needs a new model stressing interdependence, or a healthy sharing of roles and responsibilities. Those writers suggest that women have known this intuitively but have been criticized as immature in desiring meaningful relationships.

Body-Self Differentiation

As children, we think of ourselves as being our bodies. Later, especially during puberty, we come to realize that our bodies are not identical with our *selves*.[7] As the body experiences the natural changes related to the aging process, we develop a unique relationship with it, sometimes separating it from the self when it refuses to cooperate with our expectations. Often elderly patients with hesitant body parts respond to them as if they were separate human beings; for example, one bilateral amputee gave her above-knee stumps names and would call on them to perform exercises.

Florida Scott-Maxwell,[8] in her journal, *The Measure of My Days*, written when she was in her eighties, says this about her relationship with her aging body:

> Always, through everything, I try to straighten my spine, or my soul. They both ought to be upright I feel, for pride, for style, for reality's sake, but both tend to bend as under a weight that has been carried a long time. I try to lighten my burden by knowing it, I try to walk lightly, and sometimes I do, for sometimes I feel both light and proud. At other times I am bent, bent. (p. 39)

Learning Capacity Stability

Contrary to common belief, research shows that learning capacity does *not* decline as one ages. Indeed, the research indicates that "tests of language abilities were performed better by the old non brain-damaged group than they were by the young non brain-damaged group."[9] Testifying before Congress, Robert Butler[10] has said, "If you compare a group of 70-year-olds with a group of 20-year-olds, it might appear that there is a loss in intellectual function among the older people. But longitudinal studies—those which follow the same people over a long period—clearly show that intellectual abilities of healthy people grow greater through the years, not less." (p. 5)

Intelligence, however, is difficult to define, and high or low scores on intellectual function tests do not automatically predict the quality of performance one might expect from an individual.[11] The "classic aging pattern of intelligence" has been described by Botwinick.[12] Verbal abilities decline very little, if at all, over the life span, whereas psychomotor skills decline even as early as the late twenties.

Studies of learning performance indicate that a person's ability to perform new tasks is dependent on intelligence quotient (IQ), learning skills acquired over the years, and flexibility of learning style as well as such noncognitive factors as visual and auditory acuity, health status, motivation to learn, level of anxiety, the speed at which the learning is paced, and the meaningfulness of the material to be learned.[11] More will be said about the importance of these noncognitive factors when we examine the rehabilitation considerations for the elderly vis-à-vis learning ability.

Motivation

One common myth is that, as one ages, it becomes more difficult to stay motivated in seeking the things that will help assure the good life. Maslow[13] has contributed greatly to our understanding of what motivates people. He described five hierarchic stages of need (Fig. 2–1) and theorized that, as the needs of each stage are resolved, they lose their power over behavior and we move to the next higher stage. Basic physiologic and safety needs must be met before a person begins to respond to a sense of belonging or social or love needs. When one's basic needs are met, one naturally seeks out friendships. Only when we feel satisfied that we belong and are loved do we concentrate on developing feelings of self-confidence, self-worth, and self-esteem. Self-esteem is best fostered by inner beliefs about self-worth rather than by praise from others. Finally, the desire for self-fulfillment and for oneness with the universe becomes prominent at the highest level of the hierarchy: self-actualization.[14]

There is no evidence to suggest that motivation diminishes with age.[15] However, the more prominent the physical decline, the more likely that the needs of the elderly will descend to the more basic levels of Maslow's hierarchy. People with vision and hearing deficits worry greatly about their safety, and much of their behavior is controlled by that anxiety. Likewise, safety is a concern for those living in a large city amid forces that are difficult to control—even for the young. Whenever a person feels physically threatened, self-protection impulses dominate and needs revert to the level

MASLOW'S HIERARCHY OF HUMAN NEEDS

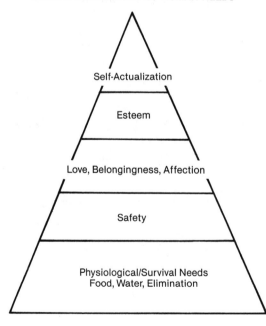

Self-Actualization

Esteem

Love, Belongingness, Affection

Safety

Physiological/Survival Needs
Food, Water, Elimination

FIGURE 2–1. Maslow's hierarchy of human needs. (From Maslow,[13] with permission.)

of safety. The reality of the threat to safety is not as relevant as a person's *perception* of fear and threat.

Rehabilitation Considerations

In the past, most health professionals concerned themselves with the elderly who were ill or disabled. Today, rehabilitation professionals must also be prepared to work with the worried well, with the chronically ill fighting the daily battle for independent function, and with those who hope to prevent disabling physical decline. Understanding the normal psychology of aging is critical to meeting the needs of *all* elderly people.

People are living longer and healthier lives, and we cannot arbitrarily place all those over age 65 in the same category. In the absence of major pathology, the physical needs of the "young old" (roughly 65 to 75 years) are significantly different from the needs of the "middle old" (76 to 85 years), and the "old old" (86 years and up) show clear differences from both these groups.

For example, the young old may visit a rehabilitation specialist only once or twice a year for a bursitis or arthritic problem. As the aging process continues, the frequency of the visits increases, and the problem becomes more central to the level of function. Rehabilitation specialists would do well to keep in mind the theories of growth and development, the body-self dialectic, and the changes in needs and motivation as essentially well and normal elderly people increasingly need rehabilitation services.

Overcoming Learning Barriers

Learning new tasks is an integral part of geriatric rehabilitation, Petersen and Orgen[11] suggest attention to the following noncognitive learning factors:

1. Individuals who are not able to see or hear well are not likely to perform at an acceptable level. Be prepared for these people to misunderstand directions, to fail to comprehend, and in general to take longer to respond.
2. Pain and poor physical health also affect performance. Concentration, stamina, and strength are also reduced.
3. Older people often benefit when new material is presented on a continuum with what they already know. Proceed in a slow and careful manner when resistance to new information is expected.
4. Older people seem to need more time to integrate new learning and to rehearse it before it settles into memory. Concentrate on one task at a time to minimize concurrent interference. Space learning experiences well enough apart.

5. Reduce the potential for distraction whenever possible in order to maximize concentration. Background noise, room conditions, and personal anxiety can be sources of distraction. Observe the person for signs of interference with concentration.
6. Allow the client to set the learning pace. This often means reducing content in a given time period to offer greater clarity, specificity, and depth. Allow adequate time for response to questions, and frame questions so that they are specific and directed. Allow adequate time for the completion of forms.
7. Provide an overview of the entire learning session so that the client can organize the material and anticipate the sequence. Outlines, summaries, and lists of facts or topics to be covered serve as guides to concentration and decrease anxiety about what is coming next.
8. Learning is facilitated when patients hear and see the same material presented at the same time. Written material assists in learning when it is very similar to what is being taught orally. However, if it differs from the spoken presentation, it tends to interfere with learning.

Overcoming Motivational Barriers

Normally, motivation does not decline with aging. However, difficulty with communication, complex prescriptions, chronic illness, and cognitive dysfunction can interfere with compliance.[15] Rehabilitation personnel should take these factors into account and plan accordingly.

Anxiety decreases motivation; therefore, providing regular corrective feedback is helpful. The manner in which feedback and instruction are given is very important. Older people, especially those with little interest in rehabilitation or with low self-esteem, typically are less able to accept negative feedback and continue to do well.[11] Paying special attention to the factors listed above will undoubtedly assist in motivation.

Kemp[16] points out that older persons receiving rehabilitation are usually more motivated by "treatment outcomes that are concrete, that are fairly immediate, and that help them to maintain their daily functioning and quality of life." (p. 50). The clinician who wants to analyze an apparent motivation problem can use a simple motivation formula developed by Kemp (Fig. 2–2). The key to helping patients overcome motivation problems is to diminish the real or imagined costs and increase the rewards. Often patients struggle with subconscious and unrealistic fears and beliefs. Helping patients to clarify these restrictive fears and beliefs can decrease the perceived cost and improve motivation.

Clarity and meaningfulness are the key factors that ensure motivated involvement. A supportive climate for learning, making the older person feel a part of the situation, and appreciating and valuing the patient regardless of achievement will undoubtedly help sustain continued involvement and progress.[11]

MOTIVATION = WANTS × BELIEFS × REWARDS
             (Clear)   (Positive) (Consistent)
             ——————————————————————
                        COSTS
                  (Real or imagined)

WANTS:
Things, actions, image (become)

BELIEFS:
What is wanted, situation or task at hand, the future, the self

REWARDS:
Pleasure to senses, success in controlling one's life, meaning in life

COSTS:
Real or imagined barriers - physical, psychological, interpersonal

TO IMPROVE MOTIVATION

1. Decrease the perceived cost.

2. Clarify the wants, goals and desires.

3. Correct of clarify critical beliefs and expectations.

4. Provide sufficient rewards to promote desired behavior.

FIGURE 2–2. The motivation formula. (From Kemp,[16] with permission.)

REHABILITATION AND ABNORMAL PSYCHOLOGIC AGING

Three key psychopathologic problems found in elderly people are hypochondriasis, depression, and dementia.

Hypochondriasis

Few things are more frustrating than a family member who is preoccupied with physical ailments. Lewis[17] suggests:

Many times the cause stems from negative feelings, guilt, depression, narcissistic pleasure, or the desire to control. Our society shuns psychological weakness, and physical illness is seen as a more acceptable excuse for nonperformance. When people no longer are able to contribute to society, they may develop physical complaints. They can thus say, "I'm sick, and I need to be taken care of." (p. 25).

The ailment is often very real to the person, and this makes treatment even more difficult, for the goal of rehabilitation is always to help the person return to as independent function as possible. The goal of the hypochondriac is to remain in need of help and attention.

Attention may be the best way for rehabilitation professionals to begin. With these elderly people, feelings of low self-esteem have been built over years of experience and faulty thinking. Thus a cure for hypochondriasis is less probable than an alteration of the elderly person's present feelings. Very often, attending to the uniqueness and importance of the person can make a difference in the person's feelings of self-worth. One way to do this is to design a written contract that clearly and completely outlines the expectations that the patient has of the rehabilitation specialist, the expectations the specialist has of the patient, and the goals that each hopes to achieve in therapy. Each should sign this contract, which is renegotiable but should be time-limited and renewable after a specified period—for example, 2 weeks. In this way, the health professional helps prevent feelings of frustration and failure on the part of both people when treatment seems not to make progress. Likewise, by signing the contract, the patient can be helped to further realize the responsibility of attending to his or her healing. If and when a standstill is reached, and if indicated, the rehabilitation specialist can then, with compassion, suggest that counseling might be in order to deal with the stress that seems to be such a critical factor in the patient's physical ailments.

Above all, it is important to treat even the most complaining of the elderly with respect and dignity, and to hold out the belief that they are not miserable by choice. Setting clear boundaries of professional responsibility lessens the frustration one feels with failure and makes it more difficult for hypochondriacs to avoid the treatment they need most: psychologic counseling.

Depression

Most hypochondriacs appear depressed, but not all depressed people are hypochondriacs. Depression is a state that has been vastly misunderstood for centuries, but recent research has enlightened us concerning its etiology and prevalence in our society. Research indicates that up to 50 percent of the elderly in the United States suffer from depression,[18] a mental state characterized by dejection, lack of hope, and absence of cheerfulness.[19] In the past, it was thought that people were depressed because of situations that occurred in their lives: struggling with loss and feelings of helplessness and profound sadness. Unlike sadness, however, depression lingers for weeks or even months.

There are people who suffer depression and undergo mood swings in regular cycles. Depression may start out as situational but is reinforced and extended by the endocrine system. These people are known to have endogenous or metabolic depression.[20]

Growing older necessitates dealing with loss. Even people with sufficient money to live well in their later years suffer losses as time alters reality: Friends die. Moving out of a house that has grown too large may result in a change of lifelong neighbors. Family members relocate, or a retired couple moves from their neighborhood of many years to the comforts of a milder climate. One's influence in the workplace decreases. Any one of these factors can trigger profound feelings of loss, and depression may ensue. Individuals who failed to keep fit physically also have to cope with the normal physical changes of aging, further threatening their feelings of independence and self-worth.

Elderly people who have a lifelong history of battling with depression often find themselves hopelessly lost as they move into the later adult years. Because few people want to be around depressed people, loneliness results. These lonely elderly people may manufacture or exaggerate physical ailments in order to get the attention they so desperately need. People who are severely depressed may not eat and drink. The resulting dehydration may cause metabolic disturbances along with profound depression, and psychomotor retardation may appear to be pseudodementia on admission[21] (Table 2–2).

Critical to the effective treatment of depression is an accurate diagnosis of all health problems. This can be achieved only with thorough physical and mental status examinations, along with as complete a history as possible. Restoring the body chemistry to normal and ruling out dementia are necessary before the depression can be treated.

Common effective approaches to the treatment of depression include medication, activity, and, less commonly, electroshock therapy. In the presence of endogenous depression, medications such as tricyclic antidepressants, monoamine oxidase (MAO) inhibitors, and lithium carbonate have proven dramatically effective.[22]

In the late 1980s, a new antidepressant medication, Prozac, was approved by the Food and Drug Administration (FDA). Renewed emphasis was placed on studying the link between the psychology and biology of depression as patients on Prozac reported alterations in their self-perceptions. As Kramer[23] notes, Prozac and its cousins Zoloft and Paxil are relatively easy to administer and have very few side effects. However, some people claimed that their loved ones became increasingly aggressive and suicidal after they took Prozac. Like the tricyclics, Prozac increases serotonin levels and activity. The higher responsivity of serotonin makes depressed individuals feel better, but it also gives them more energy to become angry, aggressive, or suicidal.

Rehabilitation professionals are especially helpful in establishing increased feelings of trust and self-worth through carefully designed activity, therapeutic exercise, and massage. Communicating with the depressed patient may be very difficult, especially at first. Maizler[24] suggests that the principal role one should play with depressed elderly patients, whether they are confused or not, is that of listener. Giving undivided attention for a specified amount of time conveys the attitude, "You are important to me." Maizler offers these guidelines:

Table 2–2. **Clinical Features Differentiating Pseudodementia from Dementia**

Pseudodementia	Dementia
CLINICAL COURSE AND HISTORY	
1. Family always aware of dysfunction and its severity	1. Family often unaware of dysfunction and its severity
2. Onset can be dated with some precision	2. Onset can be dated only within broad limits
3. Symptoms of short duration before medical help is sought	3. Symptoms usually of long duration before medical help is sought
4. Rapid progression of symptoms after onset	4. Slow progression of symptoms throughout course
5. History of previous psychiatric dysfunction common	5. History of previous psychiatric dysfunction unusual
COMPLAINTS AND CLINICAL BEHAVIOR	
1. Patients usually complain much of cognitive loss	1. Patients usually complain little of cognitive loss
2. Patients' complaints of cognitive dysfunction usually detailed	2. Patients' complaints of cognitive dysfunction usually vague
3. Patients emphasize disability	3. Patients conceal disability
4. Patients highlight failures	4. Patients delight in accomplishments, however trivial
5. Patients make little effort to perform even simple tasks	5. Patients struggle to perform tasks
6. Patients don't try to keep up	6. Patients rely on notes, calendars, etc., to keep up
7. Patients usually communicate strong sense of distress	7. Patients often appear unconcerned
8. Affective change often pervasive	8. Affect labile and shallow
9. Loss of social skills often early and prominent	9. Social skills often retained
10. Behavior often incongruent with severity of cognitive dysfunction	10. Behavior usually compatible with severity of cognitive dysfunction
11. Nocturnal accentuation of dysfunction uncommon	11. Nocturnal accentuation of dysfunction common
CLINICAL FEATURES RELATED TO MEMORY, COGNITIVE AND INTELLECTUAL DYSFUNCTIONS	
1. Attention and concentration often well preserved	1. Attention and concentration usually faulty
2. "Don't know" answers typical	2. "Near miss" answer frequent
3. On tests of orientation, patients often give "don't know" answers	3. On tests of orientation, patients often mistake unusual for usual
4. Memory loss for recent and remote events usually equally severe	4. Memory loss for recent events usually more severe than for remote events
5. Memory gaps for specific periods or events common	5. Memory gaps for specific periods unusual
6. Marked variability in performance on tasks of similar difficulty	6. Consistently poor performance on tasks of similar difficulty

Source: Adapted from Wells[21]

1. Communicate clearly about time. State exactly how much time you can spend together. At first it may be only 10 minutes, but make sure no one interrupts during that time.
2. Allow expression of feelings.
3. Communicate your understanding that sometimes we can't help feeling this way. But avoid becoming oversolicitous, overcheerful, or gushy. Have a matter-of-fact attitude.
4. Reinforce dignity. Accept anger without reacting or personalizing.
5. Be congruent with your verbal and nonverbal messages and feelings. If you don't have the time or can't give full attention, don't try half-heartedly.
6. Use touch to convey support and caring.
7. Set treatment goals that are achievable in a short period of time.

A group therapy treatment protocol for depressed patients that has proven to be useful is remotivation therapy.[25]

1. Establish a climate of acceptance. The goal is to create and maintain a warm, friendly atmosphere within the group.
2. Develop a bridge to reality; for example, discuss current events and read nonfiction.
3. Engage in sharing the events occurring in the world. Topics are developed from ideas discussed in step 2. Props often help.
4. Encourage an appreciation of work. Patients are stimulated to think about work in relation to themselves.
5. Foster a climate of appreciation. In this final stage, patients are encouraged to express their enjoyment of getting together or to express anything that they particularly enjoyed about the session.

Supervised exercise can be of great benefit in giving the depressed patient a sense of accomplishment. Specified amounts of time on a stationary bicycle, supervised ambulation (especially outdoors), and team sports all assist elderly people in forgetting their troubles for a time and help them reconnect with the larger world. Mood elevation may be facilitated by aerobic exercise, which stimulates endorphin flow.

Reynolds[26] suggests that people who are profoundly depressed must (1) move around, (2) change their environment, and (3) be encouraged to go where there are stimulating sights and sounds, not just sit in a dark room. Environments, he maintains, greatly influence who we are. Painting the walls and moving the furniture around stimulate the mind and body and encourage us to perceive ourselves and our world differently.

Dementia: Identification and Rehabilitation

A variety of terms are used to describe intellectual decline in the later years of life, including senility, delirium, acute and chronic brain syndrome, and dementia. It is important to clarify each of these terms.[27–29]

Senility is a common term that refers to a loss of mental capacity due simply to old age. Use of the term is discouraged because it is associated with the myth that as one ages, mental capacity is expected to decline. The common loss of short-term memory in some elderly people due to lack of intellectual stimulation is very often *not* a sign of developing brain disease, and it is termed *benign forgetful senescence.*

Delirium, a key symptom of acute brain syndrome, is a temporary state of clouded consciousness, drowsiness, or agitation which can also be brought on by dehydration, stress, sleeplessness, a problem with medication, or an acute infectious process. The onset is more rapid than that of dementia from chronic brain syndromes, and it is often quite reversible. But delirium is commonly misdiagnosed as irreversible dementia and often goes untreated.

Dementia, or organic brain syndrome, can be described as a global decline in intellectual function with the loss of ability to manage one's daily life because of the irreversible pathology of brain tissue. With organic brain disease, several aspects of brain function are affected: short-term memory, logic, ability to recognize familiar objects or people, and ability to carry out motor tasks. Dementia can result from untreated acute brain disease or chronic brain disease; in both instances there is cellular death. But the progression of acute brain syndrome can often be halted.

Alzheimer's disease, a chronic brain syndrome, accounts for about half of the cases of dementia. Chronic brain syndrome can also result from Parkinson's disease, cerebrovascular accident, cancer, infectious diseases such as syphilis, and autoimmune diseases such as acquired immune deficiency syndrome (AIDS).

Although the symptoms of Alzheimer's disease (AD) are well known, the definitive etiology and pathogenesis remain unknown. Current research is focused on both genetic and environmental causes. Twin studies of Alzheimer's disease are currently being conducted at Duke University and UCLA. Breitner and Murphy[30] suggest that AD is "an example of a late-onset disorder with putative genetic factors." They suggest that AD is an autosomal dominant trait with age-dependent expression. If one twin is affected, the other twin will probably have the disease, although the age of onset may vary greatly. Small and associates[31] at UCLA report on identical twins aged 81 years old. Only one twin showed signs of Alzheimer's disease; extensive brain studies confirmed the presence of the prodromes of AD in the other twin. The authors concluded that both genetic and nongenetic factors influenced the onset and expression of the disease.

Acute brain syndromes that can lead to dementia may result from thyroid dysfunction, transient ischemic attack, alcoholism, and poisoning. In sum, although both acute and chronic brain syndromes cause irreversible brain cell damage, acute syndromes can be halted, whereas chronic brain syndromes continue and are often the cause of death.

Although dementia from chronic brain disease is irreversible, many people can be helped in rehabilitation. But often we resist becoming involved with these patients and their families. Something about dementia seems to threaten or frustrate us, especially those of us who have not been trained in psychiatry. Many of us would much rather suffer from physical disability than experience "losing our minds." "At the core of this frustration," says Spiker,[32] "is the reality that, as we care for these people, we are forced to stand by and watch the life of a person disintegrate before our very eyes. . . . Personhood, of necessity, requires intact cortical structure. . . . [B]iological life prolongation becomes of secondary importance since it is only organic life that is here prolonged, not the life of a person." (p. 158)

Dementia caused by chronic brain syndromes affects over 1.5 million American adults. Sixty percent of all cases of dementia are due to Alzheimer's disease, 17 percent to multi-infarct phenomena along with Alzheimer's, and 10 percent of all cases are due to multi-infarct disease alone. According to Glenner,[29] "One family in every three will see one of their parents succumb to this disease."

Early diagnosis of chronic brain syndrome is critical in order to differentiate it from the reversible problems of depression and acute brain syndrome. The Mental Status Mini-Exam (Fig. 2–3) is especially easy and useful in this task.[33] Unfortunately, the diagnosis of chronic brain syndrome is often delayed by the patient's ability to hide symptoms from even close family members. The first signs include impairment of recent memory, common to many elderly people; but these patients soon begin to lose the higher, symbolic brain functions and become increasingly disoriented, first to time, then to place, and eventually to people. As patients begin to realize that things are somehow "not right," they become anxious and confabulate or tell lies or partial truths to hide the progression of symptoms.

Agnosia (loss of comprehension of sensation, even with sensory apparatus intact), anomia (inability to remember names and misuse of names and words), apraxia (inability to perform learned motor acts, or the carrying out of out-of-the-ordinary actions that surprise us and seem inappropriate), and aphasia (inability to express oneself appropriately due to the loss of memory of words, or the uttering of nonsense words or gibberish) begin to be manifest in everyday behavior.[27] Patients not only forget where they have put their keys, they can't figure out how to use the keys to open the door. They will stand in front of a television set, wanting to turn it off, but will be unable to figure out how. Then they might turn and say, "Turn that thing off, will you? I'm tired of it."

A phenomenon that demands attention with victims of dementia is "environmental press." Sensory overload or an increase in the number and complexity of demands on patients with dementia will frustrate them. The "press" may take place with more than one person in the room speaking or moving; with a three- or four-step request of the patient, or with voices, music, and other noises stressing the patient all at once.

Date _____

ORIENTATION

	Maximum Score	Score

ORIENTATION
What is the (year) (season) (date) (month)? — Maximum Score: 5
Where are we (state) (county) (town) (hospital) (floor) — Maximum Score: 5

REGISTRATION
Name three objects. Allow yourself one second to say each, then ask the patient to repeat all three after you have said them. — Maximum Score: 3

Give 1 point for each correct answer. Then repeat them until the patient learns all three. Count the trials and record — **Trials** _____

ATTENTION AND CALCULATION
Serial 7's. Subtract 7 from 100 and 7 from that five times. 1 point for each correct.
or
Spell the word "world" backward. — Maximum Score: 5

RECALL
Recall the three objects repeated above. 1 point for each correct. — Maximum Score: 3

LANGUAGE
Identify a pencil, identify a watch. (2 pts.)

Repeat the following, "No ifs ands or buts" (1pt.)

Follow a three-stage command. ("Take your paper in your right hand, fold it in half, and place it in your lap.") (3pts.)

Read and obey the following: "Close your eyes." (1pt.)

Write a sentence. (Grammar and spelling don't count, but must have a subject and predicate.) (1 pt.)

Copy this design. (1pt.) — Maximum Score: 9

Total _____

Level of Consciousness

Alert   Drowsy   Stupor   Coma

FIGURE 2–3. Mental Status Mini-Exam. (From Folstein et al,[33] with permission.)

Patients may refuse to cooperate. They may argue, cry, resist assistance, or even yell, scream, throw things, or move to strike those who attempt to help. This frustration response has been termed a "catastrophic reaction."[27] Family members must be helped to understand that this response is a function of the brain pathology and is not willed behavior. Restructuring the environment, diminishing the sensory overload, and acting to reduce the stress early are important factors in handling catastrophic reactions.[27]

Patients with dementia are capable of learning in spite of growing defects. Memory cues and sensory adjuncts are critical. It often takes up to 2 weeks to learn one new skill. Consistency, praise, and encouragement are important. It is never appropriate to use criticism or negative reinforcement. "You're doing it all wrong!" has no meaning to one who has lost the concept of right and wrong. We must learn to work with these patients as patiently as we would with a child, yet always respecting them as adults.[34]

Caregivers must keep in mind that, "regardless of the level of cognitive abilities, cognitive processes are maximized and behavioral responses become more effectively organized when environmental stimuli are presented to the impaired person in a manner that matches his or her level of cognitive functioning."[35] (p. 18). As the mind becomes less able to focus on certain stimuli, therapeutic interventions must be altered to fit the decline. Five- and six-step tasks should be replaced by two- and three-step tasks; symbolic reasoning and tasks including arithmetic must be replaced with concrete tasks; drawers and cabinets should be labeled with what is inside; emergency telephone numbers in large print should be kept next to the phone; car keys and checkbooks must be hidden. Finally, great attention must be paid to safety: Stair climbing must be monitored, as well as the use of hot water and knives; gates and doors should be kept locked (Table 2–3).

The goal of care is to keep the patient functioning and active for as long as possible. Confinement to bed is inevitable, however. Often pneumonia, decubitus ulcer, or urinary tract infection will cause death.

Social worker Naomi Feil[36] has developed a revolutionary approach to communicating with people struggling with the confusion, raw emotions, and rhythmic rocking of the patient with severe dementia. Validation therapy is an approach which seeks to connect to the inner person's basic human needs by respectfully mirroring his or her behavior or words. The validation worker rephrases words, with empathy, and genuinely matches the rhythmic, nonverbal gestures in order to establish a human connection when logic is no longer a communication option. Case reports indicate a high degree of success in helping patients become calm and in removing the need for medication for agitation. The key concept of validation therapy is that building trust and connection is more important than communicating to "make sense." This is especially helpful in the final stages of dementia.

SOCIOLOGIC THEORIES OF NORMAL AGING

Sociologists study groups of people in an effort to explain, understand, and predict human behavior. Here we will discuss four well-known explanations of elderly human behavior: the disengagement theory, the activity theory, the subculture theory, and the continuity theory.

Perhaps the most controversial and potentially dangerous theory is the

Table 2–3. Levels of Decline in Function with Alzheimer's Disease Progression

Level	Function	Assets	Limitations	Therapeutic Intervention
6	Normal function			
5	Beginning signs of confusion; inattentive, preoccupied, neglect basic social skills, world affairs; appointments and bills forgotten; simple decisions are forever delayed	Functions independently in manual, task-oriented activities	Unable to use symbols or abstractions or retain information to be used at a later date	No complex conversation, but no supervision required of concrete activities
4	Significant cognitive impairment, appear to be less confused while performing concrete activities. Unable to remember directions and appointments, misplace items, and will not think to ask for help when they need it	Initiates actions to produce desired result, can complete two to three-step sequences, and activities appear to be meaningful	Unable to notice mistakes or problem-solve, cannot plan beyond the immediate present	Simple, error-proof tasks that involve only two- to three-step action-oriented activities, use memory aids
3	Confused, disorganized, and utilize inappropriate gross motor patterns. Attention is oriented to own action. Repetition of actions occur to verify outcome	Easily engaged in repetitive action activities that have predictable outcomes. Imitate activities to explore the effects of their actions on objects	Unable to predict outcome or results. Learning is not possible. Activities are limited to familiar gross motor patterns	Environment should be simple and person should have consistent routine. Use one-step repetitive action-oriented activities
2	Highly disorganized, bizarre or purposeless body movements such as aimless pacing, constant disrobing and redressing, incessant searching for "lost" possessions. Attention is limited to a few minutes.	Person can initiate activity of gross motor behavior. Capable of following demonstrated directions involving familiar motor activity only. Can be diverted to more productive one-step activities for a 15 to 30 minutes	Unaware that actions affect environment. If unsupervised, use bizarre or nonproductive motor activities. Unable to carry two-step activities	Use one-step, repetitive, gross motor action. Must break down activities to step-by step process. Use simple sentences, as language skills deteriorate. Use visual cues. Maintain a predictable routine
1	No spontaneous activity. Persons are profoundly impaired and too disoriented to feed themselves. Unresponsive and stares into space. Attention is not sustained beyond a minute	Person is conscious	Unfamiliar stimuli increase agitation and confusion	Maintain consistent environment, keep sensory channels open and stimulated with familiar sensations. Change should be introduced slowly

Source: From Levy,[35] with permission. (p. 18)

disengagement theory, proposed by Cumming and Henry[37] in 1961. Based on their observations of elderly behavior, they theorized that

> When a person reaches old age, he or she begins to withdraw from society and that society, in turn, withdraws from the individual. Many examples of this can be seen in our society. Older people are less "important" in the nuclear family, in business, and in the social arena in general. According to the disengagement theory, this is a very natural occurrence. Without it, there would be havoc at the death of these people who would hold such important positions in society. For the older person, this becomes a time of freedom; there is now no emphasis on achievement or responsibility.[17] (p. 21)

Not only do theories explain behavior; especially important is the fact that they also can *prescribe* certain behavior. In terms of the disengagement theory, if the prevalent mode of responding to retirees is to expect them to disengage or disappear from our midst, pretty soon many—especially those who are depressed—will begin to do just that. As a result, elderly people get the message that they are no longer wanted or needed. They become indifferent to life and allow themselves to succumb to boredom. For many, this can foretell an early death.

Cumming and Henry have recently publicly disagreed with their own theory and have concluded that people do not naturally disengage.[38] Disengagement behavior is now seen to be an outcome of depression and is not thought of as normal but as a symptom of pathology that is in need of rapid and aggressive treatment.

An alternative to the disengagement theory is the activity theory, developed by Robert Butler,[39] author of the Pulitzer-Prize-winning book *Why Survive? Being Old in America* and former director of the National Institute on Aging. Butler maintains that

> older people must stay active and involved to continue to maintain their own integrity. The nature of the activities may change by becoming, for example, less physically stressful. However, they must be as important as other previous activities were in the person's life.[17] (p. 21).

The activity theory was further defined by others. Lemon, Bengston, and Peterson[40] tested the theory and distinguished different preferred types of activity. Informal activity (interaction with close friends, relatives, and neighbors) was preferred over formal (participation in voluntary organizations) and solitary (leisure and household activity) activities. Longino and Kart[41] repeated the study and found "that while solitary activities had no effect, and while formal activities had a negative effect, again informal activities had a positive effect on life satisfaction." (p. 713).

A third theory, the subculture theory, states that elderly people become a small group unto themselves, with their own values, mores, inside jokes, feelings, and norms that only they can understand.[42] This theory can be found in the creation of activist groups such as the Gray Panthers and the

American Association of Retired Persons. Whether elderly people constitute a minority group—thus a subculture—is debatable: Research indicates that the aged do not yet share a strong group consciousness, as measured by voting patterns or similar attitudes and values.[43]

The final theory to be discussed here is the continuity theory proposed by Neugarten.[44] This theory

> assumes that in the process of becoming adults, persons develop habits, preferences, etc. that become part of their personalities throughout their life experience. These habits and preferences are brought into old age. The continuity theory claims that neither activity nor inactivity assumes happiness. It posits that most older people want to remain engaged with their social environment and that the magnitude of this engagement varies with the person according to life-long established patterns and self-concepts. It further recognizes the interrelationships of biologic and environmental factors with psychologic preferences. Positive aging becomes an adaptive process involving interaction among all elements.[45] (p. 56)

Neugarten[46] suggests that certain tasks must be accomplished for people to age successfully, including:

1. Accepting the increasing imminence and reality of death
2. Coping with genuine—sometimes painful, severely disabling—physical ill health
3. Coordinating the necessary dependence on medical, domestic, and family support, and making an accurate estimation of the available independent choices that can still be made in order to achieve maximum satisfaction
4. Giving and obtaining emotional gratification from friends and relatives

Each of these theories informs us how we might best approach and relate to our elderly patients and clients, whether they are well, worried about chronic illness, disabled, or ill. Each theory has been debated at length and tested repeatedly by sociologists. For the purposes of this text, one theory is not better than another, but each theory informs us about the elderly people we serve and points out useful ways to respond to our elderly clients.

The disengagement theory warns us to understand but also to be suspicious of the elderly client who tells us that life no longer has meaning and that he or she just wants to be left alone to die. We now recognize these words as symptomatic of depression.

The activity theory informs us of the importance of activity that is congruent and appropriate to an elderly person's interest. It reminds us of the advantage interaction with family, friends, and neighbors has over solitary activity and formal activities.

The subculture theory instructs us that, at times, to reach our goals we may benefit from elderly persons working with other elderly persons, rather than utilizing only younger people.

Finally, the continuity theory instructs us to get to know our patients well and to provide goals that are consistent with their life activities and world view. Attention must be paid to biologic, psychologic, and environmental processes, and a balance should be emphasized.

CARE FOR THE WELL ELDERLY: PREVENTION AND FITNESS

The well elderly need our help with activities that will prevent deterioration of the body and spirit. Fitness classes that stress stretching and light aerobic activity, nutrition counseling, swimming programs, counseling about medications, and organized sports and games all help keep the elderly from experiencing disengagement and physiologic and psychologic deterioration. Health professionals have a responsibility to offer these health and wellness opportunities both within our institutions and out in the community. Likewise, reminiscence groups add to the self-esteem of the elderly and help fill in history for all who would listen. Asking the elderly to write or tape their autobiographies, and inviting one person to speak to the group, is a way to confirm the unique importance of the lives of people. Videotaping these sessions and inviting children—Brownie troops, for example—is pleasurable to many. Although not considered traditional rehabilitation, surely these measures can be included in prevention and in psychologic and spiritual fitness plans.

SPIRITUAL CONSIDERATIONS

As people enter the final stages of their lives, their thoughts tend to turn inward, and as Erikson has noted, ego integrity and despair become the forces that challenge a successful adjustment to old age. One of the most common questions pondered is, Why have I lived? This question is essentially a spiritual question. Rehabilitation professionals will often be drawn into conversations of this nature by searching patients. Cluff[47] suggests that "All persons, finally, must seek their own god or a depth of understanding that will imbue life with a sense of meaning and purpose." (p. 78).

When patients ask us these questions, most often they are asking for a chance to tell us what they've concluded. We do best to offer not a structured system of beliefs but a listening, compassionate presence and a willingness to share in their questioning. The essence of an effective spiritual response is a personal response. And the most appropriate response to a spiritual question is often, "I don't know. What do you think?"

To the patient who asks, "Why does God let me live so long when I'm no longer any use to anybody?" we might best reply that, in the story of the

Good Samaritan, there had to be a victim in order for there to be a helper. Responding to the needs of the elderly can bring great joy and satisfaction, and when it does, we would do well to assure them of that.

PSYCHONEUROIMMUNOLOGY

Many health care professionals can no longer pretend that they believe in the simplistic view of Newton and Descartes: The body is like a machine; when it's broken, it can be fixed, but over time it simply wears out.

Psychoneuroimmunology is the basic science of a new paradigm for viewing the human body. Based on Einstein's view of energy, it posits that the body and brain are inextricably meshed and that the body is an ever-changing mass that obeys the laws of energy. The mind is not encased in the cranium, but is an integral part of all of the cells of the body. Once a thought is created, the body knows it and records it in tissue. The messengers of thought are the neurotransmitters and neuropeptides. Thus, if I wake up suddenly afraid in the middle of the night, my physiology immediately responds in that thought of fear: my pupils enlarge, my heart accelerates, my hair stands on end, my muscles tense. My blood levels would reflect an outpouring of adrenalin. If I spend an idyllic afternoon walking along the ocean with a dear friend where time seems to stand still, my blood levels would reflect chemicals like interferon and the chemical indicators of joy and peace.

If I and my identical twin, whose body chemistry is generated from identical DNA to mine, both take a ride on a roller coaster, and she thinks it is thrilling and fun, and I think it is awful and frightening, our body chemistries would each reflect our perceptions. Same DNA, same experience, different neurochemistry. Why? Because our inner chemistry is entwined with our perceptions and reflects our mood and thoughts.

The implications of this theory on the process of aging are obvious. If I spend most of my life in anger and fear, adrenalin and the stress hormones will take their toll on my body much more quickly than if I spend my life largely at peace.

Deepak Chopra[48] suggests that we can delay our aging process by developing awareness and following activities that help us to perceive that life is not to be feared. Using the mind-body connection, we can reshape the aging process so that we will live longer and happier lives. Prevention of aging is linked to thoughts that are not fear-based but come from a place of peace and joy. This theory has spiritual overtones and reflects much of the ancient wisdom of the Eastern religions of Hinduism and Buddhism, as well as traditional Western neuroimmunology. It bears serious study, for it may actually replace the outdated ways in which health care views the aging process.

GROUP FORMS OF TREATMENT

Group therapy has been mentioned as an effective treatment mode in dealing with the elderly who suffer from depression and dementia. Exercise groups and therapy groups expand the abilities of one or two professionals and serve as useful modalities as patients help one another. Reality orientation groups for those who are confused and yet have the capacity to be stimulated out of their confusion; validation therapy groups for those who are confused from dementia and will never remember what day it is, or care; remotivation therapy groups for the depressed; sensory stimulation and sensory integration for those with central nervous system disabilities; group therapy for stress management, bereavement, and counseling all contribute to the psychosocial rehabilitation process.[49]

Adult day care is becoming a cost-effective and reasonable alternative to the institutionalization of patients who cannot care for themselves at home. In addition to physical, occupational, recreation, speech, and group therapy, trips to sports events, concerts, museums, and other special events, as well as picnics, meal preparation, and shopping trips, are all alternative activities.[50]

THE IMPORTANCE OF THE FAMILY

Contrary to popular myth, the family still provides the major source of support for the elderly as they age. The elderly desire, above all else, to continue being active, thriving, productive members of the community in which they live.[51] Support from the family maintains this for as long as possible. Most elderly people prefer to receive assistance from family members, and if family is not available, friends and neighbors are the next choice, followed by formal organizations.[52]

Blenkner[53] states that the family must be considered as a functional unit in the delivery of health care services to the elderly. A major task of the rehabilitation team is to assist middle-aged caregivers in performing the role of nurturer to older parents.

Rehabilitation professionals must pay special attention to the primacy of the family network as they provide care to the elderly, especially in their homes. It takes great patience and compassion, especially when one is considered an intruder or an outsider, to provide compassionate care to the patient and to attend to the needs of the rest of the family.

SUMMARY

The psychosocial needs of the well elderly and the worried well and ill elderly are complex and varied. As with all aspects of rehabilitation, individual attention and precise data collection are required in order to identify all problems adequately and to plan for interventions.

Interdisciplinarity is a must, and professionals must learn to work well with colleagues on the health team. The needs of the elderly are far too comprehensive for one person alone to understand, let alone manage.[54]

Burnout rates are high on the average among those who care for the elderly exclusively. Burnout, or professional exhaustion, however, depends on both the stress of the work environment and the personality of the individual. The keys to resisting stress in working with the elderly are the early recognition of the patient's values and goals in rehabilitation, and the setting of realistic goals within realistic time frames. With patients who attempt to manipulate, set written contracts early and emphasize the patient's responsibility for caring for his or her health.[55] Likewise, the health professional must be mature and avoid transferring unmet needs to patients regarding their own grandparents and parents.

Caring for the elderly can be very rewarding. A thorough knowledge of psychologic, sociologic, and psychoneuroimmunologic aspects of aging and a commitment to one's own ongoing professional and personal growth can only increase that enjoyment.

REFERENCES

1. Berg, J and Gadow, S: Toward more human meaning of aging: Ideals and images from philosophy and art. In Spicker, SF, Woodward, KM, and Van Tassel, DD (eds): Aging and the Elderly: Humanistic Perspectives in Gerontology. Humanities Press, Atlantic Highlands, NJ, 1978.
2. Whitehead, EE: Religious images of aging: An examination of themes in contemporary Christian thought. In Spicker, SF, Woodward, KM, and Van Tassel, DD (eds): Aging and the Elderly: Humanistic Perspectives in Gerontology. Humanities Press, Atlantic Highlands, NJ, 1978.
3. Erikson, EH: Identity: Youth and Crisis. WW Norton, New York, 1968.
4. Hall, E: A Conversation with Erik Erikson. Psychol Today, June 1983, pp 22–30.
5. Gilligan, C: In a Different Voice: Psychological Theory and Women's Development. Harvard University Press, Cambridge, 1982.
6. Miller, JB: The development of women's sense of self. Working Paper #12, Stone Center. Wellesley College, Wellesley, Mass., 1991
7. Gadow, S: Body and self: A dialectic. J Med Phil 5(3):172–185, 1980.
8. Scott-Maxwell, F: The Measure of My Days. Penguin Books, Middlesex, England, 1979.
9. Goldstein, G and Shelly, C: Similarities and differences between psychological deficit in aging and brain damage. J Gerontol 30(4):453, 1975.
10. Butler, R: Aging in America. Congressional Record—Senate, July 29, 1976, p S-12750.
11. Peterson, DA and Orgen, RA: Older adult learning. In Jackson, O (ed): Physical Therapy of the Geriatric Patient. Churchill Livingstone, New York, 1983.
12. Botwinick, J: Aging and Behavior: A Comprehensive Integration of Research Findings. Springer, New York, 1978.
13. Maslow, A: Motivation and Personality. Harper & Row, New York, 1954.
14. Ramsden, E: Compliance and motivation. Top Geriatr Rehabil 3(3):1–14, 1988.
15. Stilwell, JE: Common health problems that threaten compliance in the elderly. Top Geriatr Rehabil 3(3):34–40, 1988.

16. Kemp, B: Motivation rehabilitation, and aging: A conceptual model. Top Geriatr Rehabil 3(3):41–51, 1988.
17. Lewis, CB: Aging: The Health Care Challenge, ed 1. FA Davis, Philadelphia, 1985.
18. Blazer, D: Depression in Late Life. CV Mosby, St Louis, 1982.
19. Taber, CW: Taber's Cyclopedic Medical Dictionary, ed 16. FA Davis, Philadelphia, 1989.
20. Zung, WWF and Green, RL: Detection of affective disorders in the aged. In Eisdorfer, C and Fann, WE (eds): Psychopharmacology and Aging. Plenum, New York, 1973.
21. Wells, CE: The differential diagnosis of psychiatric disorders in the elderly. In Cole, JO and Barrett, JE (eds): Psychopathology of the Aged. Raven Press, New York, 1980.
22. Salerno, E: Psychopharmacology and the elderly. Top Geriatr Rehabil 1(2):35–45, 1986.
23. Kramer, PD: Listening to Prozac. Viking Press, New York, 1993.
24. Maizler, JS: Mourning and maturity in later life. Continuing Education, April 1982, pp 23–24.
25. Ebersole, P and Hess, P: Toward Healthy Aging: CV Mosby, St Louis, 1981.
26. Reynolds, DK: Moving out of depression. New Dimension Newsletter, Summer, 1992.
27. Mace, NL, Hardy, SR, and Rabins, PV: Alzheimer's disease and the confused patient. In Jackson, O (ed): Physical Therapy of the Geriatric Patient. Churchill Livingstone, New York, 1983.
28. Feighner, GP, et al: Diagnostic criteria for use in psychiatric research. Arch Gen Psychiatry, 26:57, 1972.
29. Glenner, GG: Alzheimer's disease (senile dementia): A research update and critique with recommendations. J Am Geriatr Soc 30:59–62, 1982.
30. Breitner, JCS and Murphy, EA: Twin studies of Alzheimer's disease. Am J Med Genetics, 44:628–634, 1992.
31. Small, GW, et al: Clinical, neuroimaging, and environmental risk differences in monozygotic female twins appearing discordant for dementia of the Alzheimer type. Arch Neurol 50(2):209–219, 1993.
32. Spicker, SF: Gerontologic mentation: Memory, dementia and medicine in the penultimate years. In Spicker, SF, Woodward, KM, and Van Tassel, DD (eds): Aging and the Elderly: Humanistic Perspectives in Gerontology. Humanities Press, Atlantic Highlands, NJ, 1978.
33. Folstein, MF, Folstein, SE, and McHugh, PR: Mini mental state. A practical method for grading the cognitive state of patients for the clinician. J Psychiatr Res 12:189–198, 1975.
34. Davis, CM: The role of the physical and occupational therapist in caring for the victim of Alzheimer's disease. In Taira, E (ed): Therapeutic Interventions for the Person with Dementia. Haworth Press, New York, 1986.
35. Levy, LL: A practical guide to the care of the Alzheimer's disease victim: The cognitive disability perspective. Top Geriatr Rehabil 1(2):16–26, 1986.
36. Feil, N: Validation therapy. Somatics, Autumn-Winter, 1991–1992, pp 48–51.
37. Cumming, E and Henry, WE: Growing Old: The Process of Disengagement. Basic Books, New York, 1961.
38. Poon, L: Aging in the 1980s: Psychological Issues. American Psychological Association, Washington, DC, 1980.
39. Butler, RN: Why Survive? Being Old in America. Harper & Row, New York, 1975.
40. Lemon, BW, Bengtson, VL, and Peterson, JA: An Exploration of the activity theory of aging: Activity types and life satisfaction among in-movers to a retirement community. J Gerontol 27:511–523, 1972.
41. Longino, CF and Kart, CS: Explicating activity theory: A formal replication. J Gerontol 37:713–722, 1982.
42. Butler, R and Lewis, N: Aging and Mental Health: Positive Psychosocial and Biomedical Approaches. CV Mosby, St Louis, 1982.
43. Streib, GF: Social stratification and aging. In Binstock, R and Shanas, E (eds): Handbook of Aging and the Social Sciences, ed 2. Von Nostrand Reinhold, New York, 1985.
44. Neugarten, BL: Adult personality: A developmental view. Human Dev 9:61–73, 1966.

45. Lipman, A and Ehrlich, IF: Psychosocial theoretical aspects of aging: Explanatory models. Top Geriatr Rehabil 1(2):46–57, 1986.

46. Neugarten, B: Middle Age and Aging. University of Chicago Press, Chicago, 1975.

47. Cluff, CB: Spiritual intervention reconsidered. Top Geriatr Rehabil 1(2):77–82, 1986.

48. Chopra, D: Ageless Body, Timeless Mind. Harmony Books, New York, 1993.

49. Maloney, CC and Daily, T: An eclectic group program for nursing home residents with dementia. In Taira, ED (ed): Therapeutic Interventions for the Person with Dementia. Haworth Press, New York, 1986.

50. Rabinowitz, E: Day care and Alzheimer's disease: A weekend program in New York City. In Taira, ED (ed): Therapeutic Interventions for the Person with Dementia. Haworth Press, New York, 1986.

51. Hawker, M: Geriatrics for Physiotherapists and the Allied Professions. Queen Square, London, 1974.

52. Cantor, MH: Neighbors and friends: An overlooked resource in the informal support system. Gerontological Society Meeting, San Francisco, 1977.

53. Blenkner, M: Social work and family relationships in later life with some thoughts on filial maturity. In Shanas, E and Streib, G (eds): Social Structure and the Family: Generational Relations. Prentice-Hall, Englewood Cliffs, NJ, 1965.

54. Davis, CM: Foundations of interdisciplinarity in caring for the elderly, or, the willingness to change your mind. Physiotherapy Pract 4:23–25, 1988.

55. Davis, CM: The "difficult" elderly patient: Stressful effects on the therapist. Top Geriatr Rehabil 3(3):74–84, 1988.

SECTION TWO

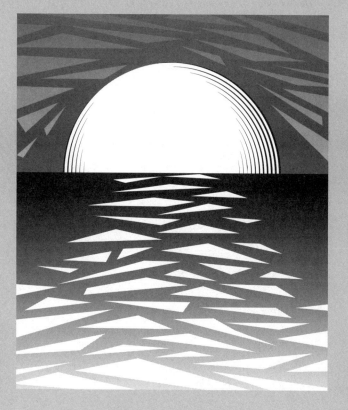

Physical Aspects of Aging

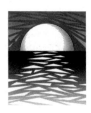

CHAPTER 3

Activities of Daily Living

Gail Hills Maguire, PhD, OTR/L, FAOTA

BEHAVIORAL OBJECTIVES

Upon completion of this chapter, the reader will be able to:

1 Identify the range of activities included under activities of daily living (ADL).
2 List methods to measure independence in ADL.
3 Describe certain ADL and instrumental ADL assessments
4 Identify the appropriateness of specific assessments in various situations.
5 Identify the categories of ADL included in the Maguire Trilevel ADL Assessment (MTAA).
6 Score a sample MTAA.
7 Describe three common functional problems of the elderly, including (1) reduced strength and endurance, (2) decreased joint mobility, and (3) increased danger of accidents.
8 Discuss a practical suggestion for each of the common functional problems.

Health status may be defined in physical, mental, or social terms[1,2] but usually has one of two meanings in relation to the elderly: (1) the absence of death, disease, disability, dysfunction, or discomfort[3,4] or (2) the degree of functional capacity or disability. This chapter is based on the latter meaning, which permits measurement in relation to departures from normal life roles or activities rather than medical or biologic criteria.[5,6] Explaining health in terms of functional design also assumes that motion is necessary in all parts of the body for functional capacity.

When we think about functional capacity, the tasks and activities of daily living come to mind. Research in this area tends to divide these essential activities into two categories: activities of daily living (ADL) and instrumental activities of daily living (IADL). ADL refers to those activities associated with self-care such as eating, dressing, grooming, toileting, and transfers. IADL includes more complex daily activities such as cooking, cleaning, using the telephone, and financial management.

Katz and Akpom[7] suggest that patients recovering from illness or disability pass through three successive stages of recovery, beginning with feeding and continence, then transferring and toileting (social and cultural aspects), followed by dressing and bathing. This pattern has some elements in common with Leering's[4] design. Pedretti[8] defines ADL to include mobility, self-maintenance, communication, and home-management tasks that enable people to be independent in their environment.

The inconsistency in defining and measuring ADL is reflected in the forms used in evaluation. The number of items included in various indexes ranges from a dozen to 85 or more. Often individual items are grouped into categories for ease of evaluation and recording, but even the categories are not uniform. The measures to determine level of performance in these categories also vary. In the past, researchers have measured functional capacity through rank-ordered descriptions such as "independent," "independent with aids," "requires some supervision/assistance," or "dependent." This approach leads to complicated decisions as to the degree of required assistance and effect of equipment.[9] For instance, how do you rate an elderly person who uses a bath rail for safety but, if necessary, could manage without it? This inconsistent use of criteria by the same or different evaluators is a potential source of unreliability.[10]

Duckworth[11] describes the characteristics of ADL indexes that provide a total score of functional ability and discusses the technical problems of developing such an instrument in terms of reliability and validity. He suggests that some reasonable instruments are available, such as the one developed by Katz and his colleagues[12] or the Barthel Index,[13] and that these should be used when total scores are needed until better indexes are available. His discussion of the influence of time and place, choice of evaluators, problems of scoring and weighing individual items, and sampling of items shows that even when an index is shown to be reproducible and valid, the total score still requires interpretation.

In a study of interrater reliability and criterion validity of gross versus specific ratings of 16 ADL tasks, it was concluded that when activities could be broken down into independent task components, specific protocols similar to the Revised Kenny Self-Care Evaluation were best.[14] When activities were composed of highly interdependent task components, such as transfer activities, a behaviorally anchored gross rating protocol that measures the total gross activity might be more effective.[15]

Some scales in both these methods are arranged in a hierarchical fashion, with tasks arranged in order of difficulty.[12,16] With hierarchical scales, assessments can be terminated at the point in the hierarchy where the patient can no longer perform. Testing can also be shortened by starting the testing at the point in the hierarchy where it is suspected that the first sign of a problem will be detected. Testing can then continue in the appropriate direction based on the results of this initial task. However, with tasks more complex than self-care, such as home-management tasks, factors other than performance ability must be considered, for instance, gender influence and the optional nature of some of the tasks. Many of the household tasks have been traditionally done by women, while men of the present cohort of elderly people have more experience than women with caring for an automobile or finances. In addition, individuals may pay to have household tasks such as cleaning done by someone else. In these instances, it is important that the health professional determine why a person does not perform an activity. It could be because of a recent performance deficit, never having learned how to perform the task, or simply a personal preference not to perform the activity. Therefore, a person may have the capacity or ability to perform an activity but does not include the activity in his or her daily life.

MEASURING INDEPENDENCE

In all the various ADL instruments, one of the following three methods has usually been used to measure independence in ADL:[17] (1) self-reports by the patient, (2) ratings based on observations of the patient's performance by a rater, attendants, or other collaterals, or (3) direct examination by a trained professional such as an occupational therapist. Examples of functional assessments using these three methods of assessment will be discussed below.

Self-Report Assessment

Researchers concerned with classification of large groups of people into similar categories have used the self-report method extensively. Self-report assessments have the advantage of being relatively easy and quick to administer through either verbal interviews or written questionnaires. Interviewers also need less expertise and training to administer self-report assessments. Self-reporting gives important information about the patients' perceptions of their reality, which may be a better indication of how they will function than the number of physical symptoms. However, the converse of this is that, because self-reporting is susceptible to the bias of respondents' perceptions of the situation, the information may not be objective. Patients may also report what they wish or what they think the tester wants to hear rather than objective reality. Responses may be influenced by factors such as the need to remain dependent or the fear that responses will affect health care services such as health insurance reimbursement, placement in an institution, etc. Self-reports can also be heavily influenced by the patient's psychological state at the time of testing.

The Activities of Daily Living Scale, which is a component of the OARS Multidimensional Functional Assessment Questionnaire,[18] was designed as part of a comprehensive interview (Fig. 3–1). The eight areas covered in the scale include eating, dressing, grooming, walking, bed transfers, bathing, continence, and availability of a helper.

The Instrumental Activities of Daily Living Scale, also part of the OARS Multidimensional Functional Assessment Questionnaire,[18] was designed as part of the same interview process as the ADL Scale (Fig. 3–2). The seven areas include activities beyond self-care: using the telephone, traveling, shopping, meal preparation, housework, medication, and money management.

A shorter screening version of an IADL Scale is the five-item Instrumental Activities of Daily Living Screening Questionnaire,[19] which covers the same areas as the OARS instrument except telephoning and medication (Fig. 3–3).

The 10-item Hebrew Rehabilitation Center for Aged Vulnerability Index[20] includes use of ambulation devices, time spent outside, and how much illness interferes with activities. This scale covers some activities and resources that may be needed by individuals with handicaps in addition to age-related problems.

A quick review of these scales shows that there are many different versions of similar assessments. This is because similar scales have been developed in response to a perceived assessment need that does not appear to be adequately or efficiently covered by the existing instruments. For example, a shorter version of a scale may be developed for an elderly population that does not have the time or endurance to complete several full scales or in response to screening for only specific targeted problems. It is up to practitioners to choose the scales that best suit their needs while also considering the validity and reliability of the instrument.

Ratings Based on Observation of Behavior

The Revised Parachek Geriatric Behavior Rating Scale[21] is an example of an assessment based on observation of behavior. (Fig. 3–4) It was designed

Activities of Daily Living (ADL)

1. Can you eat . . .
   2 without help (able to feed yourself completely),
   1 with some help (need help with cutting, etc.),
   0 or are you completely unable to feed yourself?
   - Not answered

2. Can you dress and undress yourself . . .
   2 without help (able to pick out clothes, dress and undress yourself),
   1 with some help,
   0 or are you completely unable to dress and undress yourself?
   - Not answered

3. Can you take care of your own appearance, for example combing your hair and (for men) shaving . . .
   2 without help,
   1 with some help,
   0 or are you completely unable to maintain your appearance yourself?
   - Not answered

4. Can you walk . . .
   2 without help (except from a cane),
   1 with some help from a person or with the use of a walker, or crutches, etc.,
   0 or are you completely unable to walk?
   - Not answered

5. Can you get in and out of bed . . .
   2 without any help or aids,
   1 with some help (either from a person or with the aid of some device),
   0 or are you totally dependent on someone else to lift you?
   - Not answered

6. Can you take a bath or shower . . .
   2 without help,
   1 with some help (need help getting in and out of the tub, or need special attachments on the tub),
   0 or are you completely unable to bathe yourself?
   - Not answered

7. Do you ever have trouble getting to the bathroom on time?
   2 No
   1 Yes
   0 Have a catheter or colostomy
   - Not answered
   [IF "YES" ASK a.]

   a. How often do you wet or soil yourself (either day or night)?
      1 Once or twice a week
      0 Three times a week or more
      - Not answered

8. Is there someone who helps you with such things as shopping, housework, bathing, dressing, and getting around?
   1 Yes
   0 No
   - Not answered

FIGURE 3–1. The ADL portion of the OARS Multidimensional Functional Assessment Questionnaire. (From the Older American Resources and Services Methodology, with permission.[18])

Instrumental Activities of Daily Living (IADL)

1. Can you use the telephone . . .
   2 without help, including looking up numbers and dialing,
   1 with some help (can answer or dial operator in an emergency, but need a special phone or help in getting the number or dialing),
   0 or are you completely unable to use the telephone?
   - Not answered

2. Can you get to places out of walking distance . . .
   2 without help (can travel alone on buses, taxis, or drive your own car),
   1 with some help (need someone to help you or go with you when traveling),
   0 or are you unable to travel unless emergency arrangements are made for a specialized vehicle like an ambulance?
   - Not answered

3. Can you go shopping for groceries or clothes [ASSUMING S HAS TRANSPORTATION] . . .
   2 without help (taking care of all shopping needs yourself, assuming you had transportation)
   1 with some help (need someone to go with you on all shopping trips),
   0 or are you completely unable to do any shopping?
   - Not answered

4. Can you prepare your own meals . . .
   2 without help (plan and cook full meals yourself),
   1 with some help (can prepare some things but unable to cook full meals yourself),
   0 or are you completely unable to prepare any meals?
   - Not answered

5. Can you do your housework . . .
   2 without help (can scrub floors, etc.),
   1 with some help (can do light housework but need help with heavy work),
   0 or are you completely unable to do any housework?
   - Not answered

6. Can you take your own medicine . . .
   2 without help (in the right doses at the right time),
   1 with some help (able to take medicine if someone prepares it for you and/or reminds you to take it),
   0 or are you completely unable to take your medicines?
   - Not answered

7. Can you handle your own money . . .
   2 without help (write checks, pay bills, etc.),
   1 with some help (manage day-to-day buying but need help with managing your checkbook and paying your bills),
   0 or are you completely unable to handle money?
   - Not answered

FIGURE 3–2. The IADL portion of the OARS Multidimensional Functional Assessment Questionnaire. (From the Older American Resources and Services Methodology, with permission.[18])

The Five Instrumental Activities of Daily Living

1. Can you get to places out of walking distance . . .
   1 without help (can travel alone on buses, taxis, or drive your own car),
   0 with some help (need someone to help you or go with you when traveling), or are you unable to travel unless emergency arrangements are made for a specialized vehicle like an ambulance?
   - Not answered

2. Can you go shopping for groceries or clothes [assuming she or he has transportation] . . .
   1 without help (taking care of all shopping needs yourself, assuming you had transportation),
   0 with some help (need someone to go with you on all shopping trips),or are you completely unable to do any shopping?
   - Not answered

3. Can you prepare your own meals . . .
   1 without help (plan and cook full meals yourself),
   0 with some help (can prepare some things but unable to cook full meals yourself), or are you completely unable to prepare any meals?
   - Not answered

4. Can you do your housework . . .
   1 without help (can scrub floors, etc.),
   0 with some help (can do light housework but need help with heavy work), or are you completely unable to do any housework?
   - Not answered

5. Can you handle your own money . . .
   1 without help (write checks, pay bills, etc.),
   0 with some help (manage day-to-day buying but need help with managing your checkbook and paying your bills), or are you completely unable to handle money?
   - Not answered

FIGURE 3–3. Five-item IADL questionnaire, adapted from the OARS questionnaire. (From Fillenbaum,[19] with permission.)

as a quick-screening device for use with geriatric patients. It includes 10 multiple-choice items grouped into the three categories: physical capabilities, self-care, and social interaction. The score is the sum of the individual ratings of the 10 items. The authors report that a hospital technician who is well acquainted with the patient should be able to rate the patient within 3 to 5 minutes. The patient does not need to be present.

Ratings of Performance by Direct Examination

Self-report and observation methods give an impression of the total level of independence but do not give the detailed objective profile that is often necessary to plan a specific treatment program. Therefore, even if they use self-report or observation methods, most rehabilitation specialists follow these methods with ratings of the patient's actual performance. These rat-

GERIATRIC BEHAVIOR RATING SCALE
(Revised Version)

Directions: You are to observe each patient for behavior or condition present at the time of the observation. There are ten items listed A-J. Under each item, there are five descriptive phrases. Choose the most accurate statement and mark the cumulative progress record at the crosspoint of number and letter. Be sure to use a black pen for the baseline (first) rating. Choose other colors for succeeding ratings.

PHYSICAL CONDITION

A. Ambulation
1. Deteriorative disease (Parkinson's, M.S., etc.)
2. Not ambulatory due to aging or injury
3. Partially ambulatory with walker or help
4. Ambulatory within a short range (bed to bathroom, ward to dining room)
5. Fully ambulatory (can take short walks, go on short trips)

B. Eyesight
1. Totally blind
2. Sees light and shadow (cataracts, glaucoma, aging)
3. Can see well enough to walk most places alone
4. Recognizes most people by sight alone
5. Sees well enough to read or do hand work

C. Hearing
1. Totally deaf
2. Recognizes that there is sound but cannot distinguish what is said
3. Has hearing aid or understands if voice is raised
4. Has some difficulty but usually understands what is said
5. Hears well

GENERAL SELF-CARE

D. Toilet Habits
1. Totally incontinent with no recognition of passage (urinary and anal)
2. Control of bowels but not of urination
3. Little control but notifies or signals aides when help is needed
4. Spasmodic control (sometimes remembers, sometimes not)
5. Always uses commode by self

E. Eating
1. Fed totally, requires soft foods or liquids brought to ward
2. Eats if coaxed and fed–can be taken to dining room
3. Cooperates with aide and can take liquids by self
4. Can handle tableware and feed self with minimal supervision
5. Feeds self regularly with no difficulty

F. Hygiene
1. Must be bathed by aides
2. Can have tub bath with help
3. Bathes self with help and supervision of aides
4. Bathes or washes reasonably when reminded
5. Keep self clean and bathes or washes by self

G. Grooming (hair, shaving, dressing, make-up)
1. No self-care
2. Appreciates when aide dresses hair or shaves patient
3. Asks for help and shows pride in being groomed
4. Attempts to groom self occasionally or if reminded
5. Grooms self daily without reminder

FIGURE 3–4. Revised Parachek Scale. (From Miller and Parachek,[21] p. 280, with permission.)

SOCIAL BEHAVIORS

H. Helps with work on ward (makes bed,
   folds linen, feeds others, etc.)
   1. Never–physically cannot
   2. Never–unwilling
   3. Occasionally if coaxed
   4. Generally–if coaxed
   5. Generally–self-motivated (does not have to be told what to do)

I. Individual Response
   1. Responds minimally and inappropriately to attention of aide
   2. Responds appropriately (verbal or non-verbal) to attention initiated by aide
   3. Attempts non-verbally to initiate contact with a staff member or other patient
   4. Has friendly relation with one other patient or a staff member
   5. Initiates conversations with others and is generally appropriate

J. Group Activities
   1. Shows little or no recognition of what is happening
   2. Responds minimally if attention is directed
   3. Will join group as passive participant if coaxed
   4. Participates in conversations or plans. Does not initiate ideas
   5. Initiates ideas and discusses feelings readily.

FIGURE 3–4. *Continued.*

ings are used to identify specific problem areas as a basis for therapeutic treatment. However, ratings of performance are often difficult to standardize and interpret without lengthy comments. Ratings by a trained observer are easier for simpler self-care activities such as feeding and transfers but are much more difficult for activities such as homemaking.

The Katz Index of ADL[12] was designed as a performance evaluation that has one item for each of six areas: bathing, dressing, toileting, transfers, continence, and feeding (Fig. 3–5). Evaluators select the descriptive statement that best explains the functional level ("independent," "needs assistance," or "dependent") in each of the six areas. This type of assessment gives no indication of the performance components or tasks that are problems in each of the identified areas but does give an overall picture of performance.

The Barthel Index[13] is a rating scale that was designed to obtain information on self-care from medical records or direct observation (Fig. 3–6). The 10 activities assessed include feeding, transfers from wheelchair to bed, grooming, transfers on and off the toilet, bathing, walking or wheelchair ambulation on a level surface, stair climbing, dressing, bowel continence, and bladder continence.

Granger and associates[22] compared a 15-item extended version of the Barthel Index (Fig. 3–7) with an adapted version of the PULSES Profile. The adapted PULSES profile is a scale consisting of six components, reflecting independence in the following areas: physical condition (P), upper-limb functions (U), lower-limb functions (L), sensory components (S), excretory functions

KATZ INDEX OF ADL

For each area of functioning listed below, check number of description that applies. (The word "assistance" means supervision, direction of personal assistance.)

Bathing - either sponge bath, tub bath, or shower.

1. Receives no assistance (gets in and out of tub by self if tub is usual means of bathing)

2. Receives assistance in bathing only one part of the body (such as back or a leg)

3. Receives assistance in bathing more than one part of the body (or not bathed)

Dressing - gets clothes from closets and drawers–including underclothes, outer garments, and using fasteners (including braces if worn).

1. Gets clothes and gets completely dressed without assistance.

2. Gets clothes and gets dressed without assistance except for assistance in tying shoes.

3. Receives assistance in getting clothes or in getting dressed, or stays partly or completely undressed.

Toileting - going to the "toilet room" for bowel and urine elimination; cleaning self after elimination, and arranging clothes.

1. Goes to "toilet room," cleans self, and arranges clothes without assistance (may use object for support such as cane, walker or wheelchair and may manage night bedpan or commode, emptying same in morning).

2. Receives assistance in going to "toilet room" or in cleansing self or in arranging clothes after elimination or in use of night bedpan or commode.

3. Doesn't go to room termed "toilet" for the elimination process.

Transfer -

1. Moves in and out of bed as well as in and out of chair without assistance (may be using object for support such as cane or walker).

2. Moves in or out of bed or chair with assistance.

3. Doesn't get out of bed.

Continence -

1. Controls urination and bowel movement completely by self.

2. Has occasional "accidents."

3. Supervision helps keep urine or bowel control; catheter is used, or is incontinent.

Feeding -

1. Feeds self without assistance

2. Feeds self except for getting assistance in cutting meat or buttering bread.

3. Receives assistance in feeding or is fed partly or completely by using tubes or intravenous fluids.

FIGURE 3–5. Katz Index of ADL. (From Katz, S et al,[12] p. 915, with permission.)

BARTHEL INDEX

	With Help	Independent
1. Feeding (if food needs to be cut up = help)	5	10
2. Moving from wheelchair to bed and return (includes sitting up in bed)	5-10	15
3. Personal toilet (wash face, comb hair, shave, clean teeth)	0	5
4. Getting on and off toilet (handling clothes, wipe, flush)	5	10
5. Bathing self	0	5
6. Walking on level surface (or if unable to walk, propel wheelchair) *score only if unable to walk	0*	5*
7. Ascend and descend stairs	5	10
8. Dressing (includes tying shoes, fastening fasteners)	5	10
9. Controlling bowels	5	10
10. Controlling bladder	5	10

A patient scoring 100 BI is continent, feeds himself, dresses himself, gets up out of bed and chairs, bathes himself, walks at least a block, and can ascend and descend stairs. This does not mean that he is able to live alone: he may not be able to cook, keep house, and meet the public, but he is able to get along without attendant care.

FIGURE 3–6. Barthel Index. (From Mahoney and Barthel,[13] with permission.)

(E), and support factors (S) including psychological, emotional, family, social, and financial supports. Results indicated that the scoring for both the extended Barthel Index and the adapted PULSES Profile appeared valid, reliable, and sensitive for describing functional abilities and change over a period of time.

The Performance Test of Activities of Daily Living (PADI)[23] is an operational application of Goldfarb's model,[24] which asks patients to demonstrate their ability to perform tasks considered essential for functioning at home. Sixteen activities were selected (Table 3–1), and then general items were converted into commands to demonstrate specific actions. Table 3–2 shows these activities broken down into commands of specific actions that could be demonstrated during an interview. A portable kit of all the necessary equipment for the assessment was prepared to make the administration as standard as possible.

The Revised Kenny Self-Care Evaluation[14] is designed for use in the home or sheltered environment. Six categories of self-care activities are measured, including bed activities, transfers, mobility, continence, dressing,

BARTHEL INDEX

The following presents the items or tasks scored in the Barthel index with the corresponding values for independent performance of tasks:

	"Can do "by myself"	"Can do with help of someone else"	"Cannot do at all"
Self-care Index			
1. Drinking from a cup	4	0	0
2. Eating	6	0	0
3. Dressing upper body	5	3	0
4. Dressing lower body	7	4	0
5. Putting on brace or artificial limb	0	−2	0 (not applicable)
6. Grooming	5	0	0
7. Washing or bathing	6	0	0
8. Controlling urination	10	5 (accidents)	0 (incontinent)
9. Controlling bowel movements	10	5 (accidents)	0 (incontinent)
Mobility Index			
10. Getting in and out of chair	15	7	0
11. Getting on and off of toilet	6	3	0
12. Getting in and out of tub or shower	6	0	0
13. Walking 50 yards on the level	15	10	0
14. Walking up/down one flight of stairs	10	5	0
15. IF NOT WALKING: Propelling or pushing wheelchair	5	0	0 (not applicable) _____

BARTHEL TOTAL: BEST SCORE IS 100; WORST SCORE IS 0.

NOTE: Tasks 1–9, the self-care index (including control of bladder and bowel sphincters), have a total possible score of 53. Tasks 10–15, the mobility index, have a total possible score of 47. The two groups of tasks combined make up the total Barthel index, with a total possible score of 100. We customarily prefer to use the four-level adaptation. The main difference between the two versions is that the four-level version describes independent function as either intact or with some limitation, such as the need to use an adaptive appliance. In the case of this study, review of the medical records did not consistently distinguish independent-intact from independent-limited. Therefore, the three-level version was used for this study. Both assessments of independent function receive the same Barthel scoring. Therefore, with either version, the Barthel index score sums are equivalent.

FIGURE 3–7. Modified Barthel Index. (From Granger,[22] with permission.)

Table 3–1. **Tasks in the PADL Performance Test**

Task Requests	**Props**
1. Drink from a cup	Cup
2. Use a tissue to wipe nose	Tissue box
3. Comb hair	Comb
4. File nails	Nail file
5. Shave	Shaver
6. Lift food onto spoon and to mouth	Spoon with candy on it
7. Turn faucet on and off	Faucet
8. Turn light switch on and off	Light switch
9. Put on and remove a jacket with buttons	Jacket
10. Put on and remove a slipper	Slipper
11. Brush teeth, including removing false ones	Toothbrush
12. Make a phone call	Telephone
13. Sign name	Paper and pen
14. Turn key in lock	Keyhole and key
15. Tell time	Clock
16. Stand up and walk a few steps and sit back down	

Source: Kuriansky and Gurland,[23] p. 346, with permission.

Table 3–2. **Sample Items from ADL Performance Test**

Activity	Preparation	Interviewer Instructions	Patient Performance	Rating
Eating	Place candy on spoon and put spoon on flat surface in front of patient	"Show me how you eat"	Grasps spoon by handle	0 1 9
			Keeps spoon horizontal	0 1 9
			Keeps candy balanced on spoon	0 1 9
			Aims at mouth	0 1 9
			Touches spoon to mouth	0 1 9
Grooming	Place comb on table in front of patient	"Show me how you comb your hair"	Takes comb in hand	0 1 9
			Grasps comb properly	0 1 9
			Brings comb to hair	0 1 9
			Makes combing motions	0 1 9
Dressing	Give patient jacket with sleeves	"Put this jacket on for me and then take it off"	Takes hold of jacket	0 1 9
			Slips arm in jacket	0 1 9
			Pulls jacket over shoulders and back	0 1 9
			Slips other arm into sleeve	0 1 9
			Frees one arm	0 1 9
			Frees other arm	0 1 9
			Removes jacket from body	0 1 9

Source: Kuriansky and Gurland,[23] p. 347, with permission.

and feeding. It was an attempt to give a numeric measure to observer ratings. It does not include home-management duties such as washing dishes or cooking.

The Klein-Bell ADL Scale[25] includes 170 items in six areas: dressing, elimination, mobility, bathing and hygiene, eating, and emergency telephone communication.

There is increased need to assess the functional status of patients with dementia. A full review of this area is beyond the scope of this chapter. The Direct Assessment of Functional Status (DAFS) Scale, developed by Lowenstein and associates,[26] is an example of a scale developed to examine the specific areas of functional competence that may become affected by mental impairment (Fig. 3–8).

SCREENING

Screening instruments employ a smaller number of activities to represent larger groups of activities. Screening instruments can be used in all three methods of functional assessment, that is, self-report, observation, and direct examination. Screening can be useful in identifying areas that require a more comprehensive assessment. Screening can be very helpful in initial assessments of the elderly who may present symptoms and functional problems in addition to the ones for which they were referred. However, screen-

Direct Assessment of Functional Status (DAFS)

I. Time Orientation (16 points)

	Correct (2 points)	Incorrect (0 points)
A. Telling Time		
(Use a large model of a clock)		
3:00	————	————
8:00	————	————
10:30	————	————
12:15	————	————
B. Orientation to Date		
What is the date?	————	————
What day is it today?	————	————
What month are we in?	————	————
What year are we in?	————	————

II. Communication (14 points) (Using a push-button telephone) (If at any point the patient dials, picks up, or hangs up the phone, he/she is given credit for items tapping these specific subskills.)

	Correct (1 point)	Incorrect (0 points)
A. Using the telephone	————	————
Dial operator (0)	————	————
Dial number from book	————	————
Dial number presented orally	————	————
Dial number written down	————	————
Pickup receiver	————	————
Ability to dial	————	————
Hang up phone	————	————
Correct sequence across all previous trials	————	————

	Correct (1 point)	Incorrect (0 points)
B. Preparing letter for mailing		
Fold in half	————	————
Put in envelope	————	————
Seal envelope	————	————
Stamp envelope	————	————
Address (has to be exact duplicate of examiner's copy)	————	————
Return address (has to put correct address in upper left-hand corner)	————	————

FIGURE 3–8. DAFS Scale. (From Loewenstein,[26] p. 120, with permission.)

ing is limited to the extent that the specific tasks used in the screening instrument are representative of the tasks that are relevant to the individuals who are assessed.

Activities selected for screening may be based on one or more of the following criteria: common problem areas, sampling of each category of activities, or representation of a certain level of difficulty.

MAGUIRE TRILEVEL ADL ASSESSMENT

Leering[4] has mentioned that the field of geriatrics would benefit from a uniform system to determine functional capacity. Without a structured system, the same items may be listed under many different headings, making it impossible to compare treatments and assessments worldwide.

The Maguire Trilevel ADL Assessment (MTAA) is a systems approach that divides the tasks of daily living into six categories: communication, eating, mobility, hygiene, dressing, and organization. Each category is divided into three environmental levels: personal, home or sheltered environment, and the community (Fig. 3–9).

The MTAA is an initial attempt to conceptualize a developmental analysis of components in each of the categories of activities and is not a research instrument. Categories such as "organization," which are often observed but not formally recorded, have been included. The MTAA can be used as a self-report or observed checklist. No validity or reliability studies are available, and there has been no attempt to differentiate which skills are most critical.

Most rehabilitation specialists devise simple or complex ADL evaluation procedures and forms based on the needs dictated by their environment and patient population. Individual sections of this model can be selected based on the needs of a specific patient population.

For example, the MTAA can be used for an elderly client who is living in the community, one who is independent but needs help in identifying the necessary environmental adaptations that will ensure independence as long as possible. Limited intervention with an elderly patient can make the difference between maintaining an optimal level of functioning and the steady increase in psychological and physical dependency.

Scoring the MTAA

The scoring method for the MTAA is a modification of the system used for the Revised Kenny Self-Care Evaluation.[14] The first step involves a traditional descriptive rating; the second step involves a quantitative scoring of functioning on each of three levels (self-care, home, and community). If the patient is obviously at a very high level of independence, the rehabilitation specialist can ask if he or she is totally independent in a task such as eating. If the answer is yes, mark "independent" and move to the next section. Another approach is to follow that question with a question regarding a more difficult item in the category, such as whether the patient can cut food with a knife.

In the first step, the rater assigns one of the following ratings to each task:

I = Totally independent

S = Needs any degree of supervision

MAGUIRE TRILEVEL ADL ASSESSMENT (MTAA)**

NAME _Jane Smith_   AGE _75_   DATE _2/7/85_

DIAGNOSIS _Rheumatoid Arthritis;_   DATE OF ONSET _1965_
Hypertension R Cataract Surgery c̄ Contact
DATE OF ADMISSION _2/7/85   out patient_

EYEGLASSES _✓_ SPECIAL LENS (TYPE) _R Cataract_ HEARING AIDS ___ R ___ L _✓_

SCORING

1. Rate each task under colum R as
    I = totally independent
    S = any supervision
    A = any assistance
    D = totally dependent
    NA = not applicable

2. Score each level under subtotal as
    4 = all Is in level
    3 = 1 or 2 As or Ss; Others all Is or
       equipment essential to function or safety
    2 = all other configurations
    1 = 1 or 2 As or Ss or 1 I; others all Ds
    0 = all tasks rated D

3. Transfer scores to MTAA
    Score Sheet
    Write summary of each category.

Environment	Categories	Tasks		Evaluation Date:	Progress Rounds:	Progress Rounds:
		COMMUNICATION		R	R	R
Personal	Communication	Follows verbal directions	I			
		Communicates verbally/sign language	I			
		Follows written directions	I			
		Writes name	I			
		Operates signal light	I			
		Operates TV/radio	I			
		Equipment List	✓	L Hearing Aid R Cataract Glasses		
		SCORE	3	Independent c̄ Equipment		
Home	Communication	Types/writes written communication/correspondence	I			
		Uses telephone	I	Rejected Amplifier		
		Opens and seals envelopes	I			
		Opens/locks doors	I			
		Operates light switch	I			
		Operates door bell	I			
		Equipment List	✓	See Personal		
		SCORE	3	Independent c̄ Equipment		

**(c) 1983 Maguire, G. H. Used with permission.

FIGURE 3–9. Maguire Trilevel ADL Assessment. Used with permission.

A   =   Needs any degree of assistance

D   =   Totally dependent

NA   =   Not applicable

This step of the scoring requires the rater to make only two choices regarding the patient's performance: Is the patient totally independent, or does the patient require some assistance or supervision? Does the patient

Environ-ment	Cate-gories	Tasks	Evaluation Date: 2/7/85		Progress Rounds:		Progress Rounds:	
Commu-nity	Communi-cation	Maintains personal contacts	I	MAINLY PHONE				
		Maintains business contacts	I					
		Equipment List	✓	SEE PERSONAL				
			3	INDEPENDENT ̄c EQUIPMENT				

EATING

Person-al	Eating	Finger foods	I					
		Use of utensils	I					
		Pour from container	I					
		Drink (cup/glass/straw)	I					
		Cuts with knife	I					
		Takes medication	I					
		Equipment List	N/A					
		SCORE	4					

Home	Eating-Cooking	Operates faucets	I	NEEDS NEW WASHERS				
		Lights match/gas burner	I					
		Operates appliance controls	I					
		Handles hot foods/liquids	I					
		Uses sharp utensils	I					
		Reaches and transports items to and from refrigerator/cupboards	I	NO HIGH SHELVES				
		Opens containers/pkg. foods	I					
		Opens manual/electric can opener	I					
		Opens screw jars	I					
		Breaks an egg	I					
		Peels/cuts vegetables	I	CUTS SM. PIECES AT TIME				
		Washes/dries dishes	I					

FIGURE 3–9. *Continued.*

require equipment for functioning or safety? The rater does not have to make a judgment on the degree of necessary assistance or supervision. If the patient is independent when using the equipment, an S or A is marked and the equipment is listed. If the patient is obviously on a very dependent level, the rater can give a description rating to only applicable tasks—such as communication, eating, and bed mobility on the personal level—and stop at this point. The rating of other tasks can be continued later. (*Note:* A later rating should be entered, with the date, under the progress note column.)

The next step requires the therapist to give a quantitative rating for each level (personal, home, community) of the six categories (communication through organization). The ratings are recorded on the form as follows:

3

Envi-ronment	Cate-gories	Tasks	Evaluation Date: 2/7/85		Progress Rounds:		Progress Rounds:	
Home	Eating Cooking	Uses measuring devices	I					
		Uses hand (electric) beater	I					
		*Rolls pastry	/					
		Weekly menu/shopping list	I					
		Diet (type) LOW SALT	S	DIDN'T UNDERSTAND; REFERRED TO DIETICIAN				
		Equipment List	N/A	REJECTED REACHER				
		SCORE	3	NEED SUPERVISION & DIET				
Comm-unity	Eating	Food shops	A	NEEDS TRANSPORTATION				
		Equipment List	N/A					
		SCORE	3	DAUGHTER DRIVES HER				

MOBILITY

Person-al	Moving in bed	Shift position	I					
		Turn to left side	I					
		Turn to right side	I					
		Turn to prone	I					
		Turn to supine	I					
		Equipment List	N/A					
Person-al	Rising and Sitting	Come to sitting position	I					
		Maintain sitting balance	I					
		Legs over side of bed	I					
		Move to edge of bed	I					
		Legs back onto bed	I					
		Equipment List	N/A					
Person-al	Sitting Trans-fer	Shift bed to chair	N/A					
		Shift chair to bed	N/A					
		Equipment List	N/A					

*Optional activity

FIGURE 3–9. *Continued.*

4	=	All tasks in the level rated I
3	=	One or two A's or S's; others all I's or equipment essential to function or safety
2	=	All other configurations
1	=	One or two A's or S's or one I; others all D's
0	=	All tasks rated D

After completing the rating of each level, the rehabilitation specialist should transfer the scores to the MTAA score sheet. This gives a summary of

Environ- ment	Cate- gories	Tasks	Evaluation Date: 2/7/85	Progress Rounds:	Progress Rounds:
Person- al	Stand- ing	Slide forward	*I*		
		Position feet	*I*		
		Stand	*I* GREAT EFFORT LOW SOFT CHAIR.		
	Trans- fer	Pivot	*I*		
		Sit	*I*		
		Equipment List	✓ FIRM HIGH CHAIR		
Person- al	Toilet	Position (paper sanitary supplies, etc.)	*I*		
		Manage equipment	*I*		
	Trans- fer	Transfer to commode	*I* RAISED SEAT BETTER		
		Undress	*I*		
		Dress	*I*		
		Transfer back	*I*		
		Equipment List	✓ GRAB BAR—TOILET SEAT—MUCH SAFER.		
Person- al	Bath- ing	Tub/shower approach	*I*		
		Use of grab bars	*I*		
	Trans- fer	Tub/shower entry	*I*		
		Tub/shower exit	*I*		
		Equipment List	✓ HAS STALL SHOWER SEAT + GRAB BAR— EASIER.		
		SCORE	3 INDEPENDENT ⊆ EQUIPMENT		

Home	Loco- mot- ion	Travels 30'	*I*		
		Travels 100'	*I*		
		Turns	*I*		
		Carries object	*I*		
		Opens/travels through door	*I*		
		Picks up object from floor	*I* DIFFICULT		
		Gets down/up from floor	*I* DIFFICULT		
		Stairs ___with rails ___without___ goes down/up ramp	*I* RAILS HELPFUL		

FIGURE 3–9. *Continued.*

the patient's functioning level in each category. An average score for each category may be done. For purposes of reporting, a descriptive summary of each level on completion of the MTAA might be as follows:

4 = Totally independent

3 = Mainly but not quite independent; requires equipment or extra time

2 = All other combinations; the specific degree of assistance, supervision, and equipment required should be described

5

Environ-ment	Cate-gories	Tasks	Evaluation Date: 2/7/85	Progress Rounds:	Progress Rounds:
		Equipment__w/c _✓_other (specify) CANE/SUPPORT	✓		
		SCORE	3	INDEPENDENT ē CANE	
Home	Wheel Chair Mobi-lity	Positions chair	N/A		
		Brakes on/off			
		Arm rests on/off			
		Footrests on/off			
		Positions transfer board			
		Equipment List	↓		
		SCORE	N/A		
Commu-nity	Loco-motion	Crosses street with traffic light	S	TOO SLOW TO BE SAFE	
		Operates elevator	I		
		Transfers in/out car	I		
		Transfers equipment/w/c in/out car	N/A		
		Uses public transportation	A	DIFFICULTY ē BUS STEP, FEAR	
		Operates w/c on rough surfaces	N/A		
		Equipment List	✓	CANE	
		SCORE	3	UNSAFE IN TRAFFIC/BUS	

HYGIENE

Person-al	Face Hair and Arms	Handkerchief, tissue	I		
		Wash face	I		
		Wash hands and arms	I		
		Brush teeth and dentures	I		
		Shaving/make-up	I		
		Manicure	I		
		Equipment List	N/A		
Person-al	Trunk and Peri-neum	Wash back	I	LONG-HANDLED BATH BRUSH EASIER	
		Wash buttocks	I		
		Wash chest	I		

FIGURE 3–9. *Continued.*

1 = Mainly dependent with one or two exceptions

0 = Totally dependent

Figure 3–9 shows the completed score sheet for the hypothetical client. She needs some equipment or assistance in all areas, and the tasks in the area of organization require the most assistance. A summary statement might read as follows:

The patient functions alone in her own home with the following equip-ment: hearing aid, R cataract lens, glasses, long-handled bath brush, shoe-

Environ-ment	Cate-gories	Tasks	Evaluation Date: 2/7/85		Progress Rounds:		Progress Rounds:	
Person-al	Trunk and Peri-neum	Wash abdomen	I					
		Wash groin	I					
		Equipment List	✓	LONG BRUSH EASIER, NOT NECESSARY				
Person-al	Lower Extrem-ities	Wash upper legs	I					
		Wash lower legs	I					
		Wash feet	I	LONG-HANDLED BRUSH				
		Pedicure	D	TOO PAINFUL TO STAY BENT				
		Equipment List	✓	LONG-HANDLED BRUSH HELPFUL				
Person-al	Bowel Pro-gram	Suppository	N/A					
		Digital stimulation						
		Equipment care						
		Cleaning self						
		Equipment List						
Person-al	Blad-der Pro-gram	Stimulation						
		Equipment care						
		Cleaning self						
		Catheter care						
		Equipment List						
		SCORE	3	NEEDS PEDICURE LONG HANDLED BATH BRUSH HELPFUL				
Home		Make bed	I					
		Change bed	I	LOOSE ELASTIC FITTED SHEETS				
		Dust floor	I	FLEX MOP HELPFUL				
		Wet mop floor	I	DOESN'T DO OFTEN				
		Vacuum	N/A	NO CARPET— WOOD FLOORS				
		Clean bath	I	LONG HANDLED SPONGE				
		Dust	I					
		Equipment List	✓	SEE ABOVE				
		SCORE	3	INDEPENDENT C EQUIPMENT				

Figure 3–9. *Continued.*

horn, slip-on shoes, bathroom grab bars, tub seat, raised toilet seat, 19-inch-high firm chair, railings on stairs, fleximop, and swivel sponge. She needs assistance with transportation to food store and appointments; supervision or assistance in paying bills, maintaining family contacts, heavy household tasks and repairs, and interaction with people other than her daughter. She has agreed to attend the local senior citizen center twice a week and to use their transportation for some appointments and such trips as to the library. A ride has been arranged for church activities. This should reduce her feelings of resentment and dependency on her daughter, who is busy with a job and a family. All recommendations, including energy

7

Environ-ment	Cate-gories	Tasks	Evaluation Date: 2/7/85	Progress Rounds:	Progress Rounds:
DRESSING					
Person-al	Upper Trunk and Arms	✔Hearing aid ✔eyeglasses	_I_		
		Front opening on/off	_I_		
		Pullover on/off	_I_		
		Bra on/off	_I_		
		Corset/brace on/off	N/A		
		Equipment/prosthesis on/off	N/A		
		Sweater/shawl on/off	_I_		
		Equipment List	N/A		
Person-al	Lower Trunk and Legs	Slacks/skirt on/off	_I_		
		Underclothing on/off	_I_		
		Belt on/off	_I_		
		Braces/prosthesis on/off	N/A		
		Girdle on/off	N/A		
Person-al	Feet	Stockings on/off	_I_		
		Shoes/slippers on/off	_I_ SLIP·ON SHOES LONG HANDLED SHOE HORN HELPFUL, NOT NECESSARY		
		Braces/prosthesis on/off	N/A		
		Wraps/support hose on/off	N/A		
		Equipment	✔ SEE ABOVE		
		SCORE	3 INDEPENDENT C EQUIPMENT		
Home	Laun-dry	Hand washing	_I_		
		Hang clothes rack/line	_I_		
		*Iron	N/A		
		Fold clothes	_I_		
		Washing machine	_I_		
		Dryer	_I_		
		*Polish/clean shoes	/		
	Sew-ing	*Thread needle and make knot	_I_		
		*Sew on button	_I_		
		*Mend	/		

*Optional activity

FIGURE 3–9. *Continued.*

conservation, were discussed when the patient and daughter were to-gether. Role conflicts between the two were discussed.

The patient should be reevaluated in 3 months to determine whether she is less depressed and whether she is following her low-salt diet, to check the progress of ulnar drift in her hands, and to see whether she is main-taining contacts outside the home.

Environ-ment	Cate-gories	Tasks	Evaluation Date: 2/7/85		Progress Rounds:		Progress Rounds:	
Home	Sewing	*Sewing machine	/					
		*Cut with shears	I	DIFFICULT				
		SCORE	4	INDEPENDENT				
Commu-nity		Clothes shopping/orders by phone	I	USES CATALOG, NEEDS TRANSPORTATION				
		Equipment						
		SCORE	3	NEEDS TRANSPORTATION				
ORGANIZATION								
Person-al	Plan-ning	Daily activity schedule	I					
		Identifies needed assistance	S	DENIED NEEDING ASSISTANCE INITIALLY				
		Budget/money management	I					
		Appointments - bank, medical, etc.	I	NEEDS TRANSPORTATION				
		Equipment						
			3	NEEDS TRANSPORTATION				
Home	Manage-ment	Household bills, etc.	S	DAUGHTER BAL-ANCES CHECK BOOK				
		Plans activities with families/others	S	STOPPED INITIATING				
		Fosters interpersonal rela-tionships	S	MAINTAINED PHONE CONTACT, STOPPED PERSONAL CONTACT				
		Heavy household tasks/repairs	D	FAMILY ASSISTS				
		Child care (if applicable)	N/A					
		Personal leisure activities	S	NEEDS TO LEAVE HOUSE				
		Religious activities	A	NEEDS TRANSPORTATION				
		Equipment						
		SCORE	2					
Commu-nity	Manage-ment	Job/professional affairs						
		Community leisure activities						

*Optional activity

Comments: MAINLY INDEPENDENT WITH TRANSPORTATION, EQUIPMENT AND MINIMAL ASSISTANCE. PT. REPORTS DEPRESSED BY RECENT ↑ IN R.A. RESULTED IN ↑ DEPENDENCE ON DAUGHTER + RELUCTANCE TO GO OUT. AGREED TO ACCEPT SR. CITIZEN TRANSPORTATION AND GO TO LOCAL CENTER ON TRIAL BASIS.

FIGURE 3–9. *Continued.*

Problems in Rating the MTAA

In any evaluation taken at a particular point in time, there is always the question, Am I measuring the patient's actual ability? The rehabilitation spe-cialist must always rate only the observed performance and then note on the score sheet any conditions, such as fatigue or mental state, that seemed to

MTTAA SCORE SHEET

CATEGORIES	LEVELS		LEVEL SCORES
Communication	Personal		3
	Home		3
	Community		3
			3
Food	Personal		4
Needs	Home		3
	Community		3
			3+
Mobility	Personal		3
	Home		3
	Community		3
			3
Hygiene	Personal		3
	Home		3
	Community		3
			3
Dressing	Personal		3
	Home		3
	Community		4
			3+
Organization	Personal		3
	Home		2
	Community		2
			2

FIGURE 3–9. *Continued.*

affect performance. This should be followed by a reevaluation at another session.

Some tasks or whole levels of any activity are not applicable to a given patient. Mark "NA" (not applicable) on the score sheet; it cannot be scored and is ignored in judgments. For example, under mobility, a person may do a standing transfer and not a sitting transfer. Mark items under sitting transfer NA and score only the standing transfer section.

Whenever equipment or an inordinate amount of time is essential—not just helpful—for safe performance of any tasks within a level, the score for that level is a 3 and the equipment is described under comments. This is consistent with the coverage of supervision or assistance; the patient is not totally independent in a nonadapted environment.

If there is only one item that can be scored in a level, the ratings are as follows: one I = 4, one D = 0, and one A or S = 2. This situation falls within the rules because a single I is treated as "all I's," a single D is "all D's," and an A or S falls within "all other configurations." Scoring for only two items in a level is similar: two I's = 4, two D's = 0, one I and one A or S = 3, one I and one D = 1, and one D and one A or S = 1.

COMMON FUNCTIONAL PROBLEMS FOR THE ELDERLY

A comprehensive but not exhaustive list of ADL tasks has been presented to highlight the magnitude of potential daily activities for any individual. However, the unique problem in rehabilitation of the elderly is treatment of acute or chronic conditions in the context of a gradual but continuous loss of adaptive capacity. The older the age, the more this combination of pathology superimposed on a general decline in function can lead to disability.

The purpose of the following summary of suggestions and techniques is to give you some general ideas about how to solve three of the most common functional problems of the elderly: reduced strength and endurance, joint problems, and increased safety problems.

Often the therapist must design or adapt techniques or equipment to solve individual patient problems. In fact, many of the devices presently sold by rehabilitation equipment companies were originally designed by occupational therapists or patients. Retraining in ADL is a mutual process, and clients should be freely involved in adapting situations or equipment to their particular needs.[8] The reader is referred to the references and bibliography at the end of this chapter for information about specific handicaps.

Reduced Strength and Endurance

There is a gradual decline in strength and endurance with increasing age, particularly after 75; yet most people wish to remain as independent as possible. When designing a program for an elderly patient, the rehabilitation specialist must balance the program so that the goal of maintaining full range of motion (ROM) and maximum independence is not compromised by work-simplification techniques to reduce fatigue. Work-simplification and energy-conservation techniques are often recommended for patients with rheumatoid arthritis and cardiac problems, but they can be used successfully by anyone, particularly the elderly. Individuals will make choices about adopting such techniques based on their personal and physical resources and values.

The following is a summary of energy-conservation and work-simplification techniques.[8, 11]

1. Review the normal schedule of activities and eliminate the unnecessary ones.
2. Determine whether work efficiency can be enhanced by combining, rearranging, or simplifying procedures.
3. Identify equipment or people necessary to the task.
4. Plan activities so that there is a balance of heavy and light tasks throughout the day, week, and month.
5. Alternate work sessions with sufficient rest periods to avoid overfatigue.
6. Avoid rushing, which increases tension and fatigue. A moderate, steady pace is more productive.
7. Use proper body mechanics at all times.
8. Organize storage and work areas according to function. Assemble all necessary supplies and equipment before beginning a task.
9. Maintain good posture. Sit rather than stand, and avoid bending and stooping whenever possible.
10. Use lightweight equipment and energy-saving appliances.

Decreased Joint Mobility

In addition to a decrease in strength, many elderly individuals have joint deterioration, which causes decreased mobility and discomfort. Table 3–3 lists principles of joint protection that can be used to reduce joint stress and discomfort and to preserve joint structures. These recommendations are even more crucial for conditions such as rheumatoid arthritis.

Increased Danger of Accidents

The combination of joint limitations, slowed reaction time, and decreased vision, hearing, strength, and endurance can lead to a greater risk of

Table 3–3. Joint-Protection Principles

1. Maintain full active range of motion in all joints. During daily activities, each joint should be actively moved through the full range of motion. For example, light objects can be stored at various heights to encourage full range of motion when reaching such objects. Activities such as dusting or sweeping the floor can be done in smooth, long, sweeping motions. This must be planned as part of the total program to prevent undue fatigue.
2. Avoid unnecessary pressure on joints. Use the largest joint whenever possible. For example, rather than using the fingers, use the whole palm of the hand to push off from the chair before standing. Large objects can be carried by the arms rather than by the hands. Equipment such as a jar opener, an electric can opener, and enlarged utensil handles (Fig. 3–10) can reduce stress on fingers caused by a tight grasp.
3. To reduce strain on joints, use proper body mechanics when lifting or pushing an object.
4. Avoid static motions that require sustained muscle contractions over a long period of time. Such positions are very fatiguing. For example, holders can be used for holding a book or the telephone.[7, 8, 11, 13]

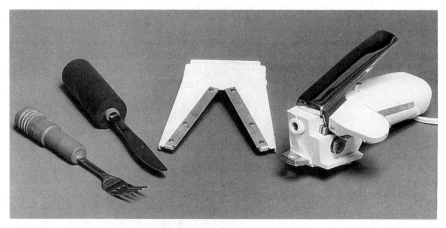

FIGURE 3–10. Adaptive equipment: *(left to right)* Large-handle fork, large-handled knife, jar opener, and one-handle can opener.

household accidents for the elderly. Slippery or uneven surfaces, stairs, or steps, the kitchen, and the bathroom are potentially hazardous areas. The elderly usually avoid icy or uneven surfaces whenever possible, but often take risks by standing on chairs to do things such as hanging curtains. Such individuals should be encouraged to identify someone who could help them with such chores. One method is to trade a service, such as baking, for jobs that are too risky. Stairs should be well lighted at all times and equipped with nonskid surfaces and handrails. A physical therapist should evaluate ambulation problems and recommend proper equipment. Canes, walkers, and crutches should not be purchased and used by the patient without fitting and training. Elderly persons should never descend stairs in stocking feet or floppy slippers with soft soles, which increase the chances of slipping. Accidents in the kitchen often involve the use of appliances. It may help forgetful persons to set a timer to remind them when stove burners or ovens need to be turned off.

The bathroom is the most common area for accidents. The rehabilitation specialist can evaluate whether the patient can transfer independently or requires supervision or assistance. The tub or shower should be measured to determine the best type and location of equipment, such as grab bars or bathtub seats (Fig. 3–11).

Because the recovery time following an injury is usually longer for the elderly than for younger people, a conservative approach to safety measures is advisable. In many families, the fear that an older member will fall and break a hip and thus become dependent is so great that family members discourage the elderly person from being as independent as possible. Anyone can have an accident while he or she is alone, but the risk is greater and the

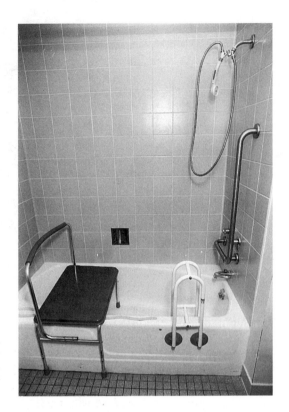

FIGURE 3–11. A bathroom with adaptive equipment: *(left to right)* Bath seat, grab bars on tub, wall grab bars, and hand-held shower head.

results can be more serious for an elderly person. Therefore, the following steps are recommended when making decisions regarding safety in performance of ADL:

1. Evaluate the patient and determine the safest method for performing an activity, including necessary equipment.
2. Give training in the method and use of equipment.
3. Determine whether the patient can consistently perform the activity in a safe manner independently, with supervision, or with assistance.
4. Arrange for someone to supervise or assist regularly with tasks the patient cannot perform safely.
5. If the patient is alone, help the patient to arrange for a family member or volunteer to check regularly on his or her welfare by telephone or visit.
6. After arrangements have been made for the safety of the patient, the individual and family should be encouraged to permit the patient to be as independent as possible within the established safety guidelines.

PRACTICAL SUGGESTIONS FOR ADL PROBLEMS

The following may be used where joint limitation and reduced strength pose problems for safety:[8, 11]

- Large buttons or fastenings
- Loose-fitting, front-opening garments
- Velcro closures
- Long-handled shoehorn and bath brush
- Slip-on shoes or elastic shoelaces
- Sock or stocking aids
- Reacher for high places
- Built-up utensil handles
- Hand-held shower head
- Safety grab bars on tub and shower
- Nonskid rubber mat or strips on tub and shower
- Bathtub or shower seat
- Raised toilet seat
- Book or telephone holder
- Lever-type faucets, doorknob extensions
- Padded handles on ambulation equipment (crutches, cane, walker)
- Suction mat to anchor dishes and bowls
- Electric typewriter or personal computer

The primary goal of health professionals working with the elderly should be to help them maintain maximum independence in ADL. This is not a simple task because the elderly are at greater risk of decreased independence through the subtle, continuous loss of adaptive capacity and the increase in chronic, disabling conditions. The expectation of reduced ability can cause both the elderly and health professionals to ignore subtle changes in functional capacity until there are major problems. It is best to identify problems early, recommend modifications in the environment or performance to maximize independence and safety, and then allow the person to function as autonomously as possible.

Chiou and Burnett[27] studied how stroke patients and their home therapists evaluated 15 ADL tasks. The results indicated that the two groups had similar perceptions of the relative importance of each of the ADLs. But they did not agree about the value of these activities to the patient. This suggests that an initial plan for determining patients' personal rehabilitative goals could increase their motivation and sense of control over their rehabilitation. Not understanding patients' motivation may explain results of studies in which comparisons of ADL evaluations by therapists to self-reported questionnaires by patients,[28] and comparisons of the results of therapists' ADL evaluations in hospitals to actual patient performance at home are made.[29,30] They usually show that patients need more assistance than projected by the therapist.

Limited intervention on an as-needed basis can encourage psychological and physical independence and the sense of control over one's life. Even though a "cure" may not always be possible, anything that will improve the quality or wholeness of the elderly person's life is worth the effort of the health professional.

REFERENCES

1. Shanas, E and Maddox, GL: Aging, health and the organization of health resources. In Binstock, RH and Shanas, E (eds): Handbook of Aging and the Social Sciences. Van Nostrand Reinhold, Toronto, 1976.
2. Stewart, A, Ware, JE, and Brook, RH: The meaning of health: Understanding functional limitations. Med Care 15:939, 1977.
3. Chappell, NL: Measuring functional ability and chronic health conditions among the elderly: A research note on the adequacy of three instruments. J Health Soc Behav 22:90, 1981.
4. Leering, C: A structural model of functional capacity in the aged. J Am Geriatr Soc 27:314, 1979.
5. Reynolds, WJ, Rushing, WA, and Miles, DL: The validation of a functional status index. J Health Soc Behav 15:271, 1974.
6. Sullivan, DF: Conceptual problems in developing an index of health. US Department of Health, Education and Welfare, Washington, DC, 1966.
7. Katz, S and Akpom, CA: Index of ADL. Med Care (Suppl)14:116, 1976.
8. Pedretti, LW: Occupational therapy practice skills for physical dysfunction. CV Mosby, St. Louis, 1985.
9. Grover, PL: Rehabilitation status index project: Executive summary. Fox Chase Cancer Center, Philadelphia, 1982.
10. Jette, A: Function status index: Reliability of a chronic disease evaluation instrument. Arch Phys Med Rehabil 61:95, 1961.
11. Duckworth, D: The measurement of disability by means of summed ADL indices. Int Rehab Med 2:194, 1980.
12. Katz, S, Ford, AB, Moskowitz, RW, et al: JAMA 185:912, 1963.
13. Mahoney, FL and Barthel, DW: Functional evaluation: Barthel Index. MD State Med J 14:61, 1965.
14. Iverson, IA, Silberberg, NE, Stever, RC, and Schoening, HA: The Revised Kenny Self-Care Evaluation. Sister Kenny Institute, Minneapolis, 1973.
15. Kerner, J and Alexander, J: Activities of daily living: Reliability and validity of gross vs specific ratings. Arch Phys Med Rehab 62:161, 1981.
16. Fillenbaum, GG: Development of a brief, internationally usable screening instrument. In Maddox, GL and Busse, EW (eds): Aging: The Universal Human Experience. Springer, New York, 1987.
17. Kuriansky, J and Gurland, B: The performance of activities of daily living. Int J Aging Hum Dev 7:343, 1976.
18. The Older American Resources and Services (OARS) Methodology: Multidimensional assessment questionnaire, ed 2. Duke University Center for the Study of Aging and Human Development, Durham, NC, 1978, pp 169–170.
19. Fillenbaum, GG: Screening the elderly: A brief instrumental activities of daily living measure. J Am Geriatr Soc 33:698, 1985.
20. Morris, JN, Sherwood, S, and Mor, V: An assessment tool for use in identifying functionally vulnerable persons in the community. Gerontol 24:373, 1984.
21. Miller, ER and Parachek, JF: Validation and standardization of a goal-oriented, quick screening geriatric scale. J Am Geriatr Soc 22:278, 1974.

22. Granger, CV, Albrecht, GL, and Hamilton, BB: Outcome of comprehensive medical rehabilitation: Measurement by PULSES Profile and the Barthel Index. Arch Phys Med Rehabil 60:145, 1979.
23. Kuriansky, J and Gurland, B: The performance test of activities of daily living. Int J Aging Hum Dev 7:343, 1976.
24. Gold, AI: The evaluation of geriatric patients following treatment. In Hoch, P and Zubin, J (eds): The Evaluation of Psychiatric Treatment. Grune & Stratton, New York, 1964.
25. Klein, RH and Bell, B: Self-care skills: Behavioral measurement with the Klein-Bel ADL Scale. Arch Phys Med and Rehabil 63:335, 1982.
26. Loewenstein, FA et al: A new scale for the assessment of functional status in Alzheimer's disease and related disorders. J Gerontol 44:P114, 1989.
27. Chiou, II and Burnett, CN: Values of activities of daily living: A survey of stroke patients and their home therapists. Phys Ther 65:901, 1985.
28. Spiegel, JS, Hirshfield, MS, and Spiegel, TM: Evaluating self-care activities: Comparison of a self-reported questionnaire with an occupational therapist interview. Br J Rheum 24:357, 1985.
29. Sheikh, K, Smith, DS, Meade, TW, Goldenberg, E, Brennan, PJ, and Kinsella, G: Repeatability and validity of a modified activities of daily living (ADL) index in studies of chronic disability. Int Rehab Med 1:51, 1979.
30. Haworth, RJ and Hollings, EM: Are hospital assessments of daily living activities valid? Int Rehab Med 1:59, 1979.

BIBLIOGRAPHY

Aniansson, A, Rundgren, A, and Sperling, L: Evaluation of functional capacity in activities of daily living in 70-year-old men and women. Scand J. Rehabil Med 12:145, 1980.
Berg, WE, Atlas, L, and Zeiger, J: Integrated homemaking services for the aged in urban neighborhoods. Gerontologist 14(5 pt 1):388, 1974.
Berrington-Jones, N: Activities for the elderly. R Soc Health J 95:96, 1975.
Clarke, M and Wakefield, LM: Food choices of institutionalized vs independent-living elderly. J Am Diet Assoc 66:600, 1975.
Cleo Living Aids Catalogue, 3957 Mayfield Rd, Cleveland, OH 44121.
Drive-Master Corporation Catalog, 16 Andrews Dr, West Paterson, NJ 07424.
Fashion-Able Catalog, Rocky Hill, NJ 08553.
Be OK Self-Help Aids Catalog, Fred Sammons, Inc., Box 32, Brookfield, IL 60513.
Functionally Designed Clothing and Aids Catalog, Vocational Guidance and Rehabilitation Services, 2239 E 55 St, Cleveland, OH 44103.
Gallo, JJ, Reichel, W, and Andersen, L: Handbook of Geriatric Assessment. Aspen, Rockville, MD, 1988.
Grauer, H and Birnbom, FA: Geriatric functional rating scale to determine the need for institutional care. J Am Geriatr Soc 23:472, 1975.
How to keep the elderly at home. Mod Health Care 3(4):29, 1975.
JA Preston Corporation Catalog, 71 Fifth Ave, New York, NY 10003.
Kaufert, JM et al: Assessing functional status among elderly patients: A comparison of questionnaire and service provider ratings. Med Care 17:807, 1979.
Klinger, JL: Mealtime Manual for People with Disabilities and Aging. Campbell Soup Co., Camden, NJ, 1978.
Lamb, HR: An educational model for teaching living skills to long-term patients. Hosp Community Psychiatry 27:875, 1976.
Lecht, S (ed): Orthotics et cetera. Baltimore, Waverly Press, 1966.
Lowman, E and Klinger, J: Aids to Independent Living. McGraw-Hill, New York, 1969.

Maddak, Inc., Catalog. Pequannock, NJ 17440.

Magid, S and Hearn, CR: Characteristics of geriatric patients as related to nursing needs. Int J Nurs Stud 18(2):95, 1981.

Malick, MH and Sherry, B: Life work tasks. In Hopkins, HL and Smith, HD (eds): Willard and Spackman's Occupational Therapy, ed 5. JB Lippincott, Philadelphia, 1978.

Manning, AM and Means, JG: A self-feeding program for geriatric patients in a skilled nursing facility. J Am Diet Asoc 66:275, 1975.

McDowell, I and Newell, C: Measuring Health: A Guide to Rating Scales and Questionnaires. Oxford University Press, New York, 1987.

Nagi, S: An Epidemiology of Adult Disability in the United States. Ohio State University, Columbus, OH, 1975.

Neubauer, H et al: Assessing functional health and sociability of aged persons: The development and validation of two Guttman scales (abstr). Aktule Gerontol 9:91, 1979.

North, AJ and Ulatowska, HK: Competence in independently living older adults: Assessment and correlates. J Gerontol (Suppl)36:576, 1981.

Pierce, CH: Recreation for the elderly: Activity participation at a senior citizen center. Gerontologist 15:202, 1975.

Rehab Aids Catalog, Box 612, Tamiami Station, Miami, FL 33144.

Salter, CL and Salter, CA: Effects of an individualized activity program on elderly patients. Gerontologist 15(5 pt 1):404, 1975.

Schlettwein-Gsell, D, et al: Guttman scales for impairment due to old age in average daily activity (abstr). Aktule Gerontol 9:87, 1979.

Sidney, KH and Shephard, RJ: Activity patterns of elderly men and women. J Gerontol 32:25, 1977.

Smith, CE, et al: Differences in importance ratings of self-care geriatric patients and the nurses who care for them. Int J Nurs Stud 17(3):145, 1980.

Staff, PH: ADL-assessment. Scand J Rehabil Med (Suppl)7:153, 1980.

Stafford, JL and Bringle, RG: The influence of task success on elderly women's interest in new activities. Gerontologist 20:642, 1980.

Sullivan, EF: Disability components for an index of health. US Department of Health, Education and Welfare, Rockville, MD 1971.

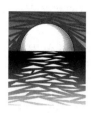

CHAPTER 4

The Effects of Aging on Communication

Leora Reiff Cherney, PhD, CCC/SLP

BEHAVIORAL OBJECTIVES

Upon completion of this chapter, the reader will be able to:

1 Identify the effects of *normal* aging on the communication process.
2 Recognize when to refer an aged individual to a speech-language pathologist or to an audiologist because of communication problems.
3 Communicate more effectively with elderly people.
4 Understand various disease processes that influence communication and are prevalent among the elderly.
5 Recognize how communicative changes in elderly people affect their lives and the lives of their families

Communication is one of the most critical human needs because it is the primary means by which people interact with their world and relate to each other. The ability to communicate effectively is especially important for the elderly person, who faces a series of lifestyle adjustments such as retirement, illness, or loss of a spouse. "Communication becomes the crucial difference between isolation and social connectedness, between dependence and independence, and between withdrawal and fulfillment."[1] (p. 339). Although certain processes important for communication diminish with age, the effects of age alone are generally subtle and should not handicap the healthy elderly individual in everyday communication. When significant alterations in communication skills are present in the elderly person, they generally are a direct result of, or are compounded by, pathologic or abnormal conditions.

This chapter discusses the components of normal communication, including speech, language, and hearing, and the effects of age on these processes. Pathologic age-related communication disorders and their effects on human interaction are also addressed. Finally, management considerations for the health care professional and specific strategies for improving communication with elderly persons are described.

COMMUNICATION CHANGES ASSOCIATED WITH NORMAL AGING

Communication is an interactive process in which verbal and nonverbal messages are sent and received by two or more specific individuals within a specific social and physical context.[2] Speech, language, and hearing are the primary communication modes through which ideas, feelings, and information are transmitted, received, and understood. In old age, these communication functions often become modified.

Elderly people are, however, heterogenous, with marked differences in their physical, mental, and social status. Communication style is related intimately to a person's individuality[3] and is dependent upon a variety of factors, including health, personality, income, education, and culture. Therefore, as a person grows old, communication skills are affected in an idiosyncratic way; some individuals may experience no problems, whereas others may begin to experience difficulties in late middle age (65 years of age). Age-related communication changes often progress slowly over an extended period of time, with the type and degree of communication difficulty varying with each individual. This section describes the complex process of normal communication and the changes that occur in this process as a result of aging.

Speech

Speech is a complex motor process involving the coordination of several physiologic systems: respiration (for the airstream), phonation (for voice production), resonance (for voice quality), and articulation (for specific sound formation and intelligibility). These components of speech production are not discrete. With advancing age, anatomic and physiologic changes in each of these systems interact to produce the characteristic speech patterns of normal older adults.[4]

Respiration

Because speech is produced on expired air, respiratory function must be sufficient to sustain phonation. A number of structural changes accompanying normal aging—such as increased rigidity of the spinal cord, vertebral column, vertebral disks, and rib cartilages—interfere with respiration by restricting rib movement and lung inflation. Other aging effects that diminish respiratory efficiency are weakening of the respiratory muscles and reduced elasticity and recoil of the lungs.[5]

Because voice production is dependent on adequate respiration, several effects on phonation can occur as a result of diminished respiration. Building up adequate subglottal air pressure may be more difficult; therefore, sustaining phonation, particularly loud voice production, may be impaired.[6] Difficulty maintaining control of the breath stream may result in intermittent or increased breathiness[6] and a tremulous, shaky voice quality. The natural flow or rhythm of speaking may be disturbed because speakers may need to pause for breath more often during periods of physical exertion.[5] In addition to the normal aging processes, respiratory function may be further compromised if the individual has been repeatedly exposed to cigarette smoke or other environmental pollutants.[6]

Phonation

During the process of phonation, the airstream generated by the lungs vibrates the vocal cords of the larynx, creating sound. Voices communicate much to the listener and are an important part of the total pattern of self-concept.[7] In voice alone, people differentiate maleness or femaleness and identify happiness or sadness, patience or irritability. The aged person's voice, however, is not necessarily reflective of the personality but, rather, may reflect the aging process.

A variety of age-related changes in laryngeal structure and physiology have an effect on voice production.[5,8,9,10] These changes include calcification or ossification of the cartilages and fatty degeneration of tissue. Bowing, atrophy, or edema of the true vocal folds may occur as well as atrophy of laryngeal mucous glands. There may be decreased blood supply to laryngeal muscles and stiffening of laryngeal ligaments.

An elderly person's voice is generally described as hoarse, tremulous, variable in pitch, rough, and breathy.[11] Male and female voices, however, change in a somewhat different manner. The pitch of the male voice rises after age 65 because there is thinning of the vocal folds, whereas it lowers in the female voice because the folds thicken and become slightly edematous.[8,11] Studies regarding changes in vocal loudness with age have been inconclusive. A few investigators have demonstrated that vocal loudness decreases with age,[12] possibly due to bowing of the vocal folds, which reduces vocal fold closure and creates breathiness and reduced loudness.[8,9]

Although drying out of the laryngeal mucosa is common in persons over 70 years of age,[5,10] many older people may suffer from certain conditions of aging, such as chronic bronchitis or allergies, that result in oversecretion of mucus from tissues in the larynx and trachea. Frequent throat clearing and hoarseness may be the result. Individuals with chronic hoarseness should always be referred to a specialist for differential diagnosis, because hoarseness is also an early symptom of laryngeal carcinoma.[13]

Resonance

Resonance, which includes aspects of nasality and denasality, is determined by the size and shape of the pharynx and the nasal and oral cavities. Although resonance is not affected significantly by normal aging, increased nasality in geriatric speakers has been noted,[5,14] possibly because of loss of dentition, changes in the structure of the lower jaw, and reduced pharyngeal function.

Articulation

In the elderly individual, a number of changes in oral-facial structure and function occur.[5,15,16] These include alterations in the facial bones, loss of teeth, and changes in the masticatory and facial muscles leading to wrinkling, sagging of the skin, and fat accumulation under the chin. Atrophy of the lips and tongue, reduced salivary gland function leading to dryness of the mouth, and reduced oral sensation also occur. Although older subjects show some slowing in their ability to reproduce rapid strings of syllables,[17,18] intelligibility of spontaneous speech of the older speaker is not affected by these age-related oral-facial changes.[5,16,19]

When a person develops articulation problems and is not intelligible, referral to a speech-language pathologist is advised. The dental status should also be checked, because missing teeth and ill-fitting dentures can create problems or compound an existing problem. The mouth changes with old age, and dentures that once fit well may no longer be comfortable. After a stroke, for example, a dental consultation to ensure proper denture fit is appropriate.[13]

Language

Language is a system of symbols that, when expressed and understood, transmit thoughts, desires, ideas, emotions, and information.[3] For descriptive purposes, language is divided into receptive and expressive processes. Reception refers to understanding what is heard or seen, and expression refers to producing what is spoken or written. Pragmatics is a third area that has recently received attention, and that overlaps both reception and expression. Pragmatics refers to how language is used in linguistic and situational contexts to communicate with others.[20,21,22]

Receptive Language

Language comprehension is a complex ability, dependent upon multiple sensory, cognitive, and linguistic factors. Intact and unimpaired sensory channels—that is, vision for written material, and hearing for verbal material—are prerequisites to receiving information for linguistic analysis. As people approach old age, these systems can deteriorate, and this deterioration contributes to subtle difficulties in understanding language. General cognitive abilities, such as memory and attention, attenuate with age and may also make comprehension more difficult; these changes are discussed further on in this chapter.

The specific components of language comprehension itself—such as understanding of vocabulary, single sentence syntax, and connected discourse—may change with normal aging. In daily conversation, these comprehension factors are not significantly affected; however, on tests of language comprehension, elderly subjects regularly do progressively worse with age. Although no age effect on understanding single word vocabulary has been demonstrated for subjects from the third to the eighth decade,[23] deficits in sentence comprehension have been identified. The elderly are slower in performing sentence comprehension tasks, with more complex syntactic sentences providing greater difficulty as age increases.[24,25] With connected discourse or paragraph level material, the elderly understand factual material but have more difficulty extracting inferential meanings.[26,27] Thus, age effects are most obvious when the information to be comprehended is new, complex, or implied and the time allowed for processing is short.

Language comprehension deficiencies can be informally detected by giving verbal directions without nonverbal cues. For example, say, "Please put the green cup next to the television, and then close the door," and observe the listener's response. By varying the length and complexity of the commands and avoiding contextual cues of facial expression or gesture, it is possible to obtain a gross measure of a person's auditory memory capability and comprehension ability.[13]

When a person exhibits mild comprehension problems, understanding can be improved by using some simple techniques.[13] Use shorter sentences and less complex language. The content of the message, however, should remain at an adult level. Comprehension can be facilitated greatly by speaking at a slightly slower rate and providing additional processing time. Facial expressions and gestures are also good comprehension facilitators. Therefore, while speaking, be sure that your face is visible at the eye level of the listener.

Expressive Language

The other major component of language is expression. The expressive language functioning of the elderly has been investigated at several levels, from analyses of single-word vocabulary skills to syntactic and grammatical usage and contextual language production. Word finding can be a problem for older people. They may not be able to retrieve from their memory storage the exact word needed to communicate a particular idea. This deficit, more commonly known as the *tip-of-the-tongue phenomenon*, is occasionally experienced by everyone and can be frustrating.

Word-finding deficits have several effects on expressive language, including the abrupt arrest of speech in midstream and the production of unfinished sentences.[28] Elderly people may react to their sudden failures in word retrieval in a number of different ways.[29] Some merely pause for a long time; others engage the listener in helping them find the word by giving clues; even if they do not remember the exact word, they do know some facts about it. Some use a word that is inexact or related, whereas others circumlocute or talk about the word without ever mentioning it. Generic substitutions such as "things" or "whatchamacallit" are frequently used; overuse of these vague words or phrases may reduce the understandability of what is being said.

Grammatical analyses of oral and written language in the elderly have demonstrated that syntax is generally preserved with aging.[30,31] In spontaneous speech, sentence length is maintained, although less complex grammatical structures may be used.[32] In contrast, the written production of older individuals is syntactically more complex and elaborate than that of younger individuals, and it is characterized by full sentences with increased numbers of words and embedded clauses.[30]

Pragmatics

The use of language in linguistic and situational contexts is known as *pragmatics*.[20,21,22] It includes the ability to evaluate a situation and to adapt language usage appropriately to that situation. It involves understanding or conveying meaning through various nonverbal communication cues, such as vocal inflection, melody, facial expression, gesture, and body posture. Pragmatics also includes the ability to organize conversation so that the message is clear to the listener, the topic is maintained, and the speaker takes turns appropriately.[20,33]

The pragmatic aspects of language have only recently received attention from researchers, with little agreement about age-related effects. Some investigators believe that "there is no evidence yet that pragmatic abilities change with healthy aging. Indeed they may be the most spared because they are learned at a young age and used throughout the life span."[29] (pp. 8–9). Others believe that the pragmatic parameter is sensitive to changes in memory and related cognitive processes, and they have discussed several pragmatic changes in elderly people's communication. These include increased verbosity, decreased organization, increased ambiguity, and changes in questioning strategies.[4,34] Internal monitoring of speech may also become less efficient with age, resulting in a variety of subtle difficulties in maintaining the topic and observing the social convention of taking turns.[13] When an individual is having difficulty staying on the subject, cues to establish the general topic can be helpful. If used in a conversational manner, these cues are nonthreatening and can often trigger an appropriate response.[13]

Hearing and Aging

Hearing is the primary way in which we receive spoken information. Sound waves collect in the outer ear. They are then conducted by vibration of the ossicles of the middle ear to the inner ear. These vibrations cause the fluid of the inner ear to vibrate in a highly systematic manner, stimulating the cochlea, where the auditory nerve is housed. It is in the inner ear that the auditory signal is converted from mechanical to electrical energy. The electrical impulses then proceed along the auditory nerve to the brain for interpretation.

Hearing loss can be divided into three main types, depending on where the lesion or pathology occurs.[35] A problem in the outer or middle ears that blocks the acoustic energy is called a conductive hearing loss. Excess wax may plug the canal; fluid in the middle ear, calcification of the ossicles, or dislocation of the bones may diminish the vibrations. Damage in the inner ear within the cochlea, or further along on the auditory nerve, results in a sensorineural hearing loss. For example, damage to the basilar membrane within the cochlea causes a frequency-specific hearing loss and interferes with the electrical impulses to the brain. A mixed hearing loss is a combination of conductive and sensorineural losses.

The incidence of hearing loss in the elderly is growing. The number of Americans over 65 years of age will grow steadily from 24 million in 1980 to nearly 48 million in 2020. The percentage of hearing loss in the over-65 age group was estimated at 43 percent in 1980; it is estimated that this percentage will increase to 46 percent by year 2000, and leap to 54 percent by 2020.[36]

Presbycusis is the name given to the most common hearing loss associated with old age. Four important characteristics of presbycusis are (1) decreased hearing sensitivity for pure tones; (2) similar hearing loss bilaterally; (3) prominent high-frequency loss, with reduced sensitivity to high-pitched sounds—*sh, s, t, ch, v, f;* and (4) greater severity in men than in women.[37] The problem may be peripherally based in the cochlea, or it may be caused by generalized deterioration in the central auditory pathways in the brain owing to aging. Probably the most vexing and handicapping aspect of presbycusis is the auditory distortion experienced by the person. The hearing loss is not simply a diminution in auditory sensitivity but a confusion and jumbling of the auditory signal. Although the person can hear someone speaking, he or she may not be able to understand exactly what has been said. When someone says "How are you?" the elderly person may answer, "Seventy-one." Clearly, such inappropriate responses can raise questions regarding mental status, so audiologic consultation is an important service.

For aged people with hearing losses, communication may become so frustrating that they lose interest in talking to people and become withdrawn and isolated. Feelings of anger and depression are common. These behavioral characteristics of hearing loss may mimic those of confusion and must be clearly differentiated for appropriate intervention. The seemingly "confused" or "uncooperative" behaviors of the person with hearing loss can lead others to limit their contact with the person and can cause further negative reactions.[38]

The management of hearing loss in the elderly involves many strategies. Early detection is an important first step in the treatment of hearing-impaired elderly persons.[39] The elderly person with a significant hearing loss often waits as long as 5 years before seeking help.[40] All elderly persons should be routinely screened for hearing and communication problems, because the progression of hearing loss in the elderly occurs in small degrees over a long period of time. Signs of possible hearing loss include inattentiveness, inappropriate responses, difficulty in following directions, speech that is unusually loud, habitually turning one ear to the speaker, turning up the volume of the television or radio, frequent requests for repetition, irrelevant comments, a tendency to withdraw from activities that require verbal communication, complaints of ringing in the ears, and a history of ear infections.[37,40] If ear discharge or ear pain is present, the patient should be referred to a physician immediately.

The communicative difficulties and subsequent psychosocial problems resulting from a hearing impairment can be reduced by the use of hearing aids and other amplification devices.[41] Many elderly individuals benefit considerably from hearing aids. However, other elderly individuals may receive only partial benefit. The function of a hearing aid is simply to amplify sound—to make it louder. It does not clarify unclear sound or unscramble distorted signals, which are the major problems of people with presbycusis. Other factors that complicate hearing aid use in elderly people are the social stigma associated with hearing aids; low tolerance for extensive testing and trial; difficulty adjusting to amplification; and inability to manipulate the small controls of the aid, particularly in those with arthritic hands and fingers.[13,41]

Hearing aids must be properly fitted, used, and cared for. The elderly person with a hearing aid may not have the memory capabilities, problem-solving skills, or manual dexterity to deal with routine problems regarding its care and use. The health care professional can help by following a few simple guidelines so that optimum benefit is attained from the aid.[35] Check to see if the battery is working by holding the hearing aid in your hand, putting the volume on high, and listening for feedback. If there is no squeal, a new battery is needed. Check the earpiece or ear mold to make sure it has not become occluded with wax, which could diminish the output of the amplified sound. Check to see that the on-off switch and volume controls are appropriately set. M stands for microphone and indicates that the hearing aid is on, and O indicates that it is off. T stands for telecoil, which is used with the telephone. The local telephone company can provide information about whether the elderly person's telephone is equipped for use with the hearing aid telecoil. If feedback is present when the aid is in the individual's ear, the ear mold may be improperly placed in the ear, or the tubing or the ear mold may be cracked and should be replaced. Remind the elderly person to remove the hearing aid when sleeping or bathing; it should not be placed on a hot surface or sprayed with hair spray. If a hearing aid becomes wet, it can be placed in an airtight glass jar with silica gel packets (obtainable from a pharmacy) for 24 hours so that excess water can be absorbed.[35]

For those individuals who do not benefit as much from conventional hearing aids, assistive listening devices that use a microphone separate from the actual hearing aid amplifier may be helpful. For example, a television listener may have a microphone near the television speaker. Sound is then transmitted from the microphone via frequency-modulated (FM) radio waves, infrared light, or hardware to a receiver that is coupled to the ear via a hearing aid.[42] Assistive listening devices are usually affordable and readily available.

Alerting devices that alert the individual to doorbells, smoke detectors, telephone rings, and alarm clocks are also readily available for the elderly hearing-impaired individual.[42] These devices convert sound to visual, somatosensory, or higher-intensity auditory signals, alerting the elderly individual by means of a flashing light, a vibrating mattress or chair, or a body-worn vibrotactile receiver.

Another important adjunctive method of treating hearing loss in the elderly is aural rehabilitation offered by a speech-language pathologist or an audiologist.[42] Most persons with a hearing loss benefit from aural rehabilitation, regardless of whether they have a hearing aid. This method of remediation helps the person maximize residual hearing and learn the use of other senses, such as vision, to aid auditory comprehension. Close attention to nonauditory language cues—body language, gestures, facial expression, contextual cues—provides additional information about what is being said and can significantly enhance a person's understanding. Speech reading (lip reading) can also be developed with practice. Aural rehabilitation addresses individual problems and provides specific instruction on the most effective means of communicating in particular environments.

A variety of techniques to enhance communication with the hearing-impaired person can be used by the health care professional and are described in the appendix to this chapter.

Nonlanguage Factors that Affect Communication

The elderly person experiences changes in vision, attention, memory, and central nervous system processing of information that can influence his or her communication skills. Medication and environment also play a part.

Visual changes in acuity are gradual, beginning in the early forties and continuing throughout the life span. Visual deficits make the perception of communication cues such as facial expressions and lip movements more difficult because they cannot be tracked easily. With age, the need for increased illumination rises; in fact, the elderly need three to four times more illumination than younger persons.[43] Proper lighting facilitates communication by enhancing acuity.

Attentional processes, including vigilance, selective attention, and divided attention, may decrease with age, with important implications for the everyday functioning of elderly adults.[44] For example, when conversing with several people, older people may find it difficult to distinguish one voice from another or to locate the person who is speaking.[29]

Memory may also decrease in healthy aging. Memory can be viewed as a multistore system.[45,46] Information is briefly held in immediate sensory memory and then processed in short-term memory, where meaning is attached. It is later encoded or cataloged into storage in long-term memory, where it is held for future retrieval and use. Although short-term memory capacity may diminish with age, it does not significantly affect language comprehension and production. With regard to long-term memory, age-related changes in storage capacity have not been found, but evidence suggests an age-related slowing of the retrieval process. The formation or encoding of new long-term memories is also affected by age because it requires organization of new information. The elderly have been found to use less effective strategies for organizing new information.[45,46] These normal age-related changes in memory do not rapidly progress in severity. It is important, therefore, to reassure healthy older individuals that some increased difficulty in remembering events and retrieving information is expected with age and does not indicate impending deterioration.[47]

With advancing age, a generalized motoric slowing has been reported.[48] Slowed central nervous system processing of information may also be evident, so the elderly may require more time to process information and to formulate appropriate responses.[29]

Some of the drugs frequently prescribed for the aged result in side effects that interfere with communication. The average older adult buys more than 13 prescription drugs a year.[49] The increased use of medications predisposes elderly patients to a much greater risk of developing adverse reactions. Depression, confusion, disorientation, slurred speech, and bizarre verbal output are some adverse drug effects that have been reported in elderly patients.[50,51] Therefore, some communication problems that are seen in the elderly may be drug-induced rather than pathologic. It is important to be aware of the potential problem of drug-induced communication deficiencies and to explore these with the physician.

The elderly person's environment may have some negative impact on his or her communication. Some elderly people are in an isolated community or institutional setting that can be characterized as "communication-impaired;" that is, an environment in which few opportunities for successful, meaningful communication are available.[1] The elderly in such environments have few reasons to talk.

Elderly people need an environment that stimulates and reinforces communication. Encourage participation in a variety of activities that can serve as the basis for conversation. Provide a socially stimulating environment with access to several communication partners. Meaningful communication, in which the elderly transmit their personal thoughts, ideas, and feelings, should be encouraged and reinforced.[52]

PATHOLOGIC AGE-RELATED COMMUNICATION DISORDERS

Aphasia

Aphasia is an acquired disturbance of language, typically a result of focal damage to the left cerebral hemisphere. Depending on the precise location of the damage, understanding, speaking, reading, writing, and symbolic gesturing may be impaired to varying degrees.

Aphasia can be caused by a wide and divergent range of neurologic disorders. The most common cause of aphasia is cerebrovascular accident (CVA) or stroke, a sudden loss of brain function resulting from interference with the blood supply to a part of the brain. Ninety percent of people who suffer strokes are 55 or older.[53] Because the incidence and prevalence of stroke increases with age, and the proportion of elderly in our society is rising, the number of aphasic patients is also increasing. Aphasia may also result from brain tumor, cerebral trauma, cerebral infections, and intracranial surgical procedures.

There are a number of behaviors frequently associated with aphasia that may occur either as a result of the aphasic person's inability to cope with the situation or as a result of damage to cerebral tissue.[54] Behaviors may include frustration, anger and hostility directed toward loved ones, or depression. A person with a stroke often shows organic emotional lability; that is, loss of emotional control, vacillating from laughter to tears for no apparent reason. Perseveration, an involuntary repetition of a word or phrase, is sometimes associated with aphasia. Inconsistent performance is also typical. Variability can be very frustrating for the aphasic person. Other people may become frustrated with the person for not performing well and may urge, "Try harder, you could do it yesterday."[13] This inconsistency in language performance should be treated with patience and support. A relaxed atmosphere facilitates communication, whereas a stressful one interferes with it.

It is important to remember that intelligence is generally maintained in aphasia. Although aphasic speech may resemble that of a child (for example, restricted vocabulary, impaired grammar, poor articulation), the patients are often very much the same as they were premorbidly. Aphasic patients should not be addressed as children or treated as if they were not present. This approach is demeaning, and it can result in anger and lack of cooperation on the part of patients. Even if the aphasic persons are not following conversations very well, often they are able to comprehend the tone and intent. Except for the early stages of the stroke, most aphasic patients are oriented, learn new information, resume many self-care activities, and exercise good judgment.[13]

Aphasia is differentiated into several types, depending on the site of the lesion and the pattern of the language disorder.[55] The two most common types are Broca's aphasia and Wernicke's aphasia.

Broca's aphasia, which generally results from an anterior lesion in the frontal lobe of the left hemisphere, is characterized by restricted vocabulary and grammar and relatively intact auditory comprehension. A person with Broca's aphasia usually knows what he or she wants to communicate, but verbal production is limited because of word-retrieval difficulties and agrammatism. Agrammatic or telegraphic speech consists of essential words only; verb endings such as -ed and -ing and small words such as is and on are omitted. A typical sentence for such a patient might be "Phone-Ruth-office-late" meaning, "Ruth called and said she might be late at the office tonight."[13] Apraxia of speech often coexists with this type of aphasia. Apraxia of speech is an impairment in motor programming, not muscle function, and causes difficulty in initiating speech and inconsistent articulation errors. Because speech is slow, labored, and halting, Broca's aphasia is also categorized as a nonfluent aphasia.

In Broca's aphasia, understanding of everyday conversation is usually relatively unimpaired, although comprehension difficulty increases as the length and complexity of conversation increase. Reading comprehension levels are similar to auditory comprehension levels. Writing is agrammatic, with frequent spelling errors. Because the patient is often forced to use the often nondominant and apraxic left hand, writing is slow and labored.

Techniques that facilitate communication with these individuals include being patient and giving the person ample time to respond.[13] Ask questions requiring yes or no or one-word responses, or provide simple multiple choices so that the aphasic person will not have to formulate a lengthy response. Keep paper and pencil available, because some aphasic persons may be able to draw the response or write part of a word that they are unable to verbalize. A listener can repeat the aphasic patient's message, which allows the aphasic person to confirm or to revise the communication and experience success.

The other major type of aphasia, Wernicke's aphasia, generally results from a posterior lesion in the temporal lobe of the left hemisphere. Language deficits of Wernicke's aphasia include impaired auditory comprehension and a fluent, flowing verbal output that is low in informational content. Word substitutions such as chair for table and sound substitutions such as flable for table are frequent. Verbal output may also include strings of nonsense words or combinations of real words that are meaningless, so that the listener hears speech but does not understand it. To illustrate, "I, my daughter, well, she's, I'll say it's really something, well, I like to, you known, well, I guess you understand."[13] The more severe the Wernicke's aphasia, the faster the rate, the longer the uninterrupted strings of words, and the more prevalent the sound and word substitutions. Sometimes a patient with Wernicke's aphasia shows a "press of speech" in that he or she talks on endlessly and is actually unable to stop talking.

People with Wernicke's aphasia usually have impaired comprehension. They cannot recognize or correct their own verbal errors because they have a failure in their monitoring systems. These patients sometimes become angry when they are not understood; they do not always perceive the communication problems as their own.

There are a variety of techniques to facilitate communication with this type of aphasic person.[13] Speech can be adjusted in rate, length, and complexity to a level at which the person responds with success. Use of more familiar and concrete vocabulary is also helpful. For example, one might hold a person's arm and say "up" instead of "lift your arm." Use of gesture and facial expression also aids comprehension. If a person does not appear to understand, rephrase the message using different words and accompany it with demonstration. Guiding a person through a task manually in combination with the verbal message often facilitates comprehension. Use of written directions, even a single word, can also be helpful to some aphasic patients. Consult the speech-language pathologist, who is familiar with the aphasic individual's level of communication and therefore can provide useful facilitating techniques for working with the patient. It is critical to know what the aphasic patient's best input level is and tailor directions and requests accordingly.[13]

There are several other aphasic syndromes. Patients with global aphasia have severe impairment of both the production and the comprehension of language. The individual may not understand what is said or written and may be incapable of meaningfully expressing himself or herself through speech, writing, or gestures.

Persons with anomic aphasia or conduction aphasia display relatively good auditory comprehension skills. Anomic aphasia is characterized by marked word-retrieval problems in the context of grammatically correct, usually fluent, easily articulated output. Conduction aphasia is characterized by impaired repetition skills, which contrast with the relative fluency of spontaneous speech. The transcortical aphasias are characterized by preserved repetition skills. In transcortical sensory aphasia, spontaneous speech otherwise resembles that of Wernicke's aphasia; in transcortical motor aphasia, there is reduced initiation and general paucity of spontaneous speech.

In terms of prognosis, although aphasic patients can improve their communication skills with speech-language pathology treatment, most will never regain their premorbid levels of communication. Complete recovery occurs in few aphasic patients. All aphasic patients, however, regardless of the severity of their communicative impairment, can benefit from a speech-language pathology treatment program. Patients with global and Wernicke's aphasia have poorer prognoses than those with Broca's aphasia. Variables that predict better improvement are younger age, good health prior to onset of aphasia, early speech and language treatment intervention, and less impaired auditory comprehension along with overall less severe initial symptoms. Recovery rates are highest during the initial 3 months when spontaneous recovery is greatest. Significant recovery also occurs in the next 3 months then slows after 6 months, and reaches a plateau after a year or more after onset.[56]

Right-Hemisphere Communication Dysfunction

When cerebral damage occurs in the right hemisphere, the nondominant side of the brain, a set of communication behaviors different from those of aphasia emerge. These behaviors are referred to as right-hemisphere communication dysfunction. Although language per se is adequate, disturbances in the attentional and perceptual mechanisms interfere with the person's ability to communicate effectively.[18,20,57] Attentional deficits include difficulty in focusing, sustaining, and shifting attention, with a reduced ability to direct attention to a task or speaker or to the left side of space.[33] Attentional deficits become more apparent as the complexity of the task and the number of competing stimuli in the environment increase. Disorientation to place and time is frequent, and memory disturbances are also often present. Perceptual deficits include difficulties in distinguishing between what is important and what is not, integrating and assessing contextual cues, and organizing information in an efficient and meaningful manner.[20,58]

These attentional and perceptual problems underlie the pragmatic deficits that characterize right-hemisphere communication dysfunction. There is generally reduced sensitivity to what is expected in a particular communication situation. Comprehension and expression of emotional tone, which is conveyed through facial expression, gesture, body language, intonation, volume, and rate of speech, are impaired. Persons with right-hemisphere communication dysfunction are often described as having flat affect, and their speech is characterized as monotonous. Literal and superficial interpretation is given to figurative language, and there may be difficulty in understanding the implied or intended meaning of a message. Reduced understanding of humor and difficulty in understanding complex instructions may be displayed. Questions are responded to with unnecessary detail and related tangential information. Patients may seem verbose, rambling, and disorganized as they address the question but do not answer it. Eye contact may not be maintained, and conversational rules may be disregarded by interrupting or by ignoring the listener's reactions. Right-hemisphere communication deficits are often overlooked by an untrained observer, although they are generally evident to the family of the person or to those interacting with the person on a regular basis.[13]

Management strategies include keeping distracting stimuli in the environment to a minimum to help a person with right-hemisphere dysfunction focus and maintain attention to a task. Establish and maintain eye contact to ensure attention to the conversation. If the person has a left-sided neglect, you may initially have to position yourself or relevant materials on the person's right side; gradually move these over to his or her left side to facilitate attention to the left side. Orienting materials such as clocks and calendars can be posted in highly visible areas. Establish consistent daily routines and provide structured rather than unstructured activities. Ask specific questions that will cue the patient to the relevant details. It is useful to ask questions during a conversation to ensure that the person remembers important details or follows topic changes. Make optimal use of the person's residual functions. A person may be able to verbalize a strategy prior to starting a task, or to talk through the sequence of a task, which will enable him or her to carry it out.[13] Verbalization also serves to regulate the patient's impulsivity in initiating an activity. Patients with right-hemisphere communication dysfunction may be difficult to work with because they are often unaware of or deny the extent of their problems.

Dementia

Dementia is another disease of the aging brain that has a language component. Dementia is a broad term describing an acquired progressive deterioration of intellectual function due to diffuse changes in the central nervous system. A variety of behavioral abnormalities may be evident, including problems with language, memory, visuospatial skills, emotion or personality, and cognition.[59]

Dementia may be caused by several different diseases. Some dementias are treatable, such as those caused by depression, drug toxicity, normal pressure hydrocephalus, vitamin deficiencies, and endocrine disorders (for instance, thyroid dysfunction). Unfortunately, most cases of dementia are irreversible. The most commonly occurring irreversible form is Alzheimer's disease, which causes approximately 50 percent of reported dementia cases in the elderly.[60] Multi-infarct dementia, which is the cumulative worsening of cognitive functioning due to repeated strokes, occurs in 14 to 20 percent of dementia cases. Another 16 to 20 percent of dementia patients suffer from a combination of Alzheimer's disease and multi-infarct dementia.[60] Other irreversible types of dementia result from disorders such as Parkinsonism, Huntington's chorea, Pick's disease, Binswanger's disease, Creutzfeldt-Jakob disease, and Korsakoff's disease.

Language impairment is present in all dementia patients.[47] The onset is slow and insidious, with the degree of the language impairment proportional to the level of mental function. Although specific language changes may vary depending on the type of dementia, there appears to be a general progression that is common to all types.[47]

In the early stages of dementing illness, the language changes are subtle and not likely to be observed in casual conversation. Articulation and syntactic rules are intact. Conversation is fluent but characterized by elaborate descriptions that are lacking in detail and information content. Word-finding difficulties are evidenced by the increased use of clichés and nonspecific terms, such as "thingamajig." Comprehension skills may be affected by the reduced attentional and memory skills, so the person may frequently request repetitions. Disorientation to time is often present. At this stage, the individual may attempt to conceal deficiencies by repeating what has already been said, blaming others for misunderstandings, and dismissing a task as trivial.

Patients in the moderate stages of dementia continue to produce fluent, well-articulated, and grammatical sentences. Yet the language impairment is readily perceived. Word-finding deficits are more pronounced, as evidenced by difficulty in naming objects and an increase in the number of verbal paraphasic errors (substitution of inappropriate words in a sentence). Perseverative responses are more frequent and are manifested as compulsive repetition of previous statements and ideas. Patients seldom initiate conversation themselves. They display difficulty in maintaining the topic of conversation and produce sequences of meaningless and unrelated utterances; self-correction is absent. These patients may be able to repeat information or read aloud fluently, but their comprehension skills are significantly compromised. Attentional deficits, disorientation to time and place, and memory problems become more severe.

In the advanced stages, persons with dementia can no longer understand or communicate effectively. Some are mute; others produce only jargon or meaningless utterances. Echolalia, that is, the repetition of words and phrases of others, may be present. Disorientation to person becomes evident, and these patients may no longer recognize family and friends.

Management strategies for the individual with dementia will differ as the dementing illness progresses. A number of techniques to facilitate increased communication with the dementia patient have been suggested.[47] Establish eye contact before addressing the patient, in order to help him or her attend to what you are saying. Avoid open-ended questions such as "What do you want to drink?" As the dementia progresses, the individual may have increased difficulty thinking of possibilities and retrieving words. Ask yes-no and either-or questions such as "Do you want milk or coffee to drink?" Use short sentences that are grammatically simple. Be concrete, direct, and brief. Avoid the use of pronouns; name the person or object. Be redundant and repeat or rephrase critical information. Keep to one topic at a time, announce any changes in the topic, and tactfully bring the patient back to the topic when he or she digresses. It is often useful to write down key words to facilitate comprehension. Provide illustrations or photographs of what you are talking about. Orientation and memory aids such as name bracelets, calendars, and clocks may also help improve daily functioning. Enhance what you say with frequent gestures or by demonstration. It is important to continue to interact even with the severely demented patient. Often a smile, a touch, or a soothing voice can be reassuring to the patient who does not understand the words themselves. The overall prognosis for improving language function is poor because the dementia is progressive. Effective communication techniques, however, can be shared with the patient's caregivers to maximize the dementia patient's ability to function in his or her environment.

Dysarthria

The dysarthrias are a group of motor speech disorders caused by damage in the central or peripheral nervous system. Consequently, the systems of respiration, phonation (voice), resonance, articulation, and prosody (the melody of speech) can be disturbed.[61] The incidence of dysarthria among the elderly has not yet been determined. However, age is closely related to neurologic conditions likely to create motor speech disorders, including strokes, tumors, and progressive neurologic disorders. Dysarthria is therefore common among older people. Dysarthric persons are often embarrassed and highly frustrated about the way they sound, because dysarthric speech can sound like drugged or drunken speech. These feelings are factors in a person's willingness to talk and in determining with whom he or she will talk.[13]

Dysarthric speech differs according to the site and extent of the lesion and the speech systems affected. The symptoms of dysarthria can range from mild, in which speech is intelligible but sounds bizarre, to severe, in which speech is completely unintelligible.[61] Clinically, five main types of dysarthria have been identified: flaccid, spastic, ataxic, hypokinetic, and hyperkinetic.[61] Each is associated with a particular neurologic site of lesion, a cluster of speech symptoms, and specific disease types. Neurologic conditions such as amyotrophic lateral sclerosis (ALS), mutliple sclerosis (MS), and Wilson's disease affect more than one site and produce a mixed dysarthria that involves multiple clusters of speech symptoms.

Flaccid dysarthria results from damage to lower motor neurons of cranial nerves V, VII, X, XI, and XII. Etiologies include strokes, tumors, viral infections, and myasthenia gravis. Speech characteristics commonly include imprecise consonants, breathy voice quality, hypernasality, and audible inhalation.

Spastic dysarthria involves bilateral upper motor neuron lesions, the cause of which may be bilateral or multiple strokes, traumatic brain injury, or multiple sclerosis (MS). Speech characteristics commonly include slow, labored articulation; imprecise consonants; strained or strangled vocal quality; low pitch; monopitch; hypernasality; and reduced patterns of stress.

Ataxic dysarthria results from damage to the cerebellum or its tracts. Possible etiologies include strokes, tumors, MS, and toxic or metabolic disorders. The cerebellum normally regulates force, speed, timing, range, and direction of movements. Dysfunction leads to speech characteristics of irregular breakdowns in articulation, imprecise consonants, distorted vowels, and inconsistent control of nasality. Scanning speech, with equal or excessive stressing of syllables, is common. Loudness variations, prolongation of sounds and the intervals between them, vocal tremor, and reduced pitch control may also be present.

Hypokinetic dysarthria results from a disorder of the extrapyramidal system and is typically associated with Parkinsonism. Hypokinetic dysarthria causes changes in muscle movements, including rigidity, reduced range and force of motion, tremor at rest, and festination of movement. Speech is characterized by a breathy or hoarse voice with reduced loudness and monopitch. The reduced excursion of articulatory movements leads to imprecise consonants and reduced stress. Intermittent short rushes of speech and involuntary repetition of syllables, words, or phrases may be present. In advanced stages of the disease, intelligibility is severely impaired. There is often difficulty in initiating speech, and reduced breath control causes many inappropriate pauses.

The hyperkinetic dysarthrias are also attributable to extrapyramidal damage and are characterized by abnormal, random, involuntary movements of the articulators. There are two subtypes of hyperkinetic dysarthria. Quick hyperkinetic dysarthrias can be found in disorders typified by myoclonic jerks, tics, and chorea. Slow hyperkinetic dysarthrias are associated with athetosis, dyskinesia, and dystonia.

Speech-language pathology treatment focuses on helping the dysarthric patient to do purposefully in speech what was once accomplished automatically.[13] Specific treatment depends on the type of disorder. In particular, the rate of speech can be manipulated for maximum intelligibility. When dysarthric persons speak slowly, using a syllable-by-syllable approach to words and exaggerating their consonants, their speech usually becomes more intelligible. When intelligibility is achieved, rate is then gradually increased. They are taught to speak in phrase lengths compatible with meaning and breath support and vary stress patterns so that speech will sound more normal. Prognosis for improved intelligibility is often good when the underlying disease process is not progressive.

When dysarthria is a symptom of a progressive neurologic disease, treatment is adjusted to the course of the disease, and early intervention is important. Speech conservation techniques can assist in maintaining a functional communication level for a longer period of time. These techniques include learning to maximize breath support and grouping words together in short phrases to ensure maximum intelligibility. Patients can also be taught to use shortened speech to convey only the most important elements of a message. Saying "toilet" is more efficient than "I would like to go to the bathroom."[13] Dysarthric patients can also be prepared for communication aids—such as language boards, gesture, or yes-no eye blinks—to be used when speech is no longer functional.

In general, the treatment program for the dysarthric person can be assisted by others.[13] Staff can be supportive by providing cues about speech rate and volume and honest feedback regarding the intelligibility of the speech. When the listener becomes familiar with the pattern of articulation errors, which are generally consistent in dysarthria, it is easier to understand the speaker. If the dysarthric person has an alternative or augmentative communication method, it is important to be familiar with it so that comfortable, efficient interactions are promoted. If dysarthria is accompanied by aphasia, the impaired language system of the patient must also be considered while conversing with the individual.

Laryngectomy

A laryngectomy is the surgical removal of the larynx because of cancer. After a laryngectomy, the individual has no voice; the person even laughs and cries silently. Respiration takes place through a permanent tracheostoma in the neck, which allows for the exchange of air from the lungs. Approximately 9000 new cases of laryngectomy occur annually, the majority in men averaging 62 years of age.[62] Prognosis for use of an alternate voice system is excellent. Therefore, if a laryngectomized patient is using writing or gesture as the chief means of communication, referral to a speech-language pathologist is indicated.[13]

Persons with laryngectomies can communicate by gesture, mouthing words, using exaggerated facial expressions, writing, or with a communication board. With the help of a speech-language pathologist, they can also be taught an alternative means of speech production. Esophageal speech is the most commonly used technique for developing voice. Air is directed into and then out of the esophagus. This action causes the sphincter at the top of the esophagus to vibrate so that it functions as a pseudoglottis and creates sound. As in the normal speaker, this sound can be shaped into intelligible speech by the vocal tract and the articulators. About half of elderly people with laryngectomies develop adequate, dependable esophageal speech for oral communication.[63]

Reconstructive surgery is another option for developing voice. A means for air to pass automatically to the esophagus is provided, and sound is produced by the vibrating pseudoglottis.[64–66] Surgical techniques have had varied success and may involve more risk for older, less healthy patients.

An electrolarynx can provide the primary means of communication for individuals who do not develop esophageal speech. It can also be used to supplement communication when a patient is learning esophageal speech or is fatigued. The electrolarynx is a portable mechanical device placed on the neck or inside the mouth to provide a buzzing sound source; this sound is then modified in a normal manner to form intelligible speech. The electrolarynx produces a mechanical-sounding voice that is reasonably intelligible. When used correctly, it is relatively simple to learn to use and it provides an immediate means of communication for some patients with laryngectomies.

Persons with laryngectomies require some special rehabilitation considerations.[13] They may feel mutilated by the operation and therefore need additional emotional support. They may also be fearful of the possibility of recurrent carcinoma. Be alert for deteriorating speech or the development of lesions about the neck or tongue. Health professionals working with these people can be an extremely valuable resource and support system.

When communicating with a laryngectomy patient, ask for repetitions and clarifications if the message is not understood. Sometimes esophageal speech is difficult for a listener to get accustomed to. Try not to be discouraged, because these patients can be quite intelligible when given the opportunity. It is easiest to listen to a laryngectomy patient in a quiet environment, inasmuch as noise and distractions can compete with the patient's message. Face-to-face positioning and lip-reading cues facilitate comprehension. The patient's facial expressions, gestures, and the situational and linguistic context will also aid understanding. Remember that the patient's comprehension of your message is not impaired in any manner.

Chronic Obstructive Pulmonary Disorder

Chronic obstructive pulmonary disease (COPD) is another disorder that occurs in aging individuals. The term COPD is used to describe the clinical phenomena resulting from the pathologic processes of emphysema, chronic bronchitis, and asthma.[67] Clinical symptoms include a chronic or recurrent productive cough and dyspnea. These people tire easily and frequently complain of difficulty in talking and walking simultaneously. Therefore, it is important for rehabilitation specialists to remember that the person's speech capability may be limited during physical exertion. Voice problems, including restricted loudness and pitch range, and chronic hoarseness are likely. Treatment procedures focus on the use of diaphragmatic breathing and pacing strategies during speech. Patients are taught to use fewer syllables per breath. Staff members can reinforce the idea of short utterances by saying, "slow down and take your time."[13]

SUMMARY

Both normal and pathologic communication changes in the aging population have been described. The effects of speech, language, and hearing disorders on aged individuals as well as on the people with whom they need to communicate can be devastating.[13] A language disorder, such as aphasia, can significantly disrupt communication and family and social life by forcing role changes, altering spousal relationships, and leading to isolation. A hearing loss, acquired gradually over time, can confuse the aged person and irritate the family. Slurred, unintelligible speech can be frustrating for both the listener and the speaker.

In terms of rehabilitation, it is important that health care professionals relate effectively to their aged patients. The way clinicians communicate with their patients can affect treatment outcome as well as patient satisfaction with their care and their lives in general.[68] Health care professionals must talk to their elderly patients to demonstrate their respect for them as well as to instruct them. Some useful management strategies have been suggested for health care professionals, along with information about potential communication difficulties that necessitate prompt referrals to ensure continued efficient, effective communication for the aged.

REFERENCES

1. Lubinski, R: Speech, language, and audiology programs in home health care agencies and nursing homes. In Beasley, DS and Davis, GA (eds): Aging: Communication Processes and Disorders. Grune & Stratton, New York, 1981.
2. Shadden, BB: Communication and aging: An overview. In Shadden, BB (ed): Communication Behavior and Aging: A Sourcebook for Clinicians. Williams & Wilkins, Baltimore, 1988.
3. Hutchinson, JS and Beasley, DS: Speech and language functioning among the aging. In Oyer, HO and Oyer, JE (eds): Aging and Communication. University Park Press, Baltimore, 1980.
4. Benjamin, BJ: Changes in speech production and linguistic behavior with aging. In Shadden, BB (ed): Communication Behavior and Aging: A Sourcebook for Clinicians. Williams & Wilkins, Baltimore, 1988.

5. Kahane, JC: Anatomic and physiologic changes in the aging peripheral speech mechanism. In Beasley, DS and Davis, GA (eds): Aging: Communication Processes and Disorders. Grune & Stratton, New York, 1981.
6. Burzynski, CM: The voice. In Mueller, HG and Geoffrey, VC (eds): Communication Disorders and Aging; Assessment and Management. Gallaudet University Press, Washington, DC, 1987.
7. Clifford, S and Gregg, JG: Considerations for the laryngectomized elderly patient. Semin Speech Lang Hear 2:3, 1981.
8. Honjo, I and Isshiki, N: Laryngoscopic and voice characteristics of aged persons. Arch Otolaryngol 106:149–150, 1980.
9. Mueller, PB, Sweeney, RJ, and Baribeau, IJ: Acoustic and morphologic study of the senescent voice. Ear, Nose Throat, 63:292–295, 1984.
10. Kahane, JC and Beckford, NS: The aging larynx and voice. In Ripich, D (ed): Handbook of Geriatric Communication Disorders. Pro-Ed, Austin, 1991.
11. Kent, RD and Burkard, R: Changes in the acoustic correlates of speech production. In Beasley, DS and Davis, GA (eds): Aging: Communication Processes and Disorders, Grune & Stratton, New York, 1981.
12. Ptacek, P and Sander, E: Age recognition from voice. J Speech Hear Res 9:273–277, 1966.
13. Pilberg, S and Hosty, K: Communication and the elderly. In Lewis, CB (ed): Aging: The Health Care Challenge. FA Davis, Philadelphia, 1985.
14. Hutchinson, JM, Robinson, KL, and Nerbonne, MA: Patterns of nasalance in a sample of normal gerontologic subjects. J Com Dis 11:469–481, 1978.
15. Somerman, MJ: Mineralized tissue in aging. Gerodontology 3:93–99, 1984.
16. Sonies, BC: The aging oropharyngeal system. In Ripich, D (ed): Handbook of Geriatric Communication Disorders. Pro-Ed, Austin, 1991.
17. Ryan, WJ and Burke, KW: Perceptual and acoustic correlates of aging in the speech of males. J Com Dis 1:181–192,1974.
18. Amerman, JD and Parnell, MM: Oral motor precision in older adults. Journal of the National Student Speech-Language-Hearing Association 10:55–67, 1984.
19. Sonies, BC, Baum, BJ, and Shawker, TH: Tongue motion in the elderly: Initial *in situ* observation. J Gerontol 39:279–283, 1984.
20. Myers, PS: Right hemisphere communication impairment. In Chapey, R (ed): Language Intervention Strategies in Adult Aphasia. Williams & Wilkins, Baltimore, 1986.
21. Hough, MS and Pierce, RS: Pragmatics and treatment. In Chapey, R (ed): Language Intervention Strategies in Adult Aphasia, ed 3. Williams & Wilkins, Baltimore, 1994.
22. Goldsmith, T: Pragmatic communication disorders following stroke. Top Stroke Rehabil 1(2):52–64, 1994.
23. Bayles, KA, Tomoeda, CK, and Boone, DR: A view of age-related changes in language function. Developmental Neuropsychology 1:231–264, 1985.
24. Feier, C and Gerstman, L: Sentence comprehension abilities throughout the adult life span. J Gerontol 35:722–728, 1980.
25. Obler, LK, Fein, D, Nicholas, M, and Albert, ML: Syntactic comprehension in aging. Presented at the annual meeting of the Academy of Aphasia, Pittsburgh, 1985.
26. Cohen, G: Language comprehension in old age. Cognitive Psychology 11:412–429, 1979.
27. Belmore, SM: Age-related changes in processing explicit and implicit language. J Gerontol 36:316–322, 1981.
28. Critchley, M: And all the daughters of music shall be brought low: Language functioning in the elderly. Arch Neurol 41:1135–1139, 1984.
29. Obler, LK and Knoefel, J: The effects of normal aging on speech, language, and communication. Top Geriatr Rehabil 1:4, 5–13, 1986.
30. Obler, L: Narrative discourse style in the elderly. In Obler, L and Albert, M (eds): Language and Communication in the Elderly: Clinical, Therapeutic, and Experimental Aspects. DC Heath, Lexington, MA, 1980.

31. Golper, LC and Binder, LM: Communicative behavior in aging and dementia. In Darby, JK (ed): Speech Evaluation in Medicine. Grune & Stratton, New York, 1981.
32. Kynette, D and Kemper, S: Aging and the loss of grammatical forms: A cross-sectional study of language performance. Language and Communication 6:65–72, 1986.
33. Burns, MS, Halper, AS, and Mogil, SI: Clinical Management of Right Hemisphere Dysfunction. Aspen, Rockville, MD, 1985.
34. Peach, RK: Language functioning. In Mueller, HG and Geoffrey, VC (eds): Communication Disorders and Aging: Assessment and Management. Gallaudet University Press, Washington, DC, 1987.
35. Washburn, AD: Hearing disorders and the aged. Top Geriatr Rehabil 1:4, 61–70, 1986.
36. Kelly, LS: Are we ready for the year 2000? The Hearing Journal 38:15–17, 1985.
37. Maurer, J: Auditory impairment and aging. In Jacobs, B (ed): Working with the impaired elderly. National Council on the Aging, Washington, DC, 1976.
38. Heller, B and Gaynor, E: Hearing loss and aural rehabilitation of the elderly. Clin Nurs 3:1, 1981.
39. Lichtenstein, MJ, Bess, FH, and Logan, SA: Screening the elderly for hearing impairment. In Ripich, D (ed): Handbook of Geriatric Communication Disorders. Pro-Ed, Austin, 1991.
40. Hull, RH: Hearing aids for the older adult: Considerations for fitting and dispensing. Sem Hear 6:181–191, 1985.
41. Stach, BA and Stoner, WR: Sensory aids for the hearing-impaired elderly. In Ripich, D (ed): Handbook of Geriatric Communication Disorders. Pro-Ed, Austin, 1991.
42. Lesner, SA and Kricos, PB: Audiologic rehabilitation: Candidacy, assessment, and management. In Ripich, D (ed): Handbook of Geriatric Communication Disorders. Pro-Ed, Austin, 1991.
43. Kenney, RA: Physiology of aging. In Shadden, BB (ed): Communication Behavior and Aging: A Sourcebook for Clinicians. Williams & Wilkins, Baltimore, 1988.
44. Kausler, DH: Cognition and aging. In Shadden, BB (ed): Communication Behavior and Aging: A Sourcebook for Clinicians. Williams & Wilkins, Baltimore, 1988.
45. Smith, AD: Age differences in encoding, storage, and retrieval. In Poon, LW, Fozard, TL, Cermak, LS, Arenberg, D, and Thompson, LW (eds): New Directions in Memory and Aging. Lawrence Erlbaum, Hillsdale, NJ, 1980.
46. Poon, LW: Differences in human memory with aging: Nature, causes and clinical implications. In Birren, JE and Schaie, KW (eds): Handbook of the Psychology of Aging. Van Nostrand Reinhold, New York, 1985.
47. Bayles, KA and Kazniak, AW: Communication and Cognition in Normal Aging and Dementia. Little, Brown, Boston, 1987.
48. Albert, ML (ed): Clinical Neurology of Aging. Oxford, New York, 1984.
49. Fisher, CR: Differences by age group in health care spending. Health Care Fin Ref 1:65–90, 1980.
50. Ronch, JL: Drugs/medication: Their impact on communication and the elderly's response to treatment. Sem Speech, Lang Hear 2:3, 1981.
51. Brandell, ME, Brandell, RK, and Hult, R: Pharmacology and the aging system. In Shadden, BB (ed): Communication Behavior and Aging: A Sourcebook for Clinicians. Williams & Wilkins, Baltimore, 1988.
52. Lubinski, R: Language and aging: An environmental approach to intervention. Top Lang Disorders 1(4):89–97, 1981.
53. Sahs, AL, Hartman, EC, and Aronson, SM (eds): Guidelines for stroke care (DHEW Publication No. 76–14017), US Government Printing Office, Washington, DC, 1976.
54. Hooper, CR and Dunkle, RE: The Older Aphasic Person: Strategies in Treatment and Diagnosis. Aspen, Rockville, MD, 1984.
55. Goodglass, H, and Kaplan, E: The Assessment of Aphasia and Related Disorders. Lee & Febiger, Philadelphia, 1983.

56. Kertesz, A: Aphasia and Associated Disorders: Taxonomy, Localization and Recovery. Grune & Stratton, New York, 1979.

57. Myers, PS: Communication disorders associated with right-hemisphere brain damage. In Chapey, R (ed): Language Intervention Strategies in Adult Aphasia, ed. 3. Williams & Wilkins, Baltimore, 1994.

58. Cherney, LR and Halper, AS: An assessment tool for evaluating cognitive-communicative problems in patients with right hemisphere damage: Preliminary findings. Top Stroke Rehabil 1(2):37–51, 1994.

59. Cummings, JL and Benson, DF: Dementia: A Clinical Approach. Butterworth, Boston, 1983.

60. Tomlinson, BE, Blessed, G, and Roth, M: Observations on the brains of demented old people. J Neurol Sci 11:205–242, 1970.

61. Darley, F, Aronson, AE, and Brown, JR: Motor Speech Disorders. WB Saunders, Philadelphia, 1975.

62. Hull, RH: Demography and characteristics of the communicatively impaired elderly in the United States. Semin Speech Lang Hear 2:3, 1981.

63. Adair, M: Communicative problems in older persons. In Jacobs, B (ed): Working with the Impaired Elderly. National Council on the Aging, Washington, DC, 1976.

64. Asai, R: Laryngoplasty after laryngectomy. Arch Otolaryngol 95:114–119, 1972.

65. Singer, MI and Blom, ED: An endoscopic technique for restoration of voice after laryngectomy. Ann Otol Rhinol Laryngol 89:529–533, 1980.

66. Sisson, GA and Krespi, YP: Voice preservation and restoration in advanced laryngopharyngeal cancer—the Northwestern experience. J Laryngol Otol (Suppl)8:30–36, 1983.

67. Zadai, CC: Pulmonary rehabilitation of the geriatric patient. In Lewis, CB (ed): Aging: The Health Care Challenge. FA Davis, Philadelphia, 1985.

68. Olson, DA: Interdisciplinary management: speech, language, and communication problems of the aged. Top Geriatr Rehabil 1(4):71–75, 1986.

Appendix

Strategies for Improving Communication

NORMAL AGING PERSON[13,52]

1. Provide meaningful opportunities for communication; encourage and reinforce communication of thoughts, ideas, and feelings.
2. Communication is easiest in a quiet, well-lighted environment.
3. Do not pretend to understand what is said; if a message is not understood, request a repeat.
4. If the older person exhibits some comprehension difficulty, use shorter sentences and a slower rate of speech.
5. Give the person time to respond.
6. If there are word-finding difficulties, give the person time to think of the word. Provide the category or topic to help cue the person to the word or politely suggest a possibility.

7. If the person goes off on a tangent while speaking, bring the person back to the topic at hand.
8. If speech and language deficits are more severe than anticipated as part of normal aging, refer the person to a physician or speech-language pathologist for evaluation.

HEARING LOSS[13,35]

1. Be alert to signs of possible hearing loss. Routine annual screenings are recommended for early detection of hearing loss.
2. Communicate in a quiet, well-lighted environment free of distraction.
3. Secure the person's attention by calling the person's name, touching the person, or making eye contact prior to speaking.
4. Speak at eye level at a distance of 3 to 10 feet to facilitate speech reading. For example, if the person with a hearing loss is in a wheelchair, the speaker should also be seated.
5. Face the person; do not cover your face with your hands; do not eat, smile, or smoke while speaking so that facial and speech reading cues can be seen.
6. Speak at a normal volume, rate, and tone, without elaborate mouthing; shouting or overarticulating distorts auditory and visual cues.
7. Ask the hearing-impaired listener to repeat directions to ensure his or her comprehension.
8. Rephrase what was said if it is not understood the first time.
9. Introduce conversation and topic changes with an orienting topic statement to cue the listener to what will be discussed.
10. Check hearing-aid batteries and earpieces regularly.
11. Check that the on-off switch and volume controls of the hearing aid are appropriately set.
12. The person should wear glasses, if prescribed, during communication.
13. Persist in the communication to let the person experience success.
14. Encourage the hearing-impaired listener to be assertive in telling others what is needed to facilitate understanding.

APHASIA[13,54]

1. Be familiar with the person's level of comprehension and adjust rate, length, and complexity of language to a level at which the person can respond with success.
2. Use concrete, familiar vocabulary in short, clear sentences.

3. Use gestures and facial expressions to augment what is said, or demonstrate the information you are trying to convey.
4. Provide written and visual cues.
5. Phrase questions for short responses, multiple choice, or yes-no responses.
6. Rephrase a message if it is not understood initially.
7. Give the person adequate time to respond.
8. Encourage the aphasic person to use gesture, facial expressions, and writing, if appropriate, to augment what is said.
9. Let the person know that you have understood the message by repeating it back conversationally.
10. Be patient and supportive to reduce any stress associated with communicating.
11. Treat the person as an adult at all times.

RIGHT-HEMISPHERE DYSFUNCTION[13,20,33,57]

1. Minimize external distractions in the environment.
2. Position yourself and any materials within the person's visual field, if he or she has a left visual field neglect.
3. Establish eye contact to ensure attention to the conversation.
4. Provide orienting materials like clocks and calendars.
5. Provide structured activities.
6. Help the person structure responses by cueing with relevant details; if the person goes off on a tangent, cue him or her back to the topic at hand.
7. Be concrete and direct in language use; avoid figurative language and sarcasm.
8. This person may not understand lengthy, complex directions, so repeat and rephrase to ensure understanding of important details.

DEMENTIA[13,47]

1. Establish eye contact prior to addressing the person, to ensure attention.
2. Use short, grammatically simple, and concrete input. Avoid the use of pronouns.
3. Keep to one topic at a time. Be redundant; repeat and rephrase critical information.
4. Provide multisensory input, both visual and tactile, to enhance comprehension. For example, provide illustrations or photographs, write down key words, or use gesture and demonstration.

5. Ask yes-no and either-or questions.
6. Provide external orientation and memory aids, such as name bracelets, reminder signs, and calendars.
7. Share successful communication techniques with the patient's caregivers.

DYSARTHRIA[13,61]

1. Communicate in a quiet, nondistracting environment.
2. Encourage the person to speak at a slower rate.
3. Have the person exaggerate production of consonants and separate syllables within words.
4. Encourage the use of shorter utterances compatible with breath support and meaning.
5. Provide honest feedback about the intelligibility of the message.
6. Provide appropriate feedback about loudness level.
7. Become familiar with the person's alternate or augmentative communication methods such as language boards and gesture.

LARYNGECTOMY[7,13]

1. Talk in a quiet environment.
2. Consider facial expressions, gestures, speech-reading cues, and situational and linguistic context, if you have difficulty in understanding the person.
3. Ask the person to repeat if a message is not understood.
4. Provide support and encouragement for the use of the new voice.

CHRONIC OBSTRUCTIVE PULMONARY DISEASE[13]

1. Encourage short utterances compatible with breath supply.
2. Encourage a reduced rate of speech.
3. Do not engage in conversation while the person is involved in physical activity.

Revision of this chapter was supported in part by a grant from The Henry Foundation, Chicago, Illinois.

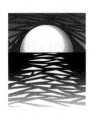

CHAPTER 5

Leisure Skills

Jerome F. Singleton, PhD, CTRS

BEHAVIORAL OBJECTIVES

Upon completion of this chapter, the reader will be able to:

1   Identify and explain the effect an institution has on an elderly individual.
2   Discuss the roles of work and leisure in an elderly person's life.
3   Summarize the planning process.
4   Identify and explain what should be encouraged in recreation.
5   Identify and explain the activity analysis process.
6   Identify how process can be applied.
7   Discuss how volunteers can be used to deliver services in an institution.

The elderly who reside in institutions relinquish many opportunities to make decisions concerning daily activities. Leisure opportunities should not further limit the individual; the elderly should be given the opportunity to control that area of life in the institution by making choices for their own leisure activities. Leisure opportunities should be planned with the individual, allowing him or her to feel some control. This chapter will illustrate how leisure services can accomplish this goal through environmental factors, development of leisure patterns, planning for the elderly, activity analysis, and volunteers.

ENVIRONMENTAL FACTORS

Most old people live in the community; but with increased life expectancy, more people may need long-term care facilities. People who live in the community can decide for themselves what kinds of recreational activities to participate in, depending on finances, accessibility, transportation, available time, health status, and previous exposure to the activity. A variety of recreational programs may be available to them—community recreation centers such as the YMCA, theaters, shows and social clubs, restaurants, bars, and universities. As shown in Figure 5–1, the degree of control that the elderly have over their environment depends on: (1) the time at their disposal; (2) available resources and finances, and (3) their physical and psychological abilities.

When the elderly enter long-term care facilities, their lives become regimented around the routine of the institution. Their choices are reduced be-

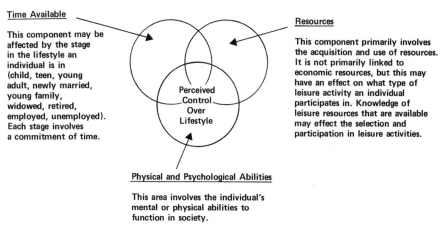

FIGURE 5–1. Schematic diagram of the extent to which an individual has control over his or her environment.

cause of both physical limitations and enforced institutional regulations. The institutional environment fosters dependence, not independence; routine and restrictions, not spontaneity; leaving the elderly individual with a narrow selection of leisure opportunities from which to choose. Goffman[1] states that an individual "comes into the establishment with a concept of himself made possible by certain stable social arrangements in his world. Upon entrance he is immediately stripped of the support provided by these arrangements." (p. 14). Large institutions often initiate and hasten a process of depersonalization in which the individual is made to conform to the regime and tyranny of the institution.

The institutional routine—breakfast, lunch, dinner, therapy hours, and so forth—forces the individual to conform to a specific lifestyle that is determined by the institution. Goffman defines a total institution "as a place of residence and work for a large number of like-situated individuals, cut off from the wider society for an appreciable period of time, [who] together lead an enclosed, formally administered round of life." (p. xiii). Hirsch[2] states that nursing homes are being criticized for operating on a pathology model of aging, viewing the individual in terms of medical management factors instead of overall human needs. Langer and Rodin[3] believe that many of the debilitating conditions of those in institutions are partially the result of their decision-free environment, and that the feeling of mastery over one's environment comes from making meaningful decisions about one's life.

Recreation and health professionals need to take into consideration these environmental factors in delivering leisure services to the elderly in long-term care facilities. McGuire[4] states that "the environmentalist's role becomes more important when older individuals are involved and the need for assistance in manipulating the environment to either eliminate or mitigate factors constraining leisure become[s] more necessary with increasing age" (p. 78). Iso Ahola[5] indicates that "it is not the recreational activity in itself that is crucial, but the extent to which such activity induces a sense of control and responsibility over one's behavior, environment and entire life" (p. 38).

DEVELOPMENT OF LEISURE PATTERNS

As the elderly move from the community into the long-term care facility, they bring with them a perception of their leisure time and their past participation patterns in recreational activities. Participation in leisure activities in adulthood is dependent on past experience in work and in leisure, finances, and the individual's health status.

Prior to retirement, work is the major focus of most people's lives. Daily activities, vacations, social engagements, and family interactions are planned around the work schedule. Work provides income to secure life's basic needs (food, shelter, clothing); from this we develop a sense of purpose, usefulness, and self-respect. A person's work establishes his or her identity and role in society. Kaplan[6] notes that "work gives order to life . . . through work, man finds his own level . . . the house in which we live and all its conveniences . . . the food we eat and the clothes we wear . . . these and indefinitely more, do we receive and give through a common bond, work" (p. 278).

As Kaplan[7] notes, the Protestant work ethic has had an effect on all of society and on our perception of leisure.

American leisure patterns reflect the history of a nation that grew up without a rigid carryover of the European or feudal principles or systems.

Leisure patterns in America have been related to the heterogeneity of our population—a factor that, in turn, is a part of the immigrant waves.

It was as hard workers that our immigrants came to this country.

The rise in mass literacy . . . becomes a . . . key element in the leisure of this country.

The social class levels of participants in community transformations are undergoing radical changes, creating new areas of significant leisure involvement.

The private business sector . . . has become a more and more important factor in . . . activities, attitudes, and tastes for leisure.

The public sector has also grown as a major instrument for leisure.

A growth has been evident in the artistic life of America (p. 278).

These variables have affected the way an individual interprets what leisure is; in addition, the historical period in which an individual lives affects that individual's perceptions of both leisure and work.

People have traditionally found a feeling of purpose, usefulness, and self-respect in work. Retirees must find another way to fulfill these needs and to fill the time that has become available. Sometimes people are forced to retire before they are ready. The central focus of their lives changes from work to the meaningful use of leisure time. Kaplan[7] feels that leisure is the social role in retirement that could provide unique opportunities for the individual to enhance self-worth in society. Like the roles of a child, which are to play and learn, the leisure roles of the elderly are to play and to teach. This can be accomplished through involvement in hobbies, clubs, senior centers, and volunteer organizations such as Vista and the Peace Corps for Action. The task of the elderly in relation to leisure is easier than that of the young person in finding a job, for at the retirement stage, each person has a lifetime of developed tasks and varied experiences upon which to draw. It is the individual's past participation in leisure activities that will determine the activities he or she will participate in once retired.[8]

Past recreation participation patterns will carry over when the elderly individual enters a long-term care facility. Therefore, the job of recreation directors and health professionals is not to find substitutes for work but to build upon the nonwork complex, *leisure*, to help the elderly maintain current recreation participation patterns and explore new activities through which they may demonstrate their skills and interests and meet their needs. This will allow the elderly to develop or renew an interest in a leisure activity that they can participate in.

Has the leisure profession allowed this to occur? Gunn[9] states, "Ironically old people and young people face many of the same crises. Neither [are] taken seriously, and both are often beset by seemingly benevolent despots intent on running programs resembling qualified playpens" (p. 27). Guadagnolo[10] elaborates further: "Through acts of commission and omission, we have witnessed a selection process which, in the final analysis, permits a very narrow spectrum of elderly with both the opportunity and ability to engage in public sponsored leisure services" (p. 5).

The aged are stereotyped in certain activities in recreation. Recreation professionals perpetuate myths of the elderly by offering passive activities. According to Verhoven:

> There have been many studies on how aging persons use their leisure. The most often mentioned leisure activities of the aged include reading, watching television, visiting, working around the yard, and going pleasure driving. These activities are strikingly similar to types of leisure activities participated in by other groups. To continue to perpetuate stereotyped activities and label them "senior citizen's" activities is a gross injustice. (p. 45).

This was verified in other studies of leisure activities participated in by the elderly.[11–15] Previous research on older individuals' activity patterns indicated that as individuals aged, their leisure times increased but they appeared to participate in fewer leisure activities. The activities that older individuals take part in appear to be primarily sedentary and homebound in nature.[16,17] These findings may be the result of the research tools and methodologies used by the investigator rather than a decline in the activity patterns of older individuals. Findings based on longitudinal data suggest that the tendency toward behavioral stability may be somewhat greater than most would imagine. Previous research indicates that both the "doing" and "nondoing" of particular activities tend to be consistent over time and that changes in roles and obligations as one moves through life.[18] Recent findings by Harvey and Singleton[19] indicate, that as a person ages, there are turning points in the use of time. These turning points may be more the result of role obligations than of age. Singleton[21] found that occupation, education, income, and gender were more relevant than age in the outdoor recreation participation patterns of the elderly. Singleton and colleagues[21] found that the vast majority of the activities participated in by the respondents were in the home environment. This finding appears to support the observation by Kelly[22] that adults in general appear to participate in a core set of activities related to the home environment. Lounsbury[23] studied the stability of leisure activities and motivation of 282 adult residents in a medium-size southeastern city in 1980, with follow-up interviews conducted in 1985 with 139 of the original sample. In a paper presented at the 10th Annual Leisure Research Symposium, Lounsberry reported that "results indicated a most encouraging, and even surprising, level of stability over 5 years for the leisure activity participation as well as, to a lesser extent, the leisure motivation variables studied. Such stabilities may reflect relatively enduring personality traits or lifestyle consistencies."

Recent research[24–26] indicates that individuals add and drop activities across the life span. Home-related activities are stable across the person's life span. The addition and deletion of activities are related to the stage of a person's life cycle and the presence or absence of children or a significant other.[27] Patterns and benefits of leisure participation appear to change with the life cycle. For example, parents may attend an event that their children participate in and enjoy the experience but cease to attend the activity when the children no longer participate.

Recreation planning should be based not on age but on the interests of the individual. Table 5–1 lists some possible recreational activities. Participation in these activities will be limited only by the person's abilities, not by his or her age or place of residence. Some people in long-term care may be able to participate in activities independently, while others may need assistance. Professionals in long-term care need to assess individual abilities and interests. Lewis and Campanelli's book, *Health Promotion and Exercise for Older Adults*,[28] provides useful tips for practitioners. Other texts and articles that illustrate how leisure contributes to the well-being of older individuals are listed at the end of this chapter.[29–47]

PLANNING RECREATIONAL OPPORTUNITIES FOR THE ELDERLY

Seleen[48] states, "If older people could spend their time as they wish, this could contribute to higher life satisfaction" (p. 57). Therefore, recreation opportunities should be designed to allow the individual to feel in control of leisure choices. This can be accomplished in the following ways:

1. Use a leisure inventory scale to assess the individual's leisure interests. Current assessment tools include the Mirenda Leisure Finder,[49] the Self Leisure Interest Profile (SLIP),[50] the Leisure Activities Blank,[51–52] and the Avocational Activities Inventory.[53]
2. Use leisure counseling to determine preferences. Gunn and Peterson[54] define leisure counseling as "a helping process that utilizes verbal facilitation techniques to promote self-awareness; awareness of leisure attitudes, values and feelings; and the development of deci-

Table 5–1. **Recreational Activities**

Sports	Games
Volleyball	Chess
Swimming	Checkers
Tennis	Bridge
Golf	Euchre
Badminton	Solo
Jogging	Poker
Bowling	Other card games
Skating	Pool, billiards
Bicycling	Horseshoes
Softball	Shuffleboard
Downhill skiing	Board games
Racquetball	Arts
Squash	Painting
Nature Activities	Photography
Hiking	Sculpture
Sailing	Creative writing
Birdwatching	Ceramics
Walking in parks	Dancing
Boating	Drama
Hunting	Playing a musical instrument
Fishing	Singing
Crafts and Hobbies	Entertainment
Sewing	Watching television
Knitting	Going to museums
Macrame	Reading for pleasure
Carpentry	Going to parks
Crocheting	Going to parties
Car repair	Dining out
Model construction	Home entertainment
Weaving	Attending church
Pottery	Going to movies
Rug making	Listening to radio
Candle making	Volunteer Work
Collecting	Member of community club
Coins, stamps, antiques, cars,	(Kiwanis, Rotary)
records, pictures	Member of church club

sion-making and problem-solving skills related to the leisure participation with self, others and the environment" (p. 214).

3. Form a committee of elderly individuals at the long-term care facility to plan leisure activities in cooperation with other health professionals (occupational therapist, physical therapist, nurses, social
workers, psychologists, health educators, doctors).[55,56]

The leisure delivery process is a component of the total team process,
dependent on, not independent of, other health professionals. The members
of the professional team need to coordinate and communicate with each
other. Singleton and associates[57] outline a systematic method for coordinating physiotherapy, occupational therapy, and therapeutic recreation services
for older individuals in a long-term care facility.

A recreation program needs to have the following goals:

1. Maintain or increase the individual's level of independence.
2. Encourage participation in new recreational activities.
3. Encourage participation in current or past recreation patterns.
4. Encourage socialization, not isolation.
5. Encourage physical activities.
6. Develop positive self-esteem and self-concept.
7. Encourage continued community involvement.

THEORETICAL FRAMEWORK FOR PROGRAM PLANNING

Programming based upon the continuity theory of aging may be appropriate to accomplish these goals.[58] Davis and Teaff[59] state that a "leisure programmer, through an assessment of the older person's biological and physiological capabilities, personal preferences and experiences, can construct situational opportunities for an individual to maintain continuity of habits, associations and preferences into later life" (p. 32). This is an important concept in planning recreational activities for the elderly once they enter the long-term care facility.

Such a model program has been developed at the Byer Activity Center, Dallas Home for Jewish Aged in Dallas, Texas. Based on interviews with each new resident, roles were created for individual participation in leisure activity. These are some of the roles created.

"The Hostess" greets and welcomes guests for a party, serves on the welcoming committee, plans refreshments for the tea, helps make decorations in the craft group for a luau. All these activities allow the continuance of the preference for hostessing.

"The Salesman" helps with the raffle for the women's group, helps run the gift shop, organizes flea markets, the annual bazaar, serves on the committee for fund-raising projects.

"The Organizer" serves as president of the council, helps on the program committee, brings helpful hints and ideas from all newspaper sources, helps call for activities, and sets up games such as bridge.

"The Entertainer," who has always enjoyed the limelight, is the bingo caller, tells jokes at social gatherings, helps provide entertainment for parties, is a member of the drama club, and is the master of ceremonies for talent shows and grandchildren's day.

"The Humanitarian" helps with service projects, cancer society bandages, crocheting for shut-ins, knitting for babies, friendly visiting with the sick, phone calling, helping with the sunshine committee, sending get-well cards, and reporting on human interest stories at the current events groups.

"The Motherer" has always had a preference for caring for others. She enjoys those activities in which she can lend a hand and take a mothering role. She bakes for others as well as for many activities and lunches. She helps with the cooking group, suggests recipes for the recipe book, and adds helpful hints to the center newsletter. She also participates in the tutoring program and children's storytelling.

"The Reporter" knows lots of information on a variety of subjects. The activities of the reporter involve announcing community events, acting as a secretary of the resident council, and interviewing members for the "mystery resident."

"The Musician" helps with all music endeavors, acts as a link to community resources for performers, helps with the choral group, plays the piano, assembles singalong books, and participates actively in music listening and music appreciation groups.

Other roles that have emerged include "The Family Man," "The Artist," "The Complainer," "The Signmaker," "The Receptionist," "The Pastor." Members may have a single role or a variety of roles within the framework of the activity program. Not all members will have an active role since some may perform the role of observer or visitor.[59]

As a result of these roles, individuals were socialized into an environment based upon predisposed activity patterns and situational opportunities. This is one method of assisting an individual to adjust to a new environment in a nonthreatening manner.

ACTIVITY ANALYSIS

Activity analysis helps recreation specialists to figure out what skills individuals have and need to develop in order to perform an activity. Activity analysis enables the professional to reduce the activity to its component parts prior to instruction.[60–62] Activity analysis has four components: assessment, planning, implementation, and evaluation.

Assessment

1. Determine what activity the person is interested in.
2. Separate the activity into its component parts, and analyze what the person needs to know, and in what order, to complete each component of the task.
3. Assess the person's basic physical skills. Are they adequate for the task? Does the person have sufficient strength, flexibility, balance,

endurance, agility, speed, and coordination? Does the person have a health condition that would affect participation in an activity—paralysis, paresis, or a heart condition, for example? Other health professionals should have input into the assessment procedure to ensure that a realistic and accurate assessment is achieved and to ensure safe and successful participation.[56,57]

Planning

Planning the activity consists of determining whether the activity needs adaptations or modifications and reducing the activity to sequential tasks or steps. Activities can be adapted or modified by changing the following: the mobility factor, the body position, boundaries or space requirements, weight and size of implements, and duration of the activity. The activity should progress from simple skills to complex skills. Planning should always include progressive increments for exercise or physical activity. Reducing an activity to its component parts consists of analyzing each step needed to perform the activity. Each task should build upon the previous task until the activity is complete. When the activity has been reduced to its component parts, select an appropriate teaching method. Three methods are listed below:

1. Present the entire activity from beginning to end to the consumer (forward chaining).
2. Present the entire activity from the last step and gradually work toward the first step (backward chaining).
3. Present the entire activity. Future trials are used to refine the activity.[60–62]

Implementation

Before the activity is performed, the elderly individual should be aware of (or educated to) his or her exercise tolerance, limitations, and emotional stress threshold.[28] The activity can be implemented using the determined adaptations and sequential tasks.

Evaluation

The evaluation process will determine whether additional modifications are required. Successful mastery of the activity will form the basis of the evaluation. Activity analysis enables an individual to determine the component of the activity that has not been mastered. Evaluation is a continual process for all activities to enhance the recreational participation of the elderly.[40–44]

ACTIVITY ANALYSIS: BOWLING

Here is an example of activity analysis using bowling.

Assessment

Strength: Does the client have enough strength in the upper body to lift a standard (10- to 16-pound) bowling ball and deliver the ball? Does the client have enough strength in the hand and fingers to grasp the ball with one hand? With two hands?

Flexibility: Does the client have enough flexibility in the shoulder (full range of motion for pendulum swing of the ball) to deliver the ball?

Balance: Does the client have adequate balance for the walking-and-slide approach?

Coordination: Can the client coordinate the approach with the delivery of the ball?

Endurance: Does the client have adequate endurance to participate (bowl 10 frames per game)?

Physical limitations: Does the client have any disability that requires adaptations or modifications?

Planning

Adaptations, Modifications

1. If the patient has difficulty in grasping the ball, adapters can be used to provide bar grip.
2. Problems with coordination, flexibility, and strength can be aided by the balance of a ball ramp.
3. Balance problems can be aided by the use of a rail such as those used by visually impaired patients.
4. Games can be shortened to five frames for those with limited endurance.
5. Bowling can be performed by the disabled with the aid of grip adapters and ball ramps.

Sequential Steps for Ball Delivery

1. Approach ball ramp.
2. Grasp ball, place second and third fingers and thumb in holes, extend first and fourth finger along contour of ball.
3. Take beginning stance facing the pins approximately four to five walking steps from the foul line.
4. Begin four-step approach to foul line with a simultaneous push-away forward motion of ball and the first step.

5. Continue approach by coordinating the next three steps with the pendulum swing. Walk straight toward the foul line.
6. The last step, executed as a slide, will be coordinated with the forward swing of the ball.
7. Release the ball by letting it roll off the palm and fingers out over the foul line.
8. Continue to lift the hand for the followthrough and hold the pose.

Tasks can be reduced further to include different grips, different stances, different approaches, and different releases. For example:

Grips: conventional, semifingertip, and fingertip
Stances: different starting positions of ball and feet
Approaches: three-, four-, and five-step approaches
Releases: hook, straight, and backup deliveries

MODIFIED ACTIVITIES

Additional instructions can also be added to improve techniques of an individual once the basic skills of any activity have been mastered. Several activities, with modifications, are listed below:

Reading	Large print books
Sewing	Large print pattern
Cards	Braille cards, large print cards, cardholders
Swimming	Flotation devices
Bowling	Ramps, rails, grip adaptors
Exercises	Chair exercises, graduated increments
Volleyball	Lower net, balloon, nerf volleyball
Dance	Wheelchair dances

The modifications of the activity depend on the abilities of the individual.

Once the mastery of this process has been accomplished, the recreation specialist can apply it to any of the following activity areas: arts, dance, drama, literature, self-improvement, sports, outdoor recreation hobbies, social recreation, volunteer services, and travel and tourism.[40] The activity analysis process allows the professional to document the client's development, no matter what his or her level of ability. The development of the program should be based on the client's—not recreation specialist's—interest.

APPLICATION OF ACTIVITY PROCESS TO PEOPLE WITH ALZHEIMER'S DISEASE

Alzheimer's is a degenerative disease of unknown etiology characterized by forgetfulness and confusion followed by a progressive downhill decline of the individual's cognitive and physiologic responses. Sevush[64] outlines the following common features of Alzheimer's-related dementia:

- Forgets recent events.
- Repeats same question.
- Forgets deadlines and appointments.
- Disorientation to time and location.
- Usually denies memory loss.
- Diminished abstract thinking, impaired judgment, and paranoid ideation.
- Neocortical dysfunction; aphasia, agnosia, and apraxia.
- Simple motor functions remain intact until late stage of the disease.
- Alzheimer's disease eventually involves all cortical functions and results in death. (p. 9).

Alzheimer's disease is progressive. At present there is no cure; the only interventions are ones of maintenance. Leisure and recreation activity can contribute to the quality of life of someone with Alzheimer's disease, but as Figure 5–2 illustrates, health professional may experi ence frustration and an inherent contradiction; the client will get progressively worse, not better. How does the professional develop a program or activity when the abilities of the client may change from week to week?

Based on the recent research findings and the continuity theory of aging, the following process was developed to help those with Alzheimer's disease to maintain their previous activity level.[65]

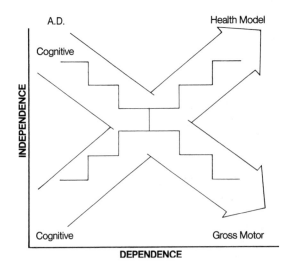

FIGURE 5–2. The ascending row represents the expectation of the rehabilitation professional that an individual will progress from dependence to independence while following a rehabilitation program. The descending arrow represents the regression from independence to dependence of an individual with Alzheimer's disease.

Task Analysis and Validation

Individuals who have Alzheimer's disease are affected in various ways. The activity selected for each individual reflects these differences. An activity should be selected based on the following steps.[68]

1. Review patient's chart, consulting especially the social history and what the patient was doing prior to admittance to the hospital. Specifically, review:
   a. **Family patterns:** possible family leisure activities.
   b. **Social patterns:** activities with spouse, friends; amount of money spent on leisure activities.
   c. **Work patterns:** type of jobs held; nature of work: shift work, labor, office job, professional?
   d. **Groups and organizations:** church, legion, card clubs.
   e. **Past interests:** person's self-report and family input, records
2. If client is able to respond, try to get him or her to identify areas of past interest.
   a. Talk about where he or she lived. Learn about the patient's former lifestyle. Did he or she live near the water? On a farm? (Where an individual lives indicates a lot about his or her leisure time and how it was spent.)
   b. Talk about jobs, employment, and various activities done around the house (for example, gardening, painting).
   c. Discuss family—parents, children, etc. What activities did the patient do with them?
   d. Attempt to explore areas of interest regarding entertainment activities. You may wish to use some activities identified in a structured form.[49–51]
3. Interview patient's family and friends about past interests. Get them to fill out SLIP or other interest finders after discussing previous activity patterns.
4. Interview staff on the present abilities of patients (check nursing notes), and ask staff if they know of any activities that the individual appears to interested in.
5. Observe patient at different intervals to note any familiar behaviors. Observation should be done daily for 1 week for 15-minute periods.
6. Try various stimuli (music, activities) and see how patient reacts based on identified interests. If that information is unavailable, expose the individual to activities related to his or her previous employment.
7. Document results:
   a. Reason for assessment
   b. Past leisure interests
   c. Current leisure activities
   d. Future potential areas (based on past interests)

e. Impressions

f. Plans to maintain level of functioning

g. Objectives: specific leisure goals and activities

This process was used with two individuals who were assessed as having Alzheimer's disease in a large eastern hospital. Results of the investigation indicate that the participants were able to complete an activity but needed reinforcement in completing the activity. Activity analyses enabled the investigators to identify the component part of the activity that caused confusion. It was found that using the individual's past experience in an activity caused less confusion for the person involved in the activity. A video entitled *Therapeutic Recreation Assessment for Persons with Alzheimer's* illustrates this process.[66]

VOLUNTEERS

Owing to budget constraints that result in greater staff-to-consumer ratio, it is often difficult to implement individual attention. Volunteers may be the solution to this problem in a long-term care facility. Volunteers have been used successfully to deliver recreation programs to the elderly in long-term care facilities. When an agency chooses to use volunteer services to deliver recreation services, the agency should be prepared to select, train, and retain volunteers just as it would employees. Koh[67] states that "screening is the quality control factor for effective volunteers" (p. 23). There is a need to interview volunteers just as you would an individual for any other type of job in the agency. Through the interview, the long-term care agency can find out where the applicant has previously worked, establish initial rapport, enforce criteria for selection, and reach a mutual decision with the applicant regarding whether he or she is suited for the agency.

Once the volunteers have been selected, an agency needs to establish a training program for them. Banes[68] indicates that during the training process "the roles, responsibilities, and parameters of authority are the most important subjects a volunteer should know, understand and accept. That same understanding and acceptance are necessary for the professionals and the elected officials involved. Too often it is assumed volunteers know what is expected, know what their limitations are and how to act" (p. 27).

If volunteers are to be a viable component to deliver services in a long-term care facility, they need to be properly oriented and trained. Schindler-Rainmann[69] suggests the following steps in training volunteers:

1. *Preservice training:* that is, training of a volunteer beginning work.
2. *Start-up support:* that is, assistance to the volunteers as they begin their volunteer work.
3. *Maintenance-of-effort training:* throughout the volunteer's period of service, regular times are needed for asking questions and gaining additional job-related knowledge.

4. *Periodic review and feedback.*
5. *Transition training:* volunteers have a need to grow and to assume more responsibility.

The development of a volunteer handbook may aid in the training of volunteers because it should outline the responsibilities of the volunteer as well as those of the agency. The handbook should include such items as a brief history of the agency, the agency program policies, the evaluation procedure used for volunteers, volunteer rights, physical aspects of aging, sexuality, and death and dying.

SUMMARY

If the elderly are to retain a degree of control of their leisure choices, the institution may need to establish the following:

1. A practicum experience with students in health-related fields (occupational therapy, physical therapy, health education, recreation) at nearby universities. This will provide the institution with individuals who are interested in the elderly. It would also allow for more one-to-one interaction between the elderly and the staff.
2. An advisory committee of patients to plan leisure activities in the institution.
3. A volunteer program that would properly select, train, and retain volunteers. Volunteers could be a benefit or a liability, depending on how well they are trained.
4. The use of existing community facilities for leisure opportunities. This will allow individuals to remain active in a community that is not age-segregated.
5. Health professionals' awareness of existing programs in the community for the elderly, as well as programs that provide activities for all ages. This ensures that the elderly people will not be segregated into one activity, but rather will be given the opportunity to participate in a variety of programs regardless of age. The only criterion should be ability.
6. Use of the activity analysis process to develop programs based on the patient's, not the staff's, interests.
7. Plans that are connected with, not for, older individuals. These encourage control of one area of an individual's life in the institution.
8. Maintenance of past recreation practices and development of new leisure opportunities.
9. Activities based on interest, not age, categories.
10. Modified activities based on the abilities of the individual, not on his or her disability.

11. Modified living environment that encourages social interaction, not isolation.
12. Communication, cooperation, and coordination of activities with other members of the health team to deliver a comprehensive program.
13. The use of the activity analysis process to determine modifications necessary for activities that are suggested by the patients.
14. Evaluation of individual's accomplishments based on the activity analysis process, not subjective criteria.

Establishing these standards may help the elderly to feel in control of their leisure lifestyle. Leviton and Campanelli[70] state that:

1. Leisure activities may contribute significantly to the older person's satisfaction with the meaning given to his or her life.
2. Leisure activities may serve as "healthy" stressors, mediators of stress, or responses to stress.
3. Empirical and scientific data offer a firm basis for the development of gerontologically oriented leisure service (p. 220).

Health professionals working with the elderly should plan with rather than for them. If they do not, they are contributing to further devaluation of the individual in the institution.

This chapter is based on the premise that an elderly person surrenders too many rights once he or she enters a long-term care facility. The individual enters an environment that encourages dependence instead of independence via such mechanisms as institutional routine (for example, meals at specific times) and administrative policies (for example, permission to attend community events). How can this issue be resolved? One answer could be based on the method outlined in this chapter, allowing an individual some control over one component of his or her lifestyle in the institution: the choice and enjoyment of leisure activities.

REFERENCES

1. Goffman E: Asylums. Doubleday, New York, 1961.
2. Hirsch, C: Integrating the Nursing Home Resident into a Senior Citizens Center. Gerontologist 17:277, 1977.
3. Langer, EJ and Rodin, J: The effects of choice and enhanced personal responsibilities for the aged: A field experiment in an institution. J Pers Soc Psychol (34):191, 1976.
4. McGuire, A: Constraints and leisure involvement in advanced adulthood. In Ray, RO (ed): Leisure and Aging. University of Wisconsin, Madison, 1978, p 78.
5. Iso Ahola, E: Perceived control and responsibility as mediators of the effects of therapeutic recreation on the institutionalized aged. Therapeutic Recreation Journal 14(1):38, 1980.
6. Kaplan, M: Leisure: Theory and Policy. John Wiley & Sons, New York, 1975.
7. Kaplan, M: Leisure: Lifestyle and Lifespan Perspective of Gerontology. WB Saunders, Philadelphia, 1979.
8. Verhoven, J: Recreation and the aging. In Stein, AT and Sessons, HD (eds): Recreation and Special Populations. Allyn & Bacon, Boston, 1977.

9. Gunn, LS: Labels that limit life. Leisure Today, October 1977, p 27.

10. Guadagnolo, B: 1000 Handmade ashtrays—meaning leisure, Leisure Today, October 1977, p 5.

11. Ekerdt, DJ, et al: Longitudinal change in preferred age of retirement. J Occup Psychol 49:161, 1976.

12. Kelly, RJ: Recreation Prediction by Age and Family Cycle. The Third Nationwide Outdoor Recreation Plan, Appendix II, Survey, Technical Report 4, 1978.

13. Baley, JA: Recreational and the aging process. Res Q Exerc Sport 26:1, 1955.

14. Cowgill, CO, and Balch, BN: The use of leisure time by old people. J Gerontol 17:302, 1962.

15. Ford, MP: An analysis of leisure time activities and interests of aged residents in Indiana. Unpublished PhD dissertation, Indiana University, 1962.

16. Szalai, A (ed): Daily activities of urban and suburban populations in twelve countries. In The Use of Time. Mouton, The Hague, 1972.

17. Bull, CN (ed): Leisure activities in Mangen: Research Instruments in Social Gerontology. University of Minnesota Press, Minneapolis, 1982.

18. Elliot, DH, Harvey, AS, and MacDonald, WS: A decade later: Stability and change in the pattern of time use in the Halifax panel. Employment and Immigration, Ottawa, 1984.

19. Harvey, AS and Singleton, JF: Canadian Activity Patterns across the Lifespan: A Time Budget Perspective. Paper presented at the 15th Annual Scientific and Education Meeting, Canadian Association on Gerontology, November 2–6, 1986.

20. Singleton, JF: Outdoor recreation participation patterns among the elderly. Activities Adaptation and Aging 6:1, 1984.

21. Singleton, JF, Mitic, W, and Farquharson, J: Activity profile of retired individuals. Activities Adaptation and Aging 9:1, 1986.

22. Kelly, RJ: Leisure styles: A hidden core. Leisure Sciences 5:4, 1983.

23. Lounsbury, WJ: Five-Year Stability of Leisure Activity and Motivation Factors. Paper Presented at the 10th Annual Leisure Research Symposium, National Recreation Park Association, New Orleans, 1987.

24. Forbes, W, Singleton, JF, and Agwani, A: Stability of activity across the lifespan. Activities Adaptation and Aging 18(1):19–27, 1993.

25. Kelly, J: Recreation demand, aging, and the life course. World Leisure and Recreation 31(2):25–28, 1989.

26. Kelly, RJ: Leisure. Prentice Hall, Englewood Cliffs, NJ, 1982.

27. Harvey, AS, and Singleton, JF: Stage of lifecycle and activity patterns across the lifespan. Paper presented at the Canadian Association on Gerontology Annual Conference, Toronto, October 25, 1991.

28. Lewis, CB and Campanelli, L: Health Promotion and Exercise for Older Adults. Aspen Publication, Rockeville, MD, 1990.

29. Moran, JM: Leisure Activities for the Mature Adult. Burgess, Minneapolis, 1979.

30. Heywood, L: Recreation for Older Adults: A Program Manual. Ministry of Culture and Recreation. Toronto, 1979.

31. Shivers, TS and Fait, HF: Recreational Services for the Aging. Lea & Febiger, Philadelphia, 1980.

32. Leitner, M and Seitner, S: Leisure in Later Life: A Source Book for the Provision of Recreational Services for Elders. Haworth Press, New York, 1985.

33. Teaff, J: Leisure Service with the Elderly. Mosby, St. Louis, 1985.

34. Burdman, GM: Healthful Aging. Prentice Hall, Englewood Cliffs, NJ, 1986.

35. MacNeill, R, Teague, M: Aging and Leisure: Vitality in Later Life. Prentice Hall Inc., Englewood Cliffs, NJ, 1987

36. Searle, SM: Leisure, aging and mental health: A review of the clinical evidence. Top Geriatr Rehabil 7(2):1–12, 1991.

37. Tabourne, ESC: The effects of a life review recreation therapy program on confused nursing home residents. Top Geriat Rehabil 7(2):13–21, 1991.

38. Weiss, RC, Blake D, and Koscianshe V: Enhancing family council members ability to relate to and reminisce with older disoriented residents: Replication and extension. Top Geriatr Rehabil 7(2):45–59, 1991.

39. Doble SE: A home-based model of rehabilitation for individuals with SDAT and their caregivers. Top Geriatr Rehabil 7(2):33–44, 1991.

40. Winslow, R: The Best of Therapeutic Recreation: Aging. National Therapeutic Recreation Society, National Recreation and Park Association. Arlington, VA, 1993.

41. Humphrey, F: The Best of Therapeutic Recreation: Assessment. National Therapeutic Recreation Society, National Recreation and Park Association. Arlington, VA, 1989.

42. Miller, M: Documentation in Long-Term Care. National Therapeutic Recreation Society, National Recreation and Park. Arlington, VA. 1989.

43. Land, C, Marmer, A, Mayfield, S, Gerski, MK, and Murphy, C: Protocols in Therapeutic Recreation. National Therapeutic Recreation Society. National Recreation and Park Association. Arlington, VA, 1989.

44. Greenwall, PH and Zeidman, B: Guidelines for the Administration of Therapeutic Recreation Services. National Therapeutic Recreation Society. National Recreation and Parks Association. Arlington, VA, 1990.

45. McGuire, AF, Boyd, KR, and Jame, A: Therapeutic Humour with Elderly. Haworth Press, Binghampton, NY, 1992.

46. Keller, JM and Woolley, SM: Designing Exercise Program with Older Adults: Theory and Practice. Activities, Adaptation and Aging. 16(2):1–17, 1991.

47. Pentland, W, McCall, M, Harvey, A, doRozario, L, Niemi, I, and Barker. The Relationships between Time Use and Health, Well-Being and Quality of Life. Queen's University, Kingston, Ont., 1993.

48. Seleen, RD: Life satisfaction and the congruence between actual and desired participation in activity by older adults. In Robert, RO (ed): Leisure and Aging. University of Wisconsin, Madison, 1979.

49. Mirenda, JJ: Mirenda Leisure Finder. In Epperson, JA, et al (eds): Leisure Counseling Kit. American Alliance for Health, Physical Education and Recreation, Washington, DC, 1973.

50. McDowell, CF: Toward a health leisure mode: Leisure Counseling. Therapeutic Recreation Journal 8(3):96, 1974.

51. McKechnie, GE: Manual for Leisure Activities Blank. Consulting Psychology Press, Palo Alto, CA, nd.

52. McKechnie, GE: Psychological foundations of leisure counseling, an empirical strategy. Therapeutic Recreation Journal 8(1):4, 1974.

53. Overs, RP: A model for avocational counseling. Journal of Health, Physical Education and Recreation 41(2):28, 1970.

54. Gunn, LS and Peterson, AC: Therapeutic Recreation Program Design Principles and Procedures, Prentice-Hall, Englewood Cliffs, NJ, 1978.

55. Humphrey, F: Communication, Cooperation, Coordination. Proceedings, Volunteer Venture, Connecticut Department of Health, 1969, p 6.

56. Hogan, DB, Hogan, JM, Ferneyhough, J, Bagley, S, Williams S, Jonstone-Chapman, C, York, M, and Tonulson, R: Interdisciplinary care in geriatric day hospital. Top Geriatr Rehabil 7(2):22–32, 1991.

57. Singleton, JF, Makrides, L, and Kennedy, M: Role of three professions in long-term care facilities. Activities, Adaptation and Aging 9(1):57, 1986.

58. Atchley, R: The Social Forces in Later Life: An Introduction to Social Gerontology. Wadsworth, Belmont, CA, 1977.

59. Davis, BN and Teaff, DJ: Facilitating role continuity of elderly through leisure programming. Therapeutic Recreation Journal 2(14):32, 1980.

60. Gold, WM and Scott, KG: Discrimination tearing. In Stephens, WB (ed): Training the developmentally young. John Day, New York, 1971.

61. Gold, WM: Task analysis of a complex assembly by retarded blind. Except Child 43:2, 1976.

62. Gold, WM: Vocational training. In Wortis, J (ed): Mental Retardation and Developmental Disabilities. Bruner/Mazel, New York, 1975.
63. Edington, RC and Williams, GJ: Productive Management of Leisure Service Organizations: A Behavioral Approach, John Wiley & Sons, Toronto, 1978.
64. Sevush, S: Alzheimer's disease: New ideas in diagnosis and therapy. Top Geriatr Rehabil 1(2):8, 1986.
65. Singleton, J, Ostiguy, L, and Riley, A: Programming for Individuals with Alzheimer's: A Systematic Approach. National Therapeutic Recreation Society. National Recreation and Park Association. Indianapolis, 1988.
66. Ritcey, A & Singleton, J: Therapeutic Recreation Assessment for Persons with Alzheimers. Camp Hill Medical Center, 1760 Robie St., Halifax, NS, B3L 3T7, 1991.
67. Koh, M: Effective use of volunteers in therapeutic settings. Therapeutic Recreation Journal 6(1):23, 1972.
68. Banes, ER: Maximizing Human Resources. Parks and Recreation, December 1975, p 27.
69. Schindler-Rainmann, E: The Volunteer Community Creative Use of Human Resources. Learning Resources Corporation, Fairfax, VA, 1975, p 75.
70. Leviton, D and Campanelli, L: Health, Physical Education, Recreation and Dance for the Older Adult: A Modular Approach. American Alliance for Health, Physical Education and Dance, Reston, VA, 1980, p 220.

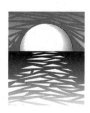

CHAPTER 6

The Changing Realm of the Senses

Gail Hills Maguire, PhD, OTR/L, FAOTA

BEHAVIORAL OBJECTIVES

Upon completion of this chapter, the reader will be able to:

1 Identify common sensory deficits in the elderly.
2 Describe compensation techniques for problems in vision, hearing, taste, smell, touch, and communication.
3 List modifications of the clinical environment to assist elderly patients with impaired hearing and vision.
4 Discuss the effects of sensory deficits on rehabilitation potential.
5 Recognize sensory deficits in the elderly.
6 Recommend modifications for the personal and physical environments of older persons.

An individual's potential for interaction with the environment is highly dependent on his or her capacity to receive and respond to information obtained through the senses. The senses that will be discussed here are what are commonly referred to as the five senses and include sight (visual), hearing (auditory), taste (gustatory), smell (olfactory), and touch (tactile). Each of these senses contributes a specific type of information necessary for a person to adapt and to adjust to the environment. Limitations in sensory input associated with aging can affect an individual's safety, functional ability, self-image, and interaction with others. The quality of life of community-dwelling elderly individuals was found to be significantly linked to sensory impairment. Mood and social relationships seemed to be particularly affected by visual impairment, while independence in daily activities seemed to be affected by hearing impairment. Either visual or hearing impairment was associated with increased risk of depression.[1] Sensory impairments, especially presbyopia, cataracts, and glaucoma, can be impediments to effective communication, especially for elderly people with senile dementia of the Alzheimer's type (SDAT).[2] Health professionals must be sensitive to the potential effects of sensory deficits on the total rehabilitation program and be prepared to modify the environment as needed.

In making recommendations for screening of the elderly, Beers and others[3] recommended vision testing for refractive error, audiometric testing for presbycusis, and surveys for hearing loss in making screening recommendations for the elderly.

Fortunately, a young person usually has sensory acuities far in excess of what is needed for normal activities. As a person ages, there is a gradual decline in the senses, and the sensory threshold levels increase. Threshold refers to the minimal degree of stimulus needed to activate the system. A higher threshold means that stronger stimuli are required to activate the sensory receptors, for example, brighter lights, louder sounds, stronger tastes and smells. Initial sensory losses are often unnoticed because of the ample margin of surplus available before normal function is affected and because of unconscious compensation techniques. However, at a certain point, depreciation of the sensory processes can become critical and seriously affect behavioral or psychologic functioning.[4]

An individual sensory process deteriorates to a greater degree over time the more it possesses one or several of the following characteristics: high specialization, greater complexity, higher discrimination, and increased articulation with other bodily systems.[4] However, this is a generalization, and aging occurs in all systems of the same individual at varying rates; and each aged individual must be approached as separate and unique.

VISION

A person may maintain nearly normal sight until well into old age. Nevertheless, the aging eye is subject to various changes and pathologies. Visual changes can be congenital or can occur throughout the life cycle. In the normal (emmetropic) eye (Fig. 6–1), the muscles (ciliary) are relaxed, and parallel light rays from distant objects are in sharp focus directly on the retina. Divergent rays from near objects require contraction of the ciliary muscles to increase the curvature of the lens so that the focal point will still fall on the retina.[5]

Common Refractive Problems

The refractive power of the eye is the ability of the lens to bend light rays. Myopia, hyperopia, and astigmatism are some of the common refractive defects of the eye that can occur at any age.

Myopia

Myopia (nearsightedness) occurs when parallel light rays from distant objects focus before the retinal surface rather than on it (Fig. 6–2) when the ciliary muscles are relaxed. This can occur when the eyeball is too long, or, less commonly, when the lens system is too strong. Only objects that are less than 20 feet from the subject are in focus. All objects beyond this distance appear blurred.[5–7]

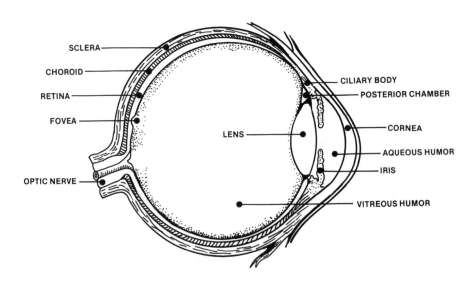

FIGURE 6–1. The eye.

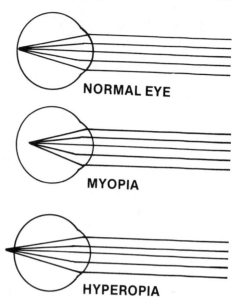

FIGURE 6–2. Parallel light rays focus on the retina in the normal eye, in front of the retina in myopia, and behind the retina in hyperopia. (Adapted from Guyton,[6] p 730.)

Hyperopia

Hyperopia (farsightedness) occurs when parallel light rays from distant objects are not refracted sufficiently by the lens system to come into focus by the time they reach the retina when the ciliary muscles are relaxed (see Fig. 6–2). The point of focus is beyond the retinal surface. This is due to an eyeball that is too short or a lens system that is too weak. Objects less than 20 feet from the subject are blurred, and objects beyond 20 feet are also blurred; in the earlier years of the developmental cycle, the lens of the eye can usually accommodate by focusing. In later years, the lens is less capable of making this accommodation, particularly with near objects.[5,6]

Astigmatism

Astigmatism is a refractive error of the lens system caused by irregularities in the curvature of the cornea or the lens. Curvature of the astigmatic lens along either the vertical or horizontal plane is less than curvature along the other plane. There will be less convergence owing to less refractive power, and the focal point of one plane will be farther from the lens than the focal point of the other plane. Rays of light are not focused equally, and both distant and near objects appear blurred.[5-7]

Age-Related Changes in Vision

Presbyopia

Presbyopia (old sight) is associated with the aging process. The lens loses its elastic nature and becomes more rigid. The ciliary muscles that hold the lens in position may become weaker, lose tone, and decrease in ability to accommodate rapidly from far to near distance (and vice versa).

Once the lens becomes unaccommodating, the eye remains permanently focused at an almost constant distance. The distance varies with individuals. In order for an older person to be able to see both near and far objects, he or she must wear bifocal glasses in which the upper segment focuses for distant objects, and the lower segment focuses for near objects, such as printed material.[5,6]

Visual acuity as well as accommodation decreases with age. In a study of 136 patients over 65, 46 (34%) were found to have a correctable undetected visual acuity deficit (CUVAD).[8] Normal vision is described as 20/20. Vision of 20/30 means that a person can identify objects at 20 feet or less that a person with normal vision can identify at 30 feet or less. Vision levels of 20/40 can still be quite functional; a person can drive a car and perform most activities. However, when vision reaches 20/50 or worse, driving is not permitted in many states. Serious problems arise at vision levels of 20/70 and less. Recognition of objects and people becomes difficult, as do reading, watching television, and seeing bus numerals and signs. Roughly one third of individuals over 80 have vision of 20/50 or less.[9,10] Strong reading glasses, magnifying glasses, and low-vision aids are available, but the tolerance for aids varies.

With reduced vision, the elderly need increased lighting that does not increase glare. Hughes and Neer[11] include a helpful discussion of the role of lighting, not only for vision but also for regulating important biochemical processes. Practical suggestions are given for lighting problems, including the advantages of full-spectrum lighting with a high color-rendering index (CRI), which simulates natural sunlight, as opposed to a conventional cool white source such as fluorescent lamps.

Hutton and others[12] reported that in 10 percent of elderly subjects they tested, restriction of vertical viewing angle ability resulted from a combination of restricted vertical eye movements and limited neck extension. This restriction, combined with the limitations of presbyopia, has important implications for architectural design and communication techniques. They suggest that communication with elderly individuals, especially those with a hearing loss, could be improved if speakers position themselves in the person's line of vision; for example, if elderly persons are seated, one would sit directly in front of them and establish eye contact rather than stand over them. Placement of important information such as fire exit signs, room numbers, and other orienting information up high in hallways and above doors should also be avoided.[12]

In a study of community elderly, Branch and others[13] found that, controlling for age and sex, vision loss was associated with unmet instrumental ADL needs such as housekeeping, grocery shopping, and food preparation. In a study of patients drawn from ophthalmologists' offices in three cities, Brenner and others[14] found that regardless of ophothalmic treatment, when vision improved, multiple quality-of-life functions were likely to improve. Conversely, when vision declined, quality-of-life indicators were also likely to decline. The greatest improvements occurred when both initial vision and quality-of-life indicators were highly impaired and considerable improvement in vision was achieved.

Hill and Hill[15] stress that a proactive lifestyle, orientation and mobility training, and strategies such as precane devices in combination with appropriate functional assessments and in-service training can increase independence and life satisfaction for the elderly with visual impairments.

Reduced Tear Flow

The research of Furukawa and Polse[16] suggests that a 40 percent reduction in tear secretion accompanies aging. The symptoms and signs, such as dryness commonly observed in older individuals, seem to be caused by altered tear chemistry and insufficient tear secretion. This condition, like all others, should be followed through regular eye examinations and treatment. Medication is available to relieve the symptoms.

Ophthalmologic Disorders

Approximately 10 percent of elderly persons have undetected eye disease or visual impairment. Because vision loss is so common in old age, both elderly persons and professionals sometimes overlook it.[17] The large proportion of elderly people with visual impairments has received little attention from educators and researchers as well. Too often, professionals fail to discriminate between changes associated with presbyopia and visual impairment resulting from age-associated disorders.[13]

The most common diseases and conditions are glaucoma, cataracts, macular degeneration, and uncorrected refractive error. The prevalence of all these conditions increases with age; persons over 85 are most likely to suffer from macular degeneration.[3] Agencies that provide services to visually impaired individuals have generally ignored older persons. This is partly due to the high cost of providing a variety of services, the pattern of institutionalizing the elderly, and the reluctance of many older people to seek services.[15] Program emphasis for the visually impaired elderly has traditionally been focused on recreational rather than rehabilitative services. Visually impaired elderly individuals are motivated to be independent; therefore, programs need to shift their emphasis from recreational to rehabilitative concerns.[18] Findings of a statewide survey of aging and blindness agencies showed that a large percentage of aging agencies were not addressing the needs of the aging blind population. Lack of interaction between the two systems was a major service delivery barrier. The authors stressed the importance of improved understanding of the resources of both systems and better communication between the two systems.[19]

Glaucoma

Glaucoma is one of the leading causes of blindness in individuals over 35 and is especially prevalent in the elderly. Between 95 and 98 percent of this blindness is preventable. The deciding factors in reducing the incidence of blindness from this often asymptomatic disease are early detection, appropriate intervention, and consistent follow-up for the rest of the patient's life.[20] Glaucoma is due to pathologically high intraocular pressure. It occurs principally in two forms: open-angle glaucoma and closed-angle glaucoma. Open-angle glaucoma is the most common and affects approximately 2 percent of people over 40. It is painless and asymptomatic until major damage and visual loss have occurred. It is insidious because the initial loss of peripheral vision is usually not noticed by the victim. Screening examinations are an important preventive measure. Acute closed-angle glaucoma is usually very sudden and painful. The entire chamber is occluded by a pushed-forward iris, leading to a rapid rise in intraocular pressure. If the pressure is not reduced, compression of the retinal artery can result in retinal atrophy and blindness. Treatment with topical eyedrops can control the disease in most cases, but surgical intervention may be necessary. Laser treatment is a noninvasive alternative to surgery. It can be done as an outpatient procedure, making it less risky and more cost-effective than traditional surgery. Many patients may resume work activities within 24 hours.[20] See Schwartz and others[21] for a good discussion of laser treatment in uncontrolled phakic open-angle glaucoma. Early diagnosis is important; the earlier treatment is begun, the easier it is to control the disease. Older people need an eye examination at least once a year and more often if indicated; it is the only way to diagnose the condition.

Cataracts

Cataracts, the most common visual problem of old age, are a developmental or a degenerative opacity of the lens of the eye, causing obstruction of the passage of light rays to the retina. Morrison and Jay[22] found that even the mildest degree of cataracts was shown to degrade optical function to the extent that it exceeded the age-related neural deterioration. Central vision is restricted first, with gradual involvement of the peripheral field (the opposite process of glaucoma). The person is bothered by glare from bright lights reflected on shiny surfaces, a gradual darkening of vision, and loss of acuity.

Myopia can develop in the early stages of nuclear cataracts, so a presbyopic individual may be able to read without glasses for a period of time. Pain is absent unless the cataract swells and produces secondary glaucoma. People vary greatly as to when they seek treatment, depending on how critical vision is to their daily activities.

Removal of the cataract (lens) is the only treatment and creates aphakia. The aphakic eye has no focusing mechanism, and the use of intraocular lens implants is the therapy of choice. Special eyeglasses, with their thick lenses and distorted vision, are rarely seen today.[23] For persons who are not candidates for lens implants, contact lenses are an option. Contact lenses greatly reduce the distortions and are preferred to glasses whenever possible. However, not everyone can wear contact lenses, and some people may not be able to wear them exclusively. The elderly person may have less tolerance for contact lenses when he or she is tired or ill.[24]

Cataract eyeglasses are less than a satisfactory substitute for the normal eye lens. Glasses cause confusing magnification of images.[25,26] The increase in the magnification makes objects appear much larger and closer than they actually are. This can cause difficulties with self-care, ambulation, and household tasks.[26] For example, a person may underestimate the distance of his or her hand from a table and thus drop and break a glass; or, when descending stairs, the person may misjudge the distance of the steps and stumble and fall.

With cataract eyeglasses, objects in the periphery are distorted, making driving a car or walking in unfamiliar surroundings frightening and hazardous if the person does not learn to accommodate. Because of the lack of focusing ability, distorted visual images occur, when the person moves his or her eyes back and forth. This results in a momentary sense of disorientation and confusion. The health professional must take these conditions into account when working with a person who wears cataract glasses and allow sufficient time for the individual to adjust visually to body movements.[24]

Belkin and others[27] reported that the results of a retrospective survey suggest that wearing sunglasses outdoors may offer some protection against solar ultraviolet radiation, which may be a contributing factor to the formation of human senile cataracts. They recommend that persons who do not routinely wear eyeglasses, including those who usually wear contact lenses, wear sunglasses. This is especially important in geographic regions where people are exposed to very high levels of ultraviolet radiation.

Macular Degeneration

This third major source of visual disability is more serious than cataracts or glaucoma because it is the least treatable at present. It is a pigmentary change of the macular area of the retina caused by small hemorrhages. Individuals see a gray shadow in the center of the visual area but can see well at the outer border. This condition is often seen in the elderly but rarely results in total blindness. However, without treatment visual loss can progress to legal blindness, making "close work" tasks difficult. Early symptoms include a slight blurring of vision in the affected eye, followed by a blind spot. Prevalence of the disease increases with age, with a 2 percent risk from ages 52 to 64 to a 28 percent risk past age 75.[28]

Compensation techniques can include wearing sun visors because vision is less acute in bright light, looking to the side to utilize peripheral vision, and the use of magnifiers. Many older individuals find such compensation techniques quite frustrating, especially because the loss of sharp central vision makes reading, watching television, and manipulation activities difficult.[5,10,25]

Retinitis Pigmentosa

Retinitis pigmentosa is a progressive pigmentary degeneration of the retina. It is more common in men than in women and is usually bilateral. Night blindness is one of the first symptoms because, unlike the situation in macular degeneration, the peripheral retina, where the rods are located, is involved first. When the person reaches 50 or 60, only 3 to 5° of central vision may remain. However, the residual central vision is often sufficient for reading until the patient reaches 70 or 80.[25,29]

Diabetic Retinopathy

Diabetic retinopathy has become the leading cause of blindness in the United States, above even glaucoma, owing to the increased life span of diabetics. The condition can occur whether or not diabetic control is good and usually takes two forms. The majority of the cases are simple diabetic retinopathy, in which microaneurysms and hemorrhages coagulate and obstruct light rays to the retina as well as damaging the retina itself. Damage is bilateral and similar in both eyes. Treatment is very difficult and unsatisfactory. Diabetes tends to have remissions and exacerbations, and therefore the course of the visual impairment may also fluctuate. Sudden changes in the eye are not uncommon. For example, the refractive status may change several diopters when changes in the blood sugar level affect hydration of the lens. Proliferate diabetic retinopathy, the second type, may be superimposed on the simple type. Large recurrent hemorrhages and retinal detachment can result in blindness.[25,29]

Retinal Detachment

Complete or partial detachment of the retina can occur as a result of trauma, as well as of diabetes. Loss of vision occurs wherever the retina is detached. Flickering flashes of light in the peripheral visual field and a sudden increase in floating specks are common symptoms, followed by a blotting out of vision if the retina becomes completely detached. The retina can often be reattached if treatment is initiated soon after it occurs. However, once detachment has progressed, extensive surgical intervention becomes necessary. The risk of recurring retinal detachment owing to strain is high.[5,9,25]

Legal Blindness

Any of these conditions can lead to sufficient visual impairment for the individual to be classified as legally blind. Legal blindness does not necessarily mean total blindness. Over 90 percent of individuals in this classification have some residual sight. The definition of legal blindness is (1) central visual acuity of 20/200 or less with the better eye with corrective lenses (that is, the individual can identify objects at only 20 feet or less that a person with normal vision can identify at 200 feet) and (2) restriction of the peripheral vision to a 20° angle or less (that is, the person sees no more than what an individual with normal vision might see through a tube or tunnel).[25]

Visual Care

Good preventive care begins with regular professional eye examinations. As a person ages, the need for such care increases. Everyone over 70 needs at least yearly professional care to correct or prevent visual problems. Yet it is estimated that the normal length of time between eye checkups for residents of nursing homes is from 5 to 7 years.[30]

As part of the initial evaluation, the nurse or therapist should check to see whether patients wear glasses and how long it has been since their last ophthalmologic examination. If it has been longer than a year, a referral should be made. In the meantime, quick screening of vision can be done with the Snellen chart. This is the common eye chart with rows of diminishing size *E*'s, beginning with a large letter E at the top. Visual acuity is recorded in the form of a fraction. The numerator 20 is the distance from the patient's eye to the chart. The denominator is the different size of the test number recorded from each line on the Snellen chart. The subject is positioned 20 feet from the chart, and vision of each eye is measured separately while vision of the opposite eye is occluded. Vision with eyeglasses is checked in a similar manner. This gives an indication of visual acuity with and without eyeglasses. A gross check of peripheral vision can be done by having the subject sit and face the evaluator. The subject is asked to fix his or her gaze on the evaluator's nose. Holding a pencil in his or her hand, the evaluator positions it behind and to the side of the patient's head. It is gradually moved into the subject's peripheral visual field. The subject is asked to indicate by word or gesture as soon as he or she first sees the pencil. The subject must maintain eye fixation during this procedure. The same process is repeated for the opposite side. It is desirable to have two evaluators, one to sit in front of the subject to be sure the subject looks straight ahead and one to move the pencil from the side. Since this is often not possible, the method described can be used.

If the visual field is imagined as a semi-circle around the front of the subject's head from the sides of the eyes, the potential visual field would be 180°. Imagine that you divide this into two equal 90° triangles, with 90° at the side of the eyes and 0° directly in front of the eyes. The subject should see the pencil on both sides of the eyes at 90°. As the pencil moves toward the center of the semicircle, the number of degrees of the visual deficit (loss) on each side can be estimated by plotting from 90° toward the center. For example, if the pencil is halfway from the sides of the eyes (90°) to the front (0°) on both sides, the remaining degrees would be 45° on each side.

If you add the remaining degrees on both sides (45° + 45°), the resulting peripheral vision is only 90°. In legal blindness, the peripheral vision is 20° (10° + 10° = 20°). This is a gross test that is reliable only to indicate the difference between eyes or monocular problems.

Poor vision that is not corrected can interfere with a total rehabilitation program. For instance, a person's difficulty with daily chores and ambulation may be greatly influenced by visual deficits.

Compensation Techniques for Visual Impairment

Several steps can be taken to compensate for visual changes associated with age or illness.[31]

1. Provide adequate light. Persons with visual problems need much more light than the average person.
2. Reduce glare. Avoid shiny surfaces, which will reflect light. Window shades, blinds, sunglasses, visors or hats with brims may reduce the glare from sunlight.
3. Avoid color coding when safety is a factor. Pastel colors, blues, greens, and very dark colors may all look alike to the elderly. Color coding should not be used for pills, marking appliances, etc. Colors used for identification and location should be strongly contrasting, such as yellow and blue.
4. Avoid abrupt changes in light. The older eye takes more time to accommodate to sudden changes. Lights should be strategically arranged, and some lights should be kept on at night in hazardous locations. For example, night lights can be left on in the bedroom, hall, and bath so that there is an even distribution of light.
5. Use large print on all signs, directions, and labels. Large print is easier for everyone to see.

6. People with cataract glasses may need assistance in crossing streets or wherever depth perception is a safety factor.
7. Low-vision aids, such as large-print books and magnifying glasses, may help.
8. Touching can be used in communication with someone of limited vision. A pat on the hand can let someone know you are listening.
9. Describe a new room or situation to a visually impaired person to help him or her locate hazards, furniture, and people who are in the room. Stay with the person until he or she is comfortably oriented.

. HEARING

The following brief discussion focuses on hearing problems as part of total sensory loss.

A review of the literature suggests that there is no general agreement on the specific effects of aging on the auditory system. However, there does seem to be a consensus that (1) auditory acuity decreases with age, and (2) the speech discrimination skills of the elderly are poorer than would be expected based on their pure tone loss.[32] Some hearing loss is usually present by 30 years of age, and the rate of loss increases as age increases.[33]

A 10-year study by Bergman and associates[34] found a noticeable decline in speech discrimination in the fifth decade of life, with a much steeper decline in the seventh decade. The reason for a greater decrement in speech discrimination scores for older listeners as compared with younger listeners in difficult situations is not understood. It may be due to a greater distortion of auditory signals.

In a study of the change in cognition over time in 38 subjects with dementia and with or without hearing impairment, hearing impairment predicted a more rapid cognitive decline only with those who had a diagnosis of Alzheimer's disease.[35]

Research is still needed on auditory problems of the elderly, particularly on measures to analyze and distinguish between peripheral and central (neural) losses. Unfortunately, most past studies did not make such distinctions and lumped all conditions under the label *presbycusis* (see subsequent text).[32]

A recent study by Cobb and others[36] examined both central and peripheral factors that may affect the hearing of elderly persons. There was a 2- to 11-fold decibel magnitude difference between elderly and younger subjects. The difference became greater with age and with short intervals between stimuli. Reductions in ganglion cell population and sensory hair cell population or function were suggested as likely explanations for increased target threshold perceptions of elderly listeners.

In a test of central auditory function of hemiplegic patients, Bergman and others[37] found differences between the two affected hemispheres. In a selective hearing test, patients with lesions in the right hemisphere generally scored 100 percent or only moderately below with the right ear but often failed to recognize speech with the left ear. It appears that this contralateral effect occurs in the apparent absence of temporal-area involvement. The patients with left-hemisphere lesions showed very different results. The contralateral effect rarely occurred. There was less difference in hearing between the two ears, with the right ear again scoring better despite being opposite the lesion. This suggests that, unlike young hemiplegic children, adults do not demonstrate a compensatory transfer of function from the usually dominant left hemisphere to the right hemisphere when there is a left-hemisphere lesion. A discrimination hearing test may identify patients who have had hemispheric lesions in addition to presbycusis. Even in someone with normal hearing, such lesions may cause difficulty in hearing others in the presence of a group.[37]

Peripheral Hearing Losses

A variety of factors can interfere with the conduction of sound waves to the inner ear, which is why such defects are often called "conduction problems."

Peripheral problems can include external ear disease and acute or chronic diseases of the middle ear.[38]

Otitis media, or inflammation of the middle ear, is one of the most common problems. In most cases the infection results when microorganisms from the nasopharynx enter via the eustachian tube. It is treated with medication but can result in permanent ear damage and hearing loss.[33]

Otosclerosis is a genetic condition characterized by a spongy bone formation around the oval window, resulting in ankylosis of the stapes. It is usually treatable with surgery, so the major problem is one of diagnosis and referral.[33]

Treatment for peripheral problems includes lowering the frequency of the sound, including the pitch of the speaking voice, and amplification through sound systems and hearing aids. People with hearing difficulties may have a very small range between the decibel (loudness) level necessary for them to hear a sound and the decibel level that may be painful or irritating. This can make adjustments of a hearing aid very difficult.[5]

A loss of hearing may interfere with receiving danger signals from the environment, such as horns or sirens, and this may impede safety.[5]

Sensorineural Losses

Central, or neural, losses in the elderly have been attributed to degeneration or changes in the neural receptors in the cochlea, the eighth nerve, the central auditory nervous system, or the central nervous system in general. Excessive noise is a common cause of hearing loss, with the most pronounced loss in the higher frequencies. Discrimination of consonants, particularly *S, Z, T, F,* and *G,* is more difficult than that of vowels.[5,31] Neural losses are usually permanent, and compensatory techniques such as lipreading may be advised.

Presbycusis

The hearing loss directly related to aging is called *presbycusis.* Presbycusis is an inner-ear loss of auditory acuity associated with aging (see Chapter 4). Previously it was thought to be a normal part of aging but now is seen as having a major genetic component. It varies tremendously in time of onset and intensity of loss.[5,33] Presbycusis may represent any one of several different types of disorders at various sites in the auditory system or a combination of these disorders. Because of the variety of conditions that may be included under presbycusis, there are various operational definitions. Pure presbycusis has been defined as the hearing loss that remains after the cumulative effects of multiple pathological processes throughout the elderly individual's life have been excluded.[39,40] Hearing impairment caused by external factors, such as the wear and tear of everyday noise, has been called *sociocusis. Nosocusis* refers to the effects of ototoxic factors and of disease.[41] Lowell and Paparella[39] grouped etiological factors as genetic (intrinsic) and nongenetic (extrinsic) factors. A longitudinal study of elderly individuals in Sweden showed a possible correlation between presbycusis and extrinsic factors, but additional study is needed.[41]

Presently there is no battery of tests that can make distinctions between the relative contributions of disease at the various neural sites. Therefore, clear-cut distinctions about pathology are difficult. It is usually characterized by a gradual progressive bilateral symmetric high-frequency sensorineural hearing loss with disproportionately poor speech discrimination occurring in old age.[5,26,33,39,42]

Tinnitus

A wide variety of "ear noises" are grouped under the general term *tinnitus.* A small percentage of the elderly suffer from this condition to varying degrees. Commonly reported noises include hissing, ringing, and buzzing. Tinnitus may be constant or intermittent and is very annoying. The condition may be due to various diseases, allergies, obstruction of the ear canal, and other causes and is often accompanied by hearing loss. Treatment of the primary etiology is essential, but many times it is unsuccessful. If relief is not obtained, stress to the elderly person can be great. Tranquilizers may help, as well as patience and consideration on the part of other people.

Assessment of Hearing Loss

Hearing loss is assessed by audiometric and nonaudiometric evaluation. Nonaudiometric assessment may include a physical examination, testing with a tuning fork, interviewing the patient and family, and self-reporting by the patient. An examination by the physician can determine if there is any evidence of structural changes or diseases of the ear. A physician often checks for hearing loss with a tuning fork as part of the examination. However, it can be done by other health professionals as a screening device, especially when medical treatment has been infrequent. The Rinne test is performed by striking the tuning fork and then placing the handle to the mastoid process (behind the ear). The patient is asked to indicate when he or she can no longer hear the sound. When this point is reached, the vibrating head of the tuning fork is immediately placed next to the external ear. The patient should continue to hear the sound because air conduction is normally greater than bone conduction. If the patient continues to hear the sound, the test is recorded as a positive Rinne test, showing that air conduction (AC) is greater than bone conduction (BC): (AC)>(BC). If the patient does not continue to hear the sound, a conduction loss is present.

Questioning the patient concerning possible problems is also helpful. (See Ebersole and Hess[43] for a comprehensive interview scale (p 217). Older people may report no difficulties because the change is very gradual or because they are sensitive about admitting losses. It is, therefore, also important to observe behavior carefully. Common behaviors that indicate hearing loss include inattentiveness, loud speech, inappropriate responses, frequent requests to repeat conversation, and consistently turning an ear to the speaker (see discussion in Chapter 4). Listening environments that can be difficult for the elderly who may or may not be wearing a hearing aid include certain common features: multiple speakers, background noise, and too great a distance between the listener and speaker.[42] If a hearing loss is suspected, it is best to recommend a referral to an otologist or otolaryngologist to identify any medical conditions, and then to an audiologist for an evaluation, which will include audiometric testing. Physical examination, interview, self-assessment, and audiometric findings are all essential to evaluate an older person's hearing fully. This is especially true with presbycusis, because the hearing loss involves confusion and jumbling of the auditory signal and not just diminution in auditory sensitivity. Treatment usually involves counseling the patient and family in communication techniques and training in the use of a hearing aid, if indicated. It may also include speech or lipreading, auditory training, speech therapy, and selection and use of special devices to facilitate training in the use of equipment such as the telephone, radio, television, doorbell, and alarm clock. Competent professional advice is needed to avoid purchasing inappropriate equipment.[44] Rupp and associates[45] have written a comprehensive review of listening devices, including frequency modulation (FM), infrared (IF), audioloop, and hardware systems. Special techniques, including self-wiring and use of a windscreen, are discussed. Frequency-modulation systems are wireless and perform like miniature radio systems. A microphone picks up the signal, and the transmitter sends it directly to the listener's personal wireless receiver. FM transmission is good for most problem environments and in the use of the telephone, radio, and television. It is unsuitable for transmitting confidential information because the transmission can be picked up by any receiver of matching frequency.

Infrared light is used with an infrared system for the indoor transmission of speech and music in small conversational groups and with use of the television and radio. One larger type of transmitter can be plugged into an existing public address system, and other types use a separate battery-powered microphone-amplifying unit. Portable battery-powered units worn by the listeners convert the light signal to an audio signal and route it to the listener's ears through attached earphones. These systems do not transmit if the light signal from the transmitter to the listener is obstructed.[45]

Hardware devices are sound sources connected by wires to the earphones of the listeners. These small portable devices consist of a microphone, amplifier, and some type of earphone. Some models are compatible with personal hearing aids. These devices are inexpensive and helpful for professionals to aid in communication with hearing-impaired clients.[45]

Compensation Techniques for Hearing Problems

Several techniques exist to compensate for hearing changes associated with age or illness.[5,31,42]

1. Before speaking, be sure you gain the attention of the hearing-impaired person: for example, address him or her by name.
2. Place yourself within 2 to 3 feet of the person, if possible, so that your speech will be louder than the background noise.
3. Face the person at eye level so that he or she does not face bright light and can read your lips.
4. Alert the person at the beginning of the conversation to topics of conversation and any changes in topics. This reduces the tendency to become paranoid or withdrawn.
5. Speak slowly and clearly, but do not shout.
6. Talk naturally, using a slower pace and a few more pauses than usual. Very rapid speech is difficult to follow.
7. If the person does not understand a statement, repeat it by using different words or paraphrasing it rather than repeating it word for word.
8. Lower the pitch of your voice if the hearing loss is in the high frequencies.
9. Include the person in small-group conversations. Ask for information, comments, or opinions.

10. Avoid background noise whenever possible. Choose a quiet environment.
11. Use nonverbal communication in your conversations, such as smiles, waving, pointing, and so forth to emphasize your "message."
12. Write any message that needs clarification.
13. Adjust the electronic or audio system so that the bass or lower tones are predominant.
14. Check to see whether the person's hearing aid is on and adjusted properly.
15. Recognize that a hearing aid does not work for all people.
16. Share in activities that require less pressure to communicate, such as cards or bowling.
17. Remember that what appears to be "selective hearing" may actually be due to factors such as high frequency, fatigue, and environmental distractions.

MODIFICATION OF THE CLINICAL SETTING FOR HEARING AND VISION PROBLEMS

Simple adaptations in the clinical environment can effectively reduce certain common problems associated with reduced hearing and vision.

1. Acoustic material such as tiles, drapes, and carpeting can be used near noisy traffic areas.
2. Locations of meeting, recreation, and treatment rooms should be away from noisy equipment such as fans, air conditioners, and appliances.
3. Noise and traffic in treatment areas should be controlled. Treatment of several people close together on a mat or in curtained cubicles can cause distracting noise and should be regulated.
4. Speak slowly in low, distinct tones when giving directions.
5. Glare from unfiltered sunlight, highly waxed floors, and shiny surfaces should be avoided.
6. Floors, railings, steps, handles on walkers, and parallel bars can be marked in a high-contrast color, such as bright yellow.

TASTE AND SMELL*

Not all studies agree,[44,46] but evidence suggests that the thresholds for taste and smell increase with age. This means that food that seems tasteless will be less appealing and may discourage the elderly from eating. This can

---

*Source: Maguire,[5] p. 32, with permission.

lead to poor nutrition and difficulty in recognizing food that is starting to spoil. In a study of nutritional health of elderly women, a relationship between dietary intake and taste perception was found.[47] Comparison of magnitude estimation for six suprathreshold concentrations of sourness and saltiness by elderly and young revealed loss of taste perception with aging. The elderly also had poorer diets than the young. The direction of the relationship between taste perception and dietary adequacy needs to be explored to determine if improved nutritional intake could improve taste perception.[47]

In a study of 50 community-dwelling elderly patients of a family physician, 39 percent were found to have olfactory dysfunction, with 18 percent being unable to detect smoke. The large percentage of elderly with olfactory dysfunction underscored the need to recognize such individuals and ensure that they use smoke detectors in their homes.[48] There is also the potential hazard that an aged person will not smell leaking gas from a stove or furnace.

Neuropathological studies of 10 confirmed cases of Alzheimer's disease (AD) indicated that the most extensive structural alterations associated with AD may occur in the olfactory system. The authors suggest that a standardized olfactory test battery could be administered to AD patients to determine if this might be an additional means to detect early manifestations of the disease, and possibly to differentiate AD from other demanding processes.[49]

Compensation Techniques

The following are possible ways to compensate for decreases in taste and smell associated with illness or age.[31]

1. The choice of foods should emphasize appearance (for those with good sight) and texture for their appeal.
2. Desirable temperatures of foods should be maintained whenever possible.
3. Condiments other than salt or other restricted items should be used liberally to enhance flavor.
4. The social aspects of mealtime, including the table settings, lighting, and pleasant company, should be emphasized whenever possible.
5. Older people themselves and their family and friends should be encouraged to check pilot lights, stored food, etc., to detect any safety problems.

TOUCH

The sense of touch, or tactile sensation, has had limited study in relation to aging. There does seem to be evidence that tactile sensation decreases with age, although this varies individually.[50] The related sense of kinesthesia is the person's awareness of his or her body in space. Information comes from receptors in muscles, joints, and the inner ear which aid movement, touch, and positioning. Decreased kinesthetic sensitivity in the elderly results in postural instability and difficulty in reacting to bodily changes in space. Dizziness and vertigo, associated with a fluid imbalance in the semicircular canals of the inner ear, are common problems in people over 50. Combined with dysfunction in kinesthetic and tactile senses, these problems increase aged individuals' vulnerability to accidental falls.[51]

Health professionals should note behaviors such as exaggerated body sway, a wide-based gait, and difficulty with balance, especially during fast movement. These may indicate compensation techniques for age-related changes in vestibular and kinesthetic senses or be symptomatic of neurologic disease.

Compensation Techniques

Compensation measures include the following:

1. Use touch as a means of communication and orientation.
2. Consider sitting closer to an elderly individual when communicating. This facilitates physical contact as well as input from the other senses, such as sight and hearing.
3. Avoid sudden, unexpected changes in body position in space.
4. Allow the individual sufficient time after he or she changes position, for example, standing from a sitting position, before beginning to walk, and so forth.
5. Incorporate sensory stimulation into all aspects of the rehabilitation program.

SUMMARY

The impact of the senses on the quality of life of an individual cannot be overemphasized. The senses are vital sources of input from one's environment; when these receptors are impaired, sensory deprivation results. This can lead to confusion, disorientation, social isolation, and the appearance of senility. Rehabilitation of the total person must include evaluation of the degree and effect of sensory impairment before planning and implementing a treatment program.

REFERENCES

1. Carabellese, C, et al: Sensory impairment and quality of life in a community elderly population. J Am Geriatr Soc 41:401, 1993.
2. Ratszan, RM: Communication and informed consent in clinical geriatrics. Intl J Aging and Hum Devel 23:17, 1986.

3. Beers, MH, et al: Screening recommendations for the elderly. Am J Public Health 81:1131, 1991.
4. Hendricks, J and Hendricks, CD: Aging in Mass Society. Winthrop, Cambridge, MA, 1977.
5. Maguire, GH: An Introduction to Aging: Module I. Howard University, Washington, DC, 1982.
6. Guyton, AC: Textbook of Medical Physiology. WB Saunders, Philadelphia, 1981.
7. Saxon, SV and Etten, MJ: Physical Change and Aging: A Guide for the Helping Professions. Tiresian Press, New York, 1978.
8. Reinstein, DZ, et al: 'Correctable undetected visual acuity deficit' in patients aged 65 and over attending an accident and emergency department. J Ophthal 77:293, 1993.
9. Wuest, FC, et al: The aging eye. Minn Med 59:540, 1976.
10. Marmor, MF: The eye and vision. Geriatrics 32:63, 1977.
11. Huges, P and Neer, R: Lighting for the elderly: A psychobiological approach to lighting. Hum Factors 23:65, 1981.
12. Hutton J, Shapiro, I, and Christians, B: Functional significance of restricted upgaze. Arch Phys Med Rehabil 63:617, 1982.
13. Branch, LG, Horowitsz, A, and Carr, C: The implications for everyday life of incident self-reported visual decline among people over age 65 living in the community. Gerontologist 29:359, 1989.
14. Brenner, MH, et al: Vision change and quality of life in the elderly. Arch Ophthalmol 111:680, 1993.
15. Hill, MM, and Hill, EW: Provision of high-quality orientation and mobility services to older persons with visual impairments. J Visual Impair & Blindness 85:402, 1991.
16. Furukawa, RE and Polse, KA: Changes in tearflow accompanying aging. Am J Optom Physiol Opt 55:69, 1978.
17. Faye, EE: Maintaining visual functions in the elderly. Bull NY Acad Med 60:987, 1984.
18. Null, R: Environmental design for the low-vision elderly. J Home Economics 80:29, 1988.
19. Biegel, DE, et al: Unmet needs and barriers to service delivery for the blind and visually impaired elderly. Gerontologist 29:86, 1989.
20. Resler, M and Tumulty, G: Glaucoma update. Am J Nurs 83:752, 1983.
21. Schwartz, A, et al: Argon laser trabecular surgery in uncontrolled phakic open-angle glaucoma. Ophthalmology 88:203, 1981.
22. Morrison, JD and Jay, JL: Changes in visual function with normal ageing, cataract and intraocular lenses. Eye 7:20, 1993.
23. Weinstock, FJ: Vision in the 1980s: A bright outlook for senior citizens. J Visual Impair & Blindness 81:313, 1987.
24. Dowaliby, M: Geriatric ophthalmic dispensing, Am J Optom Physiol OPT 52:422, 1975.
25. Caring for the Visually Impaired Older Person. Minneapolis Society for the Blind, Minneapolis, 1973.
26. Hovey, DN (ed): The Merk Manual. Merk, Rahway, NJ, 1972.
27. Belkin, M, Jacobs, DR, Jackson, SM, and Zwick, H: Senile cataracts and myopia. Ann Ophthalmol 14:49, 1982.
28. Chalifoux, LM: Macular degeneration: An overview. J Visual Impair & Blindness 85:249,1991.
29. Chalkely, T: Your Eyes: A Book for Paramedical Personnel and the Lay Reader. Charles C. Thomas, Springfield, IL, 1974.
30. Slaughter, T: Vision care for the elderly. Mod Health Care 4:47, 1975.
31. Carrol, K (ed): Compensating for Changes and Losses. Ebenezer Center for Aging and Human Development, Minneapolis, 1978.
32. Marshall, L: Auditory processing in aging listeners. J Speech Hear Disord 46:226, 1981.
33. Vernon, M, Griffin, D, and Yoken, C: Hearing Loss. J Fam Pract 12:1053, 1981.
34. Bergman, M, et al: Age-related decrement in hearing for speech: Sampling and longitudinal studies. J Gerontol 31:533, 1976.

35. Peters, CA, Potter, JF, and Scholer, SG: Hearing impairment as a predictor of cognitive decline in dementia. J Am Geriatr Soc 36:981, 1988.
36. Cobb, FE, et al: Age-associated degeneration of backward masking task performance: Evidence of declining temporal resolution abilities in normal listeners. Audiology 32:260, 1993.
37. Bergman, M, Najenson, T, Hirschc, S, and Solzi, P: Auditory perception in patients with CVA without aplasia. Scand J Rehab Med (Suppl)12:84, 1985.
38. Keim, RJ: How aging affects the ear. Geriatrics 32:97, 1977.
39. Lowell, SH and Paparella, MM: Presbycusis: What is it? Laryngoscope 87:1711, 1977.
40. Von Leden, H: Speech and hearing problems in the geriatric patient. J Am Geriatr Soc 25:422, 1977.
41. Rosenhall, U, et al: Corrections between presbycusis and extrinsic noxious factors. Audiology 32:234, 1993.
42. Olsen, W: Presbycusis: When hearing wanes, is amplification the answer? Postgrad Med 76:189, 1984.
43. Ebersole, P and Hess, P: Toward Healthy Aging: Human Needs and Nursing Response. CV Mosby, St Louis, 1981.
44. Riley, M and Foner, A: Aging and Society, vol 1. Trinity, New York, 1968.
45. Rupp, RR, Vaughn, GR, and Lightfoot, RK: Nontraditional "aids" to hearing: Assistive listening devices. Geriatrics 39:55, 1984.
46. Stevens, J and Cain, W: Smelling via the mouth: Effect of aging. Perception & Psychophysics 40:142, 1986.
47. Gee, MI, Ko, SYY, and Hawrywh, SJ: Nutritional health of elderly women: Evidence of a relationship between dietary intake and taste perception. Canadian Home Economics 38:142, 1988.
48. DeVore, PA: Prevalance of olfactory dysfunction, hearing deficit, and cognitive dysfunction among elderly patients in a suburban family practice. Southern Med J 85:894, 1992.
49. Reyes, PF, Deems, DA, and Suarez, MG: Olfactory-related changes in Alzheimer's disease: A quantitative neuropathologic study. Brain Res Bull 32:1, 1993.
50. Thornbury, JM and Mistretta, CM: Tactile sensitivity as a function of age. J Gerontol 36:34, 1981.
51. Wantz, MS and Gay, JE. The Aging Process: A Health Perspective. Winthrop, Cambridge, MA, 1981.

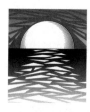

CHAPTER 7

Musculoskeletal Changes with Age: Clinical Implications

Carole Bernstein Lewis, PT, GCS, MSG, MPA, PhD

BEHAVIOR OBJECTIVES

Upon completion of this chapter, the reader will be able to:

1 Define hypokinesis.
2 List three normal and pathological causes for changes in strength, flexibility, posture, and gait.
3 Identify limitations a geriatric patient may have in a musculoskeletal rehabilitation program.
4 Suggest specific treatment modification for musculoskeletal problems encountered by older patients.
5 Describe how older patients may differ from younger patients in musculoskeletal parameters.
6 Design an evaluation and treatment protocol for a geriatric patient with a musculoskeletal disability or as a preventative measure.
7 Identify nutritional elements that play a significant role in muscle function.

There is a close similarity between the biologic changes of the musculoskeletal system attributed to the "process of aging" and those seen in the disuse phenomena. The coincidence of these two circumstances across a wide range of whole-body to subcellular changes suggests that perhaps those changes attributed to aging are correctable and ultimately preventable. Physical exercise as well as good nutrition have been found to hold promise for sustained health.[1]

Extremes of musculoskeletal functioning are clearly seen in aging. Chronologic age has little usefulness in explaining individual differences. The stereotypical institutionalized elderly person is decrepit, frail, and confused. Yet there are those like Larry Lewis, who, at age 101, broke the world's record for athletes over 100 years of age by finishing the 100-yard dash in 17.8 seconds.[2] Variability is the key in dealing with the aging musculoskeletal system. Let us look at a more typical clinical scenario:

Emily, a fragile-looking woman in her eighties, fractured her hip a week ago. She is sitting in your office for evaluation and treatment. Next to her is Rachel, a 20-year-old, athletic-looking woman. Rachel also has a week-old hip fracture. Their diagnoses are the same. Both have had this injury for the same period of time. Both are women waiting for you to provide them with the best rehabilitation program. However, they are very different.

If we were to look inside each of them, we would see different musculoskeletal pictures. Rachel is at the point in life when bone density in humans is the greatest, between ages 20 and 30 years.[3] After the age of 30, a gradual decrease in bone density occurs; this decrease is greater for women than for men. A general name for this decrease in bone mass is osteoporosis. Characteristic of osteoporosis is a decrease in total skeletal mass; however, the shape, morphology, and composition of the bone is normal. Emily is a candidate for osteoporosis simply because she is a woman over 50. Other contributing factors to this general bone condition are hormonal, nutritional, and circulatory. After menopause, women lose large amounts of bone. This is linked to the decrease in hormonal levels, specifically a lack of estrogen.[4] The older person who has a history of poor nutrition will also be a prime candidate for osteoporosis. Low-calcium, high-phosphorus diets have been implicated as causative factors of osteoporosis.[2] In addition, fasting or dieting and high alcohol consumption also contribute to the increased resorption of bony tissue. Finally, decreased circulation as a result of bed rest has been shown to cause osteoporosis in even young and healthy populations.[5] Osteoporosis is usually asymptomatic. However, it can be a major cause of pain, fractures, and posture changes.[6]

Therefore, a closer look at Emily and Rachel reveals distinct biologic differences in their seemingly similar bone structure—age being the cause of orthopedic problems. The way Emily and Rachel appear and act reveals their outward differences. The differences are a result of biologic, functional, or pathologic causes or a combination of these.

For example, Emily reaches slowly and with much effort for a magazine, but Rachel easily reaches across the table. Note the difference in their flexibility. Differences in strength become apparent when Rachel jumps from her chair to the upright posture in the parallel bars. Meanwhile, Emily methodically, cautiously, and with tremendous effort, pushes on her arms to stand upright in the parallel bars. You notice the variations in their standing postures. The two women begin their jaunt down the parallel bars for your examination. Rachel's steps are long and sure. Emily walks in a hesitating, scuffling manner. As the two pass in the adjacent parallel bars, they discuss the pain they are experiencing. Even in the area of pain, they have different outcomes and perceptions. Flexibility, strength, posture, gait, and pain are functional criteria for independence in daily living. Yet all of these criteria change considerably with age.

The changes in flexibility, strength, posture, gait, and pain are influenced internally by biologic aging and disease. In addition, functional changes in the lifestyle of the older person can also influence flexibility, strength, posture, gait, and pain. Emily demonstrated large differences in these criteria upon simple observation. Exploring these criteria in detail as to biologic, nutritional, functional, and pathologic causes, along with modifications for evaluation and treatment, will provide us with the tools to design the best rehabilitation program for someone like Emily.

LOSS OF FLEXIBILITY

The first difference we noticed in our observation of Rachel and Emily was flexibility. The change in flexibility as one ages can be the result of the change in collagen, dietary deficits, hypokinesis (decreased activity), the effects of arthritis, or a combination of these. The loss of flexibility compounds problems such as difficulty in walking, difficulties in daily activities, pain, and the ability to improve strength.

Collagen: A Biologic Cause

Collagen is defined as "the main supportive protein in skin, tendon, bone, cartilage, and connective tissue."[7] These fibers become irregular in shape owing to cross-linking, which increases as a person ages.[8] The fibers are less likely to be in a uniform parallel formation in the elderly than they are in young people. This closer meshing and decreased linear pull relationship in the collagen tissue is one reason for the decreased mobility in the body's tissues.[9] Poor nutrition may also contribute to collagen changes. For example, vitamin C has been found to be a vital component of normal collagen formation.[10,11] Fibrous elements of connective tissue, including collagen and elastin, undergo qualitative and quantitative changes in the process of biologic aging. There are changes in collagen turnover with age; less collagen is degraded and less is synthesized. A deficiency of vitamin C appears to interfere with normal tissue integrity and could therefore affect muscle functioning and collagen elastistity. Symptoms associated with vitamin C deficiency include weakness, fatigue, and stiff aching joints and muscles.[12] Muscles, skin, and tendons are not as flexible and mobile in older persons. In addition, the spine is less flexible owing to collagen changes in the annulus and decreased water content of nucleus pulposa. This results in a decrease in the disk size and a more inflexible spine. Osteoporotic changes of the vertebral bones may cause wedge fractures of the vertebrae, further increasing collagen density and scarring, thus changing the biomechanics of the spine and contributing to decreased flexibility.

Time is an important treatment consideration in working with tightness caused by collagenous adhesions. Collagen in older persons is less mobile and slower to respond to stretch, but with time it does stretch. The older person can gain flexibility with some compensation for time, just as the younger person can.[13] An effective treatment modification is to provide slow, prolonged stretching activities, either individually or in group exercise classes. Table 7–1 is a stretching protocol for contractures.[14]

Elderly people with flexibility decrements require longer rehabilitation programs than do young patients. This is not always possible. An older person with a frozen shoulder, for example, can usually gain full function range of motion if given enough time to progress slowly through an exercise program. Insurance companies do not always recognize the need for this longer rehabilitation period and limit reimbursement for services. Therefore, the basic treatment strategy should emphasize home exercise from the beginning, thus limiting the need for lengthy clinic treatment care.

Functional exercises and functional ways of measuring improvement should be the core of the home exercise program. An example of this is having the elderly person with shoulder limitations work on reaching objects in the cupboard. The method of evaluating improvement for this person would be comparing heights of objects reached. Elderly persons can also perform daily tasks that encourage their functional motion. In the case of shoulder

Table 7–1. **Protocol for Stretching Contractures**

1. Place the limb in the most lengthened position to be stretched.
2. Place hot pack on muscles to be stretched while in position 1 for 10 minutes.
3. Add weight (0.5% of patient's bodyweight) to distal part of limb in position 1 with heat still on for 5 minutes.
4. Remove heat and return part to neutral position for 1 minute.
5. Repeat steps 1–4 two more times.

Source: From Lewis, C and Bottomley, J: Geriatric Physical Therapy: A Clinical Approach. Appleton & Lange. Norwalk, CN, 1994, p. 378, with permission.

limitations, as a person is able to reach for light switches or to dust cabinets, these activities can be given as exercises.

Hypokinesis: A Functional Cause

Hypokinesis, or decreased activity, can also cause an older individual to become less flexible. Elderly people generally sit for longer periods of time than do younger people. This increase in sitting time can cause the older person to have tightness in many of the body's flexor muscles. These flexor muscles, when put into a shortened position for long periods of time, may develop the previously mentioned collagenous adhesions more easily. The hip and knee flexor muscles are commonly tight in the older person. The rotators of the hip also may become tighter because of decreased use in functional activities.

Many times older persons are thought to lose range of motion in various joints, particularly the shoulders and hips. However, on closer examination, these joints reveal a very adequate functional range of motion. This then raises the question of which joints are losing flexibility and need rehabilitation intervention. The answer is to consider functional independence in the older person and not to strive for "normal" range of motion as one would for a younger patient. Figure 7–1 is a graphic representation of lower-extremity range of motion for persons between 70 and 85 years of age.[15] Figure 7–2 shows, for several activities of daily living,[16] the smallest range of motion at which older respondents could perform with no difficulty.

An assessment of the person's daily activities and how these relate to flexibility should be noted. Although the older person may appear independent and display muscular flexibility, there may be a tightness problem that is manifesting itself in another way. A tightness in the hip rotators may be reflected in the older person's gait pattern or hip stabilization. Therefore, when these problems are seen, a simple range of motion test should be done. Gait difficulties and problems of daily inertia may relate directly to tight knee and hip flexors because of the strength needed to overcome the tightness.

Decreased flexibility occurs along any muscle that is put in its shortened state for a long period of time. The treatment for this is simply to break up the periods during which the muscles are in a shortened state. Older people need to be encouraged to stand up, walk around, lift their arms, rotate their hips, and turn and straighten their legs a minimum of thee times per day.

Decreased flexibility in an older person that is clearly a result of hypokinetics does not require intense rehabilitation measures. The rehabilitation professional should act as a consultant to activity programs that will help change the hypokinetic older person into a more active individual. Instruction to members of the health care team and family about flexibility and exercise can be the starting point for daily programs encouraging increased movement. One excellent way to encourage increased motion for home pa-

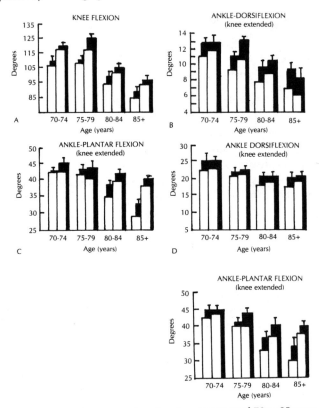

FIGURE 7–1. Lower-extremity ranges of motion for persons aged 70 to 85 years. (From Parker, JB: Active and passive mobility of lower joints in elderly men and women. Am J Phys Med Rehabil 68:162–167, 1989, with permission.)

tients is to instruct the patients to stand, stretch, and shift weight at intervals such as during every television commercial.

Finally, prevention of tightness through activity needs to be encouraged with the older person. Involvement in activities at frequent intervals in the day to maintain range of motion, along with education about the deleterious effects of a sedentary lifestyle and poor nutrition on muscular flexibility, provides important tools for intervention in this area.

Arthritis: A Pathologic Cause

There are numerous forms of arthritis that can affect any age group. Osteoarthritis, rheumatoid arthritis, and polymyalgia rheumatica are discussed here because they can frequently cause limitations in the elderly.

Osteoarthritis is an extremely common, noninflammatory, progressive disorder of movable joints, particularly weight-bearing joints, and is charac-

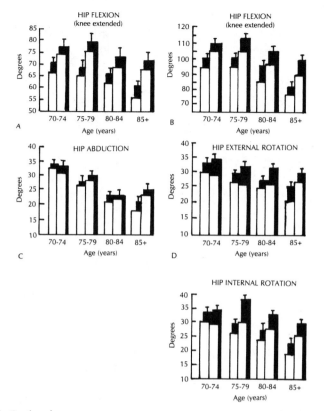

FIGURE 7–1. *Continued.*

terized pathologically by deterioration of articular cartilage and by formation of new bone in the subchondral areas and at the margins of the joint.[17] The areas most involved in older persons that affect functions are the knees, hips, and distal interphalangeal joints.

The limitations in motion observed with osteoarthritis may be caused by an acute synovitis caused by minute fragments of articular cartilage that appear in the synovial fluid or by the inability of joint surfaces to slide smoothly owing to deterioration of this particular cartilage. Muscle spasms secondary to pain can also cause limitations of motion. The physical presence of osteophytes that form at joint margins may cause limitations. These structures may also cause pain because they stretch the periosteum, which in turn limits motion. Weakness of muscles owing to disuse may also inhibit a joint's full motion.

The treatment modifications for limitation in motion owing to osteoarthritis are first to identify the source of limitation (that is, pain, weakness, or physical limitation). Pain and weakness can easily be identified with the administration of a pain questionnaire and a muscle test.

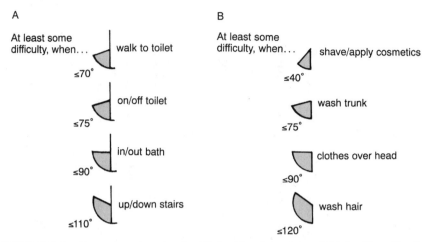

FIGURE 7–2. Smallest ranges of motion for *(A)* shoulder abduction and *(B)* shoulder adduction at which a respondent had no difficulty at performing specific ADL tasks. (From Young,[16] with permission.)

A physical limitation caused by osteophytes can be identified by a bony end feel at the point of limitation and by looking at x-ray films.

The appropriate treatment modifications for what has been described above are proper individualized exercise instruction and programming. Exercise is extremely important and should be carefully taught to the patient. Frequency of exercise rather than large numbers of repetitions is important to teach to the older person. An average program of instruction should include taking the limited joint through the range of motion two to three times a session three times a day.

Analyzing the cause of flexibility changes as a person ages and then using effective treatment planning can improve a situation that may be interfering with an older person's independent functioning. Carefully searching for the biologic, pathologic, and metabolic or functional cause may reveal a simple intervention that can give someone like Emily more independence.

LOSS OF STRENGTH

Of course, joint range of motion is a factor in independence, but strength is also necessary to perform motion.

Biologic Causes

The obvious decrease in muscular hypertrophy and change in muscular function that occur in the elderly are a result of complex interactions among a variety of factors. There is a reduction in strength with advanced age due to a decrease in the number and size of muscle fibers.[18] The number of muscle motor units also declines with age, influencing functional patterns by decreasing coordination and speed of muscle contraction. There is a reduced ability of the cardiovascular system to deliver raw materials to the working muscles, and there are subsequent alterations in the chemical composition of the muscle fibers.[2]

The cardiovascular system loses some of its efficiency with age.[2] As a consequence, important elements, such as various proteins, are not delivered to the muscle tissues in the same quantity as with younger persons. Glycoproteins are small molecules that produce an osmotic force important in maintaining the fluid content of tissues. The reduction of this molecule (as in aging) results in an increased difficulty for the tissues to retain their normal fluid content.[19] This results directly in muscle hypertrophy differences in older persons.

In a study of younger and older men in a strength-training program of the quadriceps muscle, it was found after 2 months that both groups had increased in strength to the same level. The interesting point is that the older group increased in girth by only 1 to 2 percent, whereas the younger group increased by 12 percent.[20]

The clinical implications of this concept are twofold. First, the rehabilitation specialists need to be aware that the older person does have the potential to increase significantly in strength as a result of treatment intervention. Second, in the elderly, increasing muscle measurement is not a good indicator of improved muscle strength. Assessment of an individual's ability to carry out functional activities without muscle fatigue or evaluation of workload achieved in an exercise program (that is, measuring increase in weight per exercise) is a better indicator of the older person's performance.

Chemically, the greatest change with age is a decrease in efficiency of the muscle cells' selectively permeable membrane.[20] Certain chemicals—particularly potassium, magnesium, and phosphate ions—are in high concentration in the sarcoplasm, but other materials—such as sodium, chloride, and bicarbonate ions—are largely prevented from entering the cell under resting conditions. A characteristic feature of senescent muscle is a shift from this normal pattern. The concentration of potassium is particularly reduced. Lack of potassium ions in aging muscles reduces the maximum force of contraction that the muscle is capable of generating. Tiredness and lethargy in elderly persons may result from reduction of potassium ion content in the tissue. The clinical implication of this is to check for potassium deficiencies if a patient complains of excessive tiredness or lethargy. Attempting exercises with someone who has potassium depletion will only fatigue the patient more. Therefore it is imperative to check the tired person's electrolytes before beginning exercises.

The nutritional status of the muscle is rarely considered in exercise or activity prescriptions. Little is known about the nutritional needs of the aging muscle.

Aging involves distortions and deteriorations in the integrative homeo-static mechanisms that stimulate and sustain a human being.[21,22] In considering the effects of nutrition on functional activity capabilities, it is important to remember that aging may change nutrient intake, increase the need for specific nutrients, and interfere with absorption, storage, and utilization of specific nutrients.

There is no concrete information identifying nutritional factors as influencing selective erosion of muscle tissue with aging. Several elements, however, have been shown to promote overall health and homeostasis of muscle tissue.

Nutritionally, vitamin C is of interest; in vitro studies with frog muscle have shown that vitamin C enhances contraction and delays the onset of fatigue.[23] Subsequent studies using human muscle tissue revealed the same result.[24] Vitamin C appears to be important in maintaining the physiologic health of muscle tissue while clearly not functioning independently. It is considered an important energizer and assists the body's tolerance of both heat and cold, a mechanism that declines with age and results in a poor tolerance to physical demands.[25]

Zinc, a nutritional element often found to be deficient in the aged population, functions in muscle homeostasis for needed growth and normal muscles longevity.[26] High concentrations of zinc have been found in muscles following physical exertion,[26,27] and recent research suggests its importance in enhancing muscle function and strength of muscle contraction.[28,29]

Although this chapter does not allow intensive study of the effects of nutrition on muscle function, these examples clearly support the need for proper nutritional consideration in exercise and activity prescriptions for aged patients.

Functional Causes

Numerous studies show a decline in strength as a person ages, especially after 60. Some studies have shown a loss of up to 40 percent of maximum force by age 65, whereas others indicate losses of up to 18 to 20 percent.[30]

The areas most likely to show a decrease in muscle strength are the active antigravity muscles, such as the quadriceps, hip extensors, ankle dorsiflexors, latissimus dorsi, and triceps.[31] These muscles are used frequently in daily activity; however, they are used to a much greater extent when a person is engaged in vigorous work or athletic activities. The older person may no longer engage in these strenuous activities and therefore may have comparatively less maximum strength in these muscles.

Strength norms are difficult to obtain for older persons because they are written in terms that are not as functional as the range-of-motion norms. A good screening tool that is more functional for lower-extremity strength and balance is the one-legged standing balance test, developed by Richard Bo-

Table 7–2. **The Time Needed to Stand 10 Times from an 18-Inch Chair Seat**

Age (years)	Women (sec)	Men (sec)
65	18.4	17.6
70	19.3	18.5
75	20.1	19.5
80	20.9	20.5
85	21.8	21.5

Source: From Csuka and McCarty,[34] with permission.

hannon.[32] Bohannon found that people over 70 are able to stand for 14.2 seconds on one leg with their eyes open and 4.3 seconds with their eyes closed. This 14.2-second norm will give therapists a general idea as to whether this person has strength and balance deficits or not.[32,33]

Another good screening tool for lower-extremity strength is the time needed to stand 10 times from a standard chair without armrests. Csuka and McCarty have reported the norms listed in Table 7–2.[34] Although both of these tests may be too advanced for the very frail patient, standing on one leg or rising from a chair without armrests may be considered when using functional strength measures.

An effective approach to evaluating the functional limitations caused by a decrease in strength is to evaluate the person in a situation that closely resembles the difficult functional activity. The muscles involved can then be strengthened in a close resemblance of the functional activity. Specificity of exercise for functionally strength-training an older person is extremely important because, in many older persons, tolerance for activity is decreased. It is imperative not to waste the older person's ability to improve in strength with meaningless exercises.

The following is an example of how to evaluate and to train functionally for strength in an older person. If the person has difficulty in getting up from a chair, he or she should be evaluated for the phase that is most difficult. The treatment will work on that particular stage and integrate it into the entire activity.

If traditional progressive resistive exercise is the preferred method for strength training, considerations for isometric and isotonic strength training in the aged are listed in Table 7–3.[35,36]

Pathologic Causes

Numerous strength-altering diseases affect all segments of the population. These causes of muscle weakness may contribute to an older person's loss of strength. One strength-altering disease of older people that has no

Table 7–3. **How to Train Strength in the Aged**

ISOMETRIC

1. Near maximum effort
2. 6–10 second hold (to recruit all fibers)
3. 5–10 repetitions
4. At least three times a day for maximum of 5 weeks
5. 10-second rest in between

ISOTONIC

1. Determine 1 RM (maximum amount a person can lift)
   Exercise at 60–80% of 1 RM
   Reevaluate RM each week
2. Three sets of 8–10 reps
3. 1–2 minute rest between sets
4. Three times a week for minimum of 8 weeks

neurologic basis, that can be detected easily, and that can be treated effectively is polymyalgia rheumatica.

Polymyalgia rheumatica is a syndrome occurring in older individuals and is characterized by pain, weakness, and stiffness in proximal muscle groups along with fever, malaise, weight loss, and very rapid erythrocyte sedimentation rate. The areas most affected in these persons are the neck, back, pelvis, and shoulder girdle.[37]

The origin of this disease is not known, and it affects both men and women, mostly those over 65. The most important aspect of this disease is that it responds dramatically and almost completely to corticosteroid therapy.[37] Therefore, this is not only the best treatment modality but also a diagnostic tool.

The rehabilitation professional should be aware of this disease as a possible cause for weakness, limitation, and pain in the older person. The professional should also realize that the only effective treatment in the acute phases is cortisone. Stretching and strengthening exercises may be useful later, along with heat (after the acute phase), if the older person has any residual weakness or limitation. When weakness is related to pathological causes, additional symptoms may be present. Table 7–4 lists clues to diagnosing the cause of weakness in the elderly.[38]

POOR POSTURE

A decline in strength and flexibility will lead to poor posture. One of the most noticeable orthopedic changes with age is in the area of posture. Normal or good posture traverses a plumb line of the individual in the standing

Table 7–4. **Clues to Diagnosing the Cause of Weakness in the Elderly**

Symptoms	Diagnostic Possibilities
Shortness of breath	Painless myocardial ischemic disease
	Interstitial pulmonary disease
	Subclinical bronchospastic disease
Pain	Arthritis
	Peripheral vascular disease
Paresthesia	Neuromuscular disorder: subdural hema-
Dizziness	toma; cerebral TIAs; amyotrophic lateral
Visual impairment	sclerosis; peripheral neuropathy due to
Asymmetry of neuromuscular symptoms	diabetes mellitus or alcoholism; Shy-
	Drager syndrome
	Drug reaction
	Autoimmune disorder
	Vasculopathy
Depression	Temporal arthritis with polymyalgia rheu-
Weight loss	matica
Muscle aches and pains	
Fever	
High ESR	
Gait disturbance	Parkinsonism
Inability to turn and rise from chair	
Weakness of arms when reaching over head	Myasthenia gravis
Excessive fatigue when walking	
Poor visual accommodation	
Fear of fainting or falling	Occult cardiac arrhythmia
Lack of motivation or interest in surroundings	Medication
Loss of appetite	Depression
Difficulty sleeping	
Weakness with cough	Tuberculosis
	Other causes of weakness: medication, in-
	teraction, overdoses, side effects; hypo-
	adrenalism; hypo- or hyperthyroidism;
	unrecognized or uncontrolled diabetes
	mellitus

Source: Gordon,[38] with permission.

position (Fig. 7–3).[39] The lateral view of normal posture has the ear, acromion, greater trochanter, posterior patella, and lateral malleolus in a straight line. In an older person, these landmarks and various body curves change their position around the line (Fig. 7–3). The older person's head tends to extend forward; shoulders may be rounded, and the upper back will have a slight kyphosis. Populations of older persons who tend to sit for longer periods of time overall have flatter lumbar spines. The lordotic curve may be flatter or more accentuated. The knees and hips will be in slight flexion. There are two major reasons for these changes: the changing structure of the intervertebral disk (IVD) and hypokinetics.[40] The REEDCO posture score sheet is an excellent tool for evaluating the posture of older persons (Fig. 7–4).[41,42]

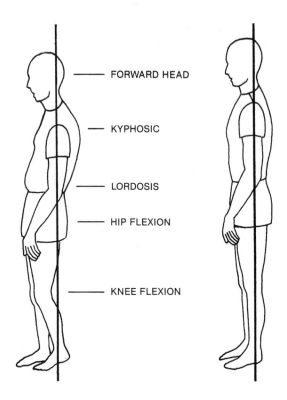

FORWARD HEAD

KYPHOSIC

LORDOSIS

HIP FLEXION

KNEE FLEXION

FIGURE 7–3. Posture changes with age.

Biologic Causes

The IVD is composed of two parts: the annulus fibrosis and the nucleus pulposus. The nucleus pulposus is composed mainly of water. In the sixth and seventh decades, intracellular water is decreased by 30 percent.[40] the annulus is composed of collagen, which becomes less elastic as a person ages. The decreased water in the nucleus and the increased fibrousness of the annulus cause the older person to have a flatter and less resilient disk. This structurally different disk can cause the spine's natural curves to become accentuated or more flexed due to the less-resistant disk succumbing to the continued forces of gravity and muscle pull of the spine, along with the osteoporotic vertebrae crumbling as a result of pressure.

The treatment modifications of improving posture in the older person are based on exercise and education. The older person must learn the components of good posture. The patient should then receive information on how his or her posture deviates from this model. Simple stretching exercises can be given along with instruction in adapting daily activity for improving posture. A simple exercise for a forward head is axial extensions (Fig. 7–5).[43] These exercises should be done three to five times twice daily. Trunk strengthening, specifically of the extensor groups and abdominal muscles, can be

POSTURE SCORE SHEET	Name _____			SCORING DATES				
	GOOD-10	FAIR-5	POOR-0					
HEAD LEFT RIGHT	HEAD ERECT GRAVITY LINE PASSES DIRECTLY THROUGH CENTER	HEAD TWISTED OR TURNED TO ONE SIDE SLIGHTLY	HEAD TWISTED OR TURNED TO ONE SIDE MARKEDLY					
SHOULDERS LEFT RIGHT	SHOULDERS LEVEL (HORIZONTALLY)	ONE SHOULDER SLIGHTLY HIGHER THAN OTHER	ONE SHOULDER MARKEDLY HIGHER THAN OTHER					
SPINE LEFT RIGHT	SPINE STRAIGHT	SPINE SLIGHTLY CURVED LATERALLY	SPINE MARKEDLY CURVED LATERALLY					
HIPS LEFT RIGHT	HIPS LEVEL (HORIZONTALLY)	ONE HIP SLIGHTLY HIGHER	ONE HIP MARKEDLY HIGHER					
ANKLES	FEET POINTED STRAIGHT AHEAD	FEET POINTED OUT	FEET POINTED OUT MARKEDLY ANKLES SAG IN (PRONATION)					
NECK	NECK ERECT, CHIN IN, HEAD IN BALANCE DIRECTLY ABOVE SHOULDERS	NECK SLIGHTLY FORWARD, CHIN SLIGHTLY OUT	NECK MARKEDLY FORWARD, CHIN MARKEDLY OUT					
UPPER BACK	UPPER BACK NORMALLY ROUNDED	UPPER BACK SLIGHTLY MORE ROUNDED	UPPER BACK MARKEDLY ROUNDED					
TRUNK	TRUNK ERECT	TRUNK INCLINED TO REAR SLIGHTLY	TRUNK INCLINED TO REAR MARKEDLY					
ABDOMEN	ABDOMEN FLAT	ABDOMEN PROTRUDING	ABDOMEN PROTRUDING AND SAGGING					
LOWER BACK	LOWER BACK NORMALLY CURVED	LOWER BACK SLIGHTLY HOLLOW	LOWER BACK MARKEDLY HOLLOW					
		TOTAL SCORES						

FIGURE 7–4. REEDCO Posture sheet. (From REEDCO Research,[42] with permission.)

helpful in increasing lordosis and preventing the "flexed" posture associated with aging.

Hyperextension exercises can be tried for a decrease in lordosis. Because the elderly population spends so much time in flexed positions, resulting in kyphotic or decreased lordotic curves, these exercises may prove beneficial

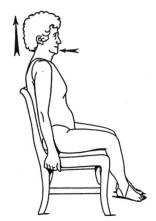

Gently pull chin in while
lengthening back of neck.
Hold this position
for _____ seconds.

REPEAT: _____ Times
_____ Times a Day.

FIGURE 7–5. A simple stretching exercise can help reduce "forward neck." (From Lewis and Campanelli,[43] with permission.)

(Figs. 7–6 and 7–7). For the wheelchair-bound person, a towel roll in the lumbar area or a Mckenzie pillow can help restore the lumbar curve and decrease pain.[44] Pectoral stretches can also be very beneficial in stretching muscles that are commonly tight in the older person (Fig. 7–8).[43]

Recreation classes should encourage good posture in their exercise programs. Rehabilitation professionals should not assume that recreational specialists or activity directors understand the components of good posture. Often a rehabilitation professional can visit these classes as a guest lecturer on the topic of good posture.

Functional Causes

Hypokinesis affects posture. Older persons sit for longer periods of time, whether in job situations or during leisure-time activities. The body's flexor muscles shorten because sitting requires bent hips and knees, decreases lordosis, and increases kyphosis. A clear relationship has been established between osteoporosis and inactivity. Increased stress on bone stimulates bone growth; lack of stress results in decreased bone formation and increased resorption. This is hypothesized to be the result of the piezo-electric effect of stress on crystals. In the case of human bone, weight bearing produces stress, and the collagen acts as the crystal that transforms the stimulus into an osteoblastic effect. Bone tissue is laid down along the lines of stress. Lack of muscular stress on bone, as well as of a weight-bearing stimulus, will facilitate osteoporosis. Fracture of vertebral bodies will add to the postural deformities associated with aging.[3]

Treatment considerations are obvious. Increased activity in positions other than sitting are mandatory. Weight-bearing activities should be encouraged to obtain and to maintain extensor strength and bone health. The suggestions for hypokinesis presented earlier in both the strength and flexibility sections can be implemented here.

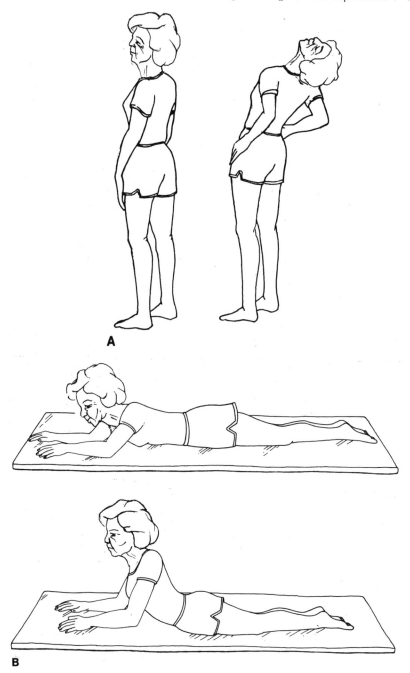

FIGURE 7–6. Hyperextension exercises. *(A)* Place hands in small of the back and gently bend backward from the waist. Hold 10 seconds and stand up straight. Repeat five times. *(B)* Lying on the stomach, slowly raise the trunk and head and prop on the elbows. Hold 10 seconds, then return to starting position. Repeat five times.

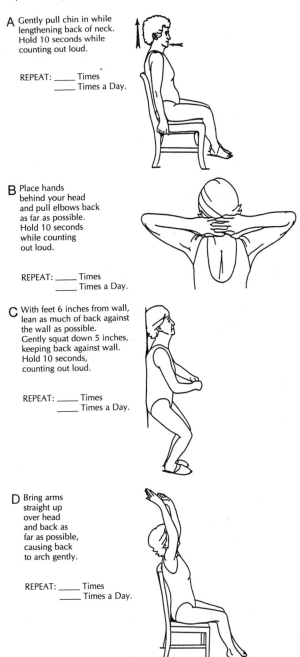

A Gently pull chin in while lengthening back of neck. Hold 10 seconds while counting out loud.

REPEAT: _____ Times
_____ Times a Day.

B Place hands behind your head and pull elbows back as far as possible. Hold 10 seconds while counting out loud.

REPEAT: _____ Times
_____ Times a Day.

C With feet 6 inches from wall, lean as much of back against the wall as possible. Gently squat down 5 inches, keeping back against wall. Hold 10 seconds, counting out loud.

REPEAT: _____ Times
_____ Times a Day.

D Bring arms straight up over head and back as far as possible, causing back to arch gently.

REPEAT: _____ Times
_____ Times a Day.

FIGURE 7–7. Other extension exercises for improving posture. *(A)* The chin tuck helps improve axial extension. *(B)* The elbows-back exercise can help in combating postural effects of osteoporosis as can *(C)* Back wall slides and *(D)* Arm reaches. (From Lewis and Campanelli,[43] with permission.)

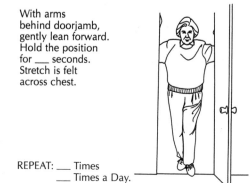

With arms
behind doorjamb,
gently lean forward.
Hold the position
for ___ seconds.
Stretch is felt
across chest.

REPEAT: ___ Times
___ Times a Day.

FIGURE 7–8. Pectoral stretch exercises can help stretch muscles commonly found tight in older individuals. (From Lewis and Campanelli,[43] with permission.)

Pathologic Causes

Any neurologic disease, arthritic involvement, or cardiopulmonary decrement may affect posture. Muscle imbalance caused by neurologic disease can be evaluated and treated. Pain and joint limitation caused by arthritis can be evaluated and treated, as well as chest cavity limitations caused by cardiopulmonary complications. Any disease entity may cause a postural change in the older person; therefore, contributing factors of multiple disease should be analyzed and corrected.

Even though poor posture may not directly impede an older person's functional activity, it is worth the small effort required for evaluation, instruction, and treatment intervention. The approach of decreasing postural abnormalities not only has the possibility of preventing increased disability but also encourages improved self-image, body awareness, and body language.

The human body is most efficient in its upright state, allowing maximum length and contraction of its muscles and joints.

CHANGES IN GAIT

The functional application of motion is gait. Just as balance, strength, and flexibility provide for proper posture, so do these three elements provide the background to ensure adequate walking in a person of any age. Figure 7–9 depicts the normal gait cycle. Within this cycle are numerous changes with age as follows:

1. Mild rigidity, proximal greater than distal (there will be less body motion)
2. Fewer automatic movements, decreased in amplitude and speed (e.g., arm swing will be less)

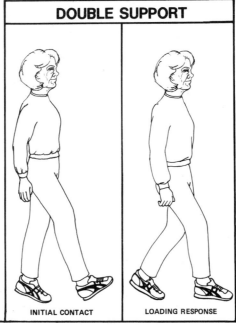
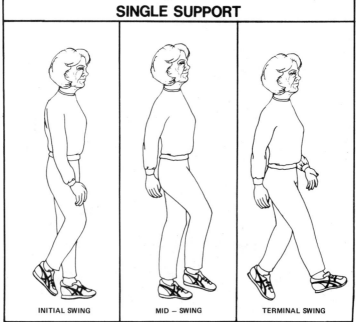

FIGURE 7–9. The normal gait cycle.

3. Less ability to use gravity, thus increasing muscle work
4. Less accuracy and speed, especially seen in the hip muscles
5. Shorter steps, to ensure safety
6. Stride width broader for a more stable base, to ensure safety
7. Decrease in swing-to-stance ratio (this, too, improves safety by allowing more time in the phase of double support)
8. Decrease in vertical displacement (this is usually secondary to stiffness)
9. Decrease in excursion of leg during swing phase (the free leg extends to a lesser degree)
10. Decrease in heel-to-floor angle (this may be due to the lack of flexibility of the plantarflexor muscles)
11. Slower cadence (a slower gait is also another assurance of safety)
12. Decrease in rotation of the hip and shoulder (the person appears to have a very stiff, unidimensional gait)
13. Decrease in velocity of limb motions (arms and legs move at a slower rate when walking)[45]

Gait is simply the manner or style of walking. Momentum and the use of gravity are important aspects of effective, effortless walking. Many gait problems due to loss and recovery of balance among the elderly are related to the inability to maximize momentum and the use of gravity.

Biologic Causes

A combination of biologic causes of flexibility, strength, and posture limitations is involved in gait changes with age. Stiffness caused by decreased collagen mobility in joint and muscles will cause shorter strides, decreased ancillary limb movements, and less efficient use of gravity and momentum.[45] Decreased strength caused by chemical or circulatory deficiencies causes a shuffling gait with a dangerously decreased heel-to-floor angle that may cause an older person to fall and thus sustain a fracture.[46] Poor posture caused by changes in the internal structure of the bones or disks enhances the decreased vertical displacement as well as the slower cadence.[45]

These biologic changes can be treated by stretching, strengthening, and positioning techniques that closely resemble the deficient phase of gait. For example, standing someone with shortened hip flexors in a position of exaggerated hip extension will help increase the range of hip extension in the push-off phase of the gait cycle.

Functional Causes

Functional causes are related directly to hypokinesis. Gait can be affected by ill-fitting, nonsupportive shoes as well as by bony changes in the foot influencing the normal biomechanics of the foot during gait. As the elderly person shuffles along and becomes less confident of the base of support owing to balance, flexibility, and strength changes, the entire gait pattern becomes less than efficient. Proper-fitting shoes and orthotics should be used to maximize the stability of the foot. Foot comfort can greatly affect the amount and intensity of ambulation activities. Starting with the foot and working up the kinetic chain during evaluation, addressing muscle imbalance and loss of flexibility, will improve efficiency and enhance activity. Tightness and weakness in the flexor muscles compound the inefficient gait of the elderly.

Daily routines of exaggerated hip extension, hip rotation, and arm movements practiced regularly will enhance the gait pattern.

Pathologic Causes

"By supporting a newborn infant on his feet, steppage movements can be elicited; however, the mechanism of antigravity support, postural function, and control of equilibrium takes time to develop. These responses depend on the integrity of many interrelated neurological mechanisms and final integration at the cerebral cortical level. Therefore, it is not surprising that performance in this area deteriorates with age and that this deterioration is accelerated by pathology changes."[46] (For specific information on nervous and sensory effects on gait, see Chapter 8.)

The particular type of patient that will be discussed here is the geriatric amputee patient. The geriatric amputee patient is considered to be any amputee over 55 years of age. These special patients stand out because they are more likely than their younger counterparts to have complications or associated problems. Some common complications are stump contractures, atrophy, skin breakdown, and difficulties with the other limb. Problems that the geriatric amputee may have to cope with are financial problems, general weakness, arteriosclerosis, diabetes, and cardiovascular and neurologic deficits, in addition to decreased sensory input, difficulty with balance, and a change in posture. This type of patient poses a tremendous challenge and is a prime candidate for continuous evaluation and prevention measures.

Ninety percent of amputees over 55 have had the amputation as a result of a disease.[47] Seventy percent of the same population have had limbs amputated as a result of arterial disease.[47] These statistics point out how important it is in the rehabilitation process to consider the entire person with all the concurrent diagnoses and intervening variables.

The following are some treatment modifications for working with someone who is older and has had an amputation. If you are lucky and are able to see the patient before surgery, an evaluation should be done to establish a baseline. The patient should not be allowed to drop below the baseline after surgery. In the case of lower-extremity amputation, the person should be checked in this evaluation and taught transfer skills and three-point ambulation with the walker in preparation for postoperative programming.[47]

In prosthetic fitting, there are several rules to follow. The therapist should be careful of any belts or straps because of the possibility of rubbing on various scars or pressure areas. The older person's skin is more fragile, especially if the patient is diabetic, and breaks down quickly. Remember also that, owing to the older person's decreased reporting of pain, the patient may not report the pain until a sore has already developed.[47]

The prosthesis itself should be easy to maneuver in gait and application. Many times arthritis of the hands can lead to difficulties with buckles and straps. Therefore, alternative methods of fastening, such as Velcro or a suction socket, may be needed. The prosthesis should be as light as possible because of the decreased strength found in the older population; however, this should not be at the risk of security.

It has been found that the most critical phase of the geriatric amputee patient in the gait cycle is at the point of heel contact and immediately following. This relates directly to the stability of the knee. Two factors can cause instability of the knee in a prosthesis. One is the loss of extensor power. This can be compensated for by

1. Exercising to increase the quadriceps strength
2. Redesigning the prosthesis
3. Changing the body alignment
4. Attaching elastic to help pull the knee into extension
5. Using a knee lock[48]

The second factor causing instability at heel contact is too much plantarflexion. This can be alleviated by using a soft-sach heel or a single-axis heel.

The energy expenditure in using a prosthesis for the older person is also an important variable. It has been shown that the energy expenditures required for an elderly patient to walk with an above-knee prosthesis is 55 percent greater than for a normal elderly person.[48] It is also important to remember that a large portion of this energy is being expended by the upper extremities. Any time the upper extremities are used in an activity, there is a tendency for systolic blood pressure to rise.[46] If the patient already has difficulties with cardiovascular compromise, an upper-extremity stress test should be done to evaluate the person's ability to ambulate successfully with the prosthesis.

Finally, in working with the geriatric amputee patient, it is extremely important to have a team approach. Encourage frequent and intensive follow-ups and define success of prosthetic wear in terms of its functional usage and psychosocial support for the older person. Ideally, the internist should be part of the rehabilitation process because of the numerous complications this patient may face. The team is extremely useful if it can encourage and perpetuate ongoing patient groups. There are numerous psychologic and social problems that are faced by an amputee patient at any age. The ability to participate, learn, and share with others who may have similar problems can be very helpful. Frequent and intensive follow-ups are very important in this population because of the continual change in status. Such problems as arthritis, cerebrovascular accidents, weight change, and vascular problems can cause severe complications if not assessed frequently.

The success of the prosthesis must be judged not only in terms of functional ambulation but also in terms of quality of life. If wearing the prosthesis while in the wheelchair enhances the person's self-esteem and social participation, it is not only functional but, in the long run, cost-effective. In many instances, because the person has "two legs," he or she will do his or her own dressing, feeding, and daily hygiene without fear of social rejection. Using this independent functioning instead of costly personnel to help with these endeavors can be very cost-effective. It is obvious that providing a prosthetic device to someone without adequate mentality, motivation, or vigor is inappropriate; however, if the person can appreciate how this device improves the quality of life, its worth is unquestionable.

The geriatric amputee is a very special patient who requires very special care. Modifying the evaluation procedure to include specific aging variables, along with altering the treatment programs to fit the pace and complications commonly seen in these older persons, is essential. The most important aspect of treatment, however, is a team approach that probes and encourages individual maximum functional independence.

PAIN

In all the functional criteria previously mentioned, pain can be a limiting factor of each or the cause for functional limitations themselves.

Biologic Causes

There are two major causes of pain differences in the older person. One is the difficulty that an older person has in localizing pain.[49] Clinically, this should alert the practitioner to be very specific when asking the older person about pain. The elderly person should also be encouraged to point to the exact location of the pain.

The second difficulty involves the pain pathways. Associated with the pathway that sends most of the chronic pain messages, the spinothalamic pathway, are a number of cells that secrete enkephalin. Enkephalins are the body's own opiates, or painkillers. In older subjects, the production and liberation of enkephalin is reduced, and chronic discomfort becomes more of a problem.[49]

Clinically, techniques for relieving chronic pain should be attempted before resorting to acute interventions. Such programs as visual imagery, relaxation, and biofeedback transcutaneous electric nerve stimulation (TENS) can be very effective with older clients in the treatment of chronic pain.[50]

Functional Causes

The primary functional difference in pain between younger and older clients is of social origin. The older person does not want to complain about pain. Older people as well as younger people hold the stereotype of "the complaining old crock." To avoid fitting into this mold, they tend not to report pain as often as their younger counterparts.

Any complaints of pain expressed by an older person should receive very serious attention from the health professional. Knowing that the older person complains of pain less should encourage the practitioner to solicit responses from the older person about his or her feeling of pain through specific questioning techniques.

Pathologic Causes

The two most common disease-induced causes of pain in elderly persons are fractures and arthritis. Fractures in the older person are more common for a number of reasons. On the physiologic level, the osteoporotic bone fractures with significantly less force. The older person's equilibrium and vision may be poorer. These decrements make daily activities less safe in older people and make these people more likely candidates for falls.[51]

The most common areas for fractures in the older person are the hips and wrists.[51] The increased incidence of fracture in these areas is directly related to falls. The wrist fracture occurs because the older person attempts to catch himself on the extended wrist. The increased incidence of hip fractures occurs because of the position of the fall and the less efficient kinesiologic leverage at the hip joint.

A fracture in an older person differs from that in a younger person for several reasons. First, the older person heals more slowly. Second, the older person is more prone to complications during the healing process.[51] Some common complications are pneumonia, osteoporosis, decubiti, and mental status complications. The older person may also have fewer support systems (family and friends) to aid in the rehabilitation process.

The evaluation of the elderly person with a hip fracture should include very specific questions about complaints of pain. The evaluation should also include assessment of the person's equilibrium, five senses, strength, flexibility, posture, and gait.

Pain in a fractured hip should subside in a few days, or at the most in a week. If a person still complains of pain, the problem should receive additional consideration to determine the source of the pain. Pain in a fractured hip, for example, could be nonunion, osteomyelitis, aseptic necrosis, displaced fixation device, bursitis, referred pain from the hip or spine, or fibrositis.[52] This list has specific implications for modifications of treatment.[53] For example, the person may need an additional treatment modality for bursitis that developed as a result of a new gait compensation.[54] It is important that the underlying cause of pain be found and treated so that the person can resume exercise and ambulation activities.

Stress fracture can occur easily with daily activities. The signs of stress fracture are:

1. Unusual complaints of pain after an exercise
2. Local tenderness
3. Local swelling[40]

In working with an older person who is suspected of having a stress fracture, encourage activity as long as it does not cause pain from the suspected fracture site. It is important that the older person stay as active as possible to avoid future complications. Caution must be taken, however, in an activity to avoid any undue strain on the possible fracture site. In other words, the elderly person can exercise as long as no pain is elicited from the suspected fracture site. (This last bit of information may be very helpful for persons working in facilities that seem to take forever to get the needed physician services.)

Arthritis can cause pain by the presence of osteophytes, which stretch the periosteum and may stretch, pinch, or wear nerve endings. Finally, muscle spasms can compound the effects of this pain.[53]

Modalities for the treatment of osteoarthritis begin by incorporating some of the drugs prescribed by the physician. These drugs do not cure osteoarthritis, but they can relieve the symptoms. The modalities that can be used by the older person in a home program with instruction from a rehabilitation professional are heat, cold, and exercise. Heat can be applied in the most simple forms of relief of pain and for relaxation. Caution should be stressed in checking for burns. Heat pads should never be turned above low for home use. The older person should be warned about the dangers of sleeping with heat on a body part. Bandages may be advantageous as a form of superficial heat. They are easy for an older person to apply and they keep in the body heat. The bandages should be checked to ensure enough looseness so that there is no restriction of motion or compromise of the venous system. Many older persons also use liniments as a form of heat. This practice need not be discouraged if the person receives benefits. Many times liniments act as a counterirritant and may work as well as more expensive treatment modalities. If the older person can tolerate its application, cold works to decrease pain and in many cases allows better joint mobilization than heat.

When exercise is treated as a modality, it can do more than just increase range of motion. Increasing strength around a weight-bearing joint can help decrease the shock on that joint during weight bearing. A study done by Radin[54] found that active contraction of a muscle against tension can absorb tremendous amounts of stress. Therefore, strengthening programs are very important, especially in the weight-bearing joints, to aid in relieving stress and improve function.

Mobilization techniques can be used with the older person who has osteoarthritis; however, care should be used. There should be careful consideration of the person's ability to assess and report pain accurately. Inaccurate reporting of pain can lead to possible damage of fragile joint structure during a mobilization technique.

Some additional treatment comments on osteoarthritis are specific to the different body parts. Osteoarthritis of the shoulder in the older person is usually rare.[55] There is not much degeneration in the shoulder joint, but there is frequently degeneration of the rotator cuff muscles and capsulitis, which may be the cause of pain and limitation. These pathologies respond extremely well to a program of ultrasound, exercise, and mobilization.

The problem of hip pain should instantly alert the rehabilitation professional to make a thorough investigation of the person's daily activities. Too often, older people do not complain of their hip pain and continue to walk beyond their pain limits. This actually aggravates the pain, degeneration, and limitation associated with osteoarthritis. The person is putting more stress on an already stressed joint and should be instructed in an incremental ambulation program along with non-weight-bearing exercises. Older persons can also be victims of bursitis. The intertrochanteric bursa is a very common place for inflammation. Many times bursitis around the hips mimics deep joint pain; therefore, careful assessment is needed. Hip bursitis responds well to a decrease in usage along with heat, ultrasound, and cold applications.

Osteoarthritis in the knee relates strongly to a person's past or present weight and occupation.[56] It is usually very localized. Ultrasound and cold applications for 20 minutes three times a day, along with exercises to strengthen muscles and decrease stress, may be very helpful. Weight reduction is imperative to help decrease the stress on the knee joint.[56] Again, non-weight-bearing exercises are extremely beneficial in providing the shock-absorbing mechanism discussed earlier.[57]

The cervical area in the older person presents quite an enigma in many instances. Lehman[58] claims that there is no such thing as disk herniation in the older person, and yet there are frequent reports of older persons complaining of radiculitis. Because osteoarthritis of the cervical spine is a continuous process beginning at maturity, it is common to see osteophyte formation at the apophyseal joints that may impinge on the intervertebral foramina or any other pain-sensitive structure in the cervical spine. There may also be hyperostosis at the vertebral margins, especially at C-5 and C-6, which may cause neurologic involvement.[58] Any of the above schemes can be exacerbated by a recent injury, such as whiplash. A recent trauma may also bring out an asymptomatic spondylosis in the cervical spine. If the person's pain relates to an acute incident, then rest, positioning, and the use of a collar are indicated until the acute episode subsides. Once the person has received some mild relief or is in a chronic stage, such modalities as heat, ultrasound, traction (beginning gently), and slow range-of-motion exercises are indicated. When the older person finally has little or no pain, a strengthening and posture program done regularly and gradually should be taught before discharge. The strengthening exercises will aid in providing strong muscles to prevent future injuries and complications. The common hyperostosis in the cervical area needs special mention in regard to a very common problem in the elderly—falling. Because disks are smaller and the vertebral margins are larger, owing to the hyperostosis, the vertebral arteries begin to pursue a very tortuous path. These arteries can be compromised by even a simple motion, such as neck extension or rotation. One of these motions with its effect on the artery can cause decrease of blood flow to the brain, and a person may fall or become dizzy. The therapist should check supine head movements in extension and rotation to be sure that a patient who falls subsequent to head movements is not a victim of the vertebral artery syndrome.

SUMMARY

Looking back on our meeting of Emily and Rachel, we now see two patients at two stages of aging. We understand how and where they differ on some functional criteria. Now we can not only modify our treatment and evaluation strategies accordingly but also become more adept at outlining the best plan of care for the geriatric patient.

REFERENCES

1. Wilmore, J: The aging of bone and muscle. Clinics in Sports Medicine. 10(2):231–243, 1991.
2. Nelson, CL and Dwyer, AP (eds): The Aging Musculoskeletal System. Physiological and Pathological Problems. DC Health, Lexington, MA 1984.
3. Ross, P, et al: Pre-existing fractures and bone mass predict vertebral fracture incidence in women. Ann Intern Med 114(11):919–923, 1991.
4. Barrett-Connor, E: Post-menopausal estrogen and prevention bias. Ann Intern Med 115(6):455–456, 1991.
5. Bloomfield, SA, Williams, NI, Lamb, DR, and Jackson, RD: Non-weight-bearing exercise may increase lumbar spine bone mineral density in healthy postmenopausal women. Am J Phys Med Rehabil, 72:204–209, 1993.
6. Napier, K and Dunkin, M: Osteoporosis: Resisting the silent crippler. Arthritis Today. March–April; 18–24, 1994.
7. Agnew L (ed): Dorland's Illustrated Medical Dictionary, ed 24. WB Saunders, Philadelphia, 1965.

8. Smith, E and Serfass, R: Exercise and Aging: The Scientific Basis. Enslow Publishers, Hillside, NJ, 1981.
9. Bick, EM: Aging in the connective tissues of the human musculoskeletal system. Geriatrics 11:445, 1971.
10. Robertson, WVB: The biochemical role of ascorbic acid in connective tissue. Ann NY Acad Sci 258:159–167, 1975.
11. Schneider, WL: Nutrition: Basic Concepts and Applications. McGraw-Hill, New York, 1983.
12. Roe, DA: Geriatric Nutrition, Prentice Hall, Englewood Cliffs, NJ, 1983.
13. Leslie, D and Frekaney, G: Effects of an exercise program on selected flexibility measurements of senior citizens. Gerontologist, 15:182, 1975.
14. Lentell, G, Hetherington, T, Eagan, J, and Morgan, M: The use of thermal agents to influence the effectiveness of low-load prolonged stretch. JOSPT 16(5):200–207, 1992.
15. James, B and Parker, AW: Active and passive mobility of lower limb joints in elderly men and women. Am J of Phys Rehabil 68:162–167, 1994.
16. Young, A: Exercise in geriatric practice. Acta Med Scand 711:227–232, 1986.
17. Rodman, G: Primer on the rheumatic diseases. J Am Geriat Soc 224:5, 1973.
18. Mitolo, M: Electromyography on aging. Gerontology 14:54, 1968.
19. Carlson, KE, Alston, W, and Feldman, DJ: Electromyographic study of aging in skeletal muscle. Am J Phys Med 43:141, 1964.
20. Gutmann, E and Hanzlikova V: Fast and slow motion units in aging. Gerontology 22:280, 1976.
21. Fries, JF: Aging, natural death and the compression of morbidity. N Engl J Med 309:130–135, 1980.
22. Schneider, EL and Brody, JA: Aging, natural death, and the compression of morbidity: Another view. N Engl J Med 309:854–856, 1983.
23. Basu, NM and Biswas, P: The influence of ascorbic acid on contractions and the incidence of fatigue of different types of muscles. Indian J Med Res 28:405–417, 1940.
24. Basu, NM and Ray, GK: The effect of vitamin C on the incidence of fatigue in human muscle. Indian J Med Res 28:419–426, 1940.
25. Riccitella, ML: Vitamin C therapy in geriatric practice. J Am Geriartr Soc 20(1):34–42, 1972.
26. Kutsky, RJ: Handbook of Vitamins, Minerals and Hormones, ed 2. Van Nostrand Reinhold, New York, 1981.
27. Hamilton, EM and Whitney, E: Nutrition: Concepts and Controversies, ed 2. West, 1982.
28. Isaacson, A and Sandow, A: Effects of zinc on responses of skeletal muscle. J Gen Physiol 46:655–677, 1978.
29. Krotkiewki, M, Gudmundson, M, Backstrom, P, and Mandovlas, K: Zinc's relationship to muscle strength and endurance. Acta Physiol Scand, 116:309–311, 1982.
30. Murray, P: Strength of isometric and isokinetic contractions in knee muscles of men aged 20 to 86. Phys Ther 60:4, 1980.
31. Browse, N: The Physiology and Pathology of Bed Rest. Charles C Thomas, Springfield, IL, 1965.
32. Bohannon, RW, Larkin, PA, Cook, AC, Gear, J, and Singer, J: Decrease in timed balance test scores with aging. Physical Therapy 649(7):1067–1070, 1984.
33. Newcomer, KL, Krug, HE, and Mahowald, ML: Validity and reliability of the timed-stands test for patients with rheumatoid arthritis and other chronic diseases. J Rheumatol 20:21–27, 1993.
34. Csuka, M and McCarty, DJ: Simple method for measurement of lower extremity muscle strength. Am J Med 78:77–81, 1977.
35. Atha, J: Strengthening Muscle. Exercise and Sport Science in Review, 9:1–73, 1981.
36. Fonterra, WR, et al: Strength training and determinants of VO_2 max in older men. J of Applied Physiol 68(1):329–333, 1990.
37. Hicks, J: Exercise in patients with inflammatory arthritis and connective tissue disease. Rheumatic Disease Clinics of North America 16(4):845–876, 1990.

38. Gordon, M. Differential diagnosis of weakness: A common geriatric symptom. Geriatrics 41(4):75–80, 1986.
39. Kendall, H and Kendall, F: Posture and Pain. Williams & Wilkins, Baltimore, 1980.
40. Borenstein, DG and Burton, JR: Lumbar spine disease in the elderly. J Am Geriatr Soc 41(2):167–175, 1993.
41. O'Neil, M, et al: Physical therapy assessment and treatment protocol for nursing home residents. Physical Therapy 72(8):596–603, 1992.
42. REEDCO Research: REEDCO Posture Score Sheet. Auburn, NY, 1974.
43. Lewis, C and Campanelli, L: VHI Geriatric Exercise and Rehabilitation: Exercise Kit. Visual Health/Stretching Charts, Takoma, WA, 1993.
44. McKenzie, R: The Lumbar Spine, Spinal Publications, Waekanae, New Zealand, 1981.
45. Imns, F and Edholm, F: The assessment of gait and mobility in the elderly. Age and Aging 8:261, 1979.
46. Adams, G: Essentials of Geriatric Medicine. Oxford University Press, New York, 1977.
47. Pedersen, H: The Geriatric Amputee: Principles of Management. Government Printing Office, Washington, DC, 1971.
48. Ebert, H: The Geriatric Amputee. National Academy of Sciences, National Research Council, Washington, DC, 1961.
49. Herr, K and Mobly, PR: Complexities of pain assessment in the elderly: Clinical considerations. J Geront Nurs 17:12–19, 1991.
50. Ziebell, B: Wellness; An Arthritis Reality. Kendall/Hunt, Dubuque, 1981.
51. Kalchthaler, T, Bascon, R, and Quintos, V: Falls in the institutional elderly. J Am Geriatric Soc 26:424, 1978.
52. Sweezy, R: Pseudoradiculpathy in subacurte trochantive bursites of subgliteus maximum bursa. Arch Phys Med Rehabil 57:387, 1976.
53. Adams, P, Eyre, H, and Muir, H: Biochemical aspects of development and aging of the human lumbar intervertebral disks. Rheumatol Rehabil 16:22, 1979.
54. Radin, E: Mechanical effects of osteoarthritis. Bull Rheum Dis 26:7, 1976.
55. Stecher, R: Osteoarthritis and old age. Geriatrics 16(4):167, 1961.
56. Felson, DT, et al: Weight loss reduces the risk of symptoms of osteoarthritis in women. Ann Int Med 115:535–539, 1992.
57. Kriendler, H, et al: Effects of three exercise protocols on oesteoarthritis of the knee. Top Geriatr Rehabil 2(3):32–44, 1989.
58. Lehman, L: Cervical spondybolic myelopathy: A diagnostic challenge in aging patients. Postgrad Med 88:240–243, 1990.

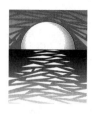

CHAPTER 8

Clinical Implications of Neurologic Changes during the Aging Process

Richard W. Bohannon, EdD, PT, NCS

BEHAVIORAL OBJECTIVES

Upon completion of this chapter, the reader will be able to:

1   Identify changes in muscle performance, perception, and balance that occur with increasing age and stroke.
2   Describe the relationship between functional performance and muscle performance, perception, and balance in the elderly and in patients with stroke.
3   Select interventions appropriate for reducing impairments in muscle performance, perception, and balance in the elderly or in patients with stroke.

Functional performance is limited by an individual's underlying physiologic capacity. Although the degree and rate may vary, both physiologic status and functional performance tend to diminish with age. When such decreases are compounded by the sequelae of diseases that sometimes accompany aging, the results can be devastating. Among the more common physiologic performance deficits and diseases that occur with aging are those typically classified as neurologic. In this chapter we will (1) describe the deterioration of selected neurologic capabilities and related functional deficits that go along with aging, (2) indicate how the same neurologic and functional performances are compromised further in individuals with a specific disease, stroke, and (3) outline an approach for treating individuals with neurologic and functional limitations resulting from age and stroke.

DETERIORATION OF NEUROLOGIC AND FUNCTIONAL PERFORMANCES WITH AGE

A myriad of neurologic and functional performances have been shown to diminish with age. Selected for attention in this chapter are a limited number of neurologic performances that have particular importance to function in the elderly. Specifically discussed are muscle, perceptual, and balance performance.

Muscle Performance

The body and its various segments have masses, the controlled movements of which are dependent on the body's muscles. Specifically, it is the muscles that create the force that accelerates and decelerates the masses and allows an individual to deal appropriately with the objects and forces encountered in the environment. The maximum resultant short-duration force or torque that an individual can bring to bear on the environment under specific test conditions is referred to as *muscle strength.*

Numerous studies have shown that muscle strength in adults declines with age.[1-6] The decline is present in both men and women, tends to increase with age,[1] and is greater in some muscles than others.[2] Although less than 50 percent of the variance in muscle strength can be attributed to age,[3,4] age remains a significant independent predictor of muscle strength even when the effects of other important variables are controlled in regression analysis.[3-5]

The decreases in strength that accompany aging may go unnoticed for a considerable time because most daily activities do not place a particularly heavy demand on the muscular system. When, however, an individual's strength approaches the force threshold required for an activity, strength limitations may become apparent. This is particularly true for women, who tend to be weaker than men anyway.[1,5,7] Functional activities such as rising from a floor or bathtub, standing from a low chair, or climbing stairs require a relatively high output from some of the muscles of the lower extremity.[8-13] Such activities, therefore, may prove increasingly difficult for some individuals as they age.[1,14-17]

Research examining the association between lower-extremity muscle strength and functional performance in the elderly, though limited, does exist. Most such research has addressed walking, which like strength deteriorates with age.[18-21] The research has shown a positive correlation between the strength of the ankle plantarflexor[21] and knee extensor[22,23] muscles and walking speed. As adequate walking speed is important for community ambulation,[24-26] such correlations are important. A nongait function with which shoulder and knee muscle strength have been shown to relate is the ability to get up from the floor after a noninjurious fall.[14]

Perceptual Performance

Perception is defined by Wilson[27] as the "process of integrating and organizing information" received by the senses. Just as individuals possess senses to receive visual, auditory, positional, or tactile information, they have a perceptual mechanism for interpreting each type of sensory information. Although problems can arise with the interpretation of any type of sensory input, impairments in visual perception are probably the most widely recognized. Such problems have been categorized by Lincoln[28] as visuoperceptive, visuospatial, or visuoconstructive.

Notable problems with visual perception in the elderly have been revealed by clock drawings and visual judgments of vertical or horizontal. An individual's clock-drawing performance, though thought to be a function of numerous neuropsychologic factors, is considered to be guided by visual perception.[29] Abnormalities in clock drawing have been demonstrated by elderly individuals with "dementia and related disorders," and to a lesser degree by "well elderly in a seniors' residence."[29] Huntziger and associates,[30] who tested 431 medical-surgical outpatients over the age of 55, found clock-drawing errors "suggestive of moderate to severe cognitive impairment" among 42.7 percent of the patients. Measurements of visual perception of vertical or horizontal obtained with rod-and-frame or lighted-rod tests have shown the elderly to err in their judgments of rod position.[31,32] The errors tend to be small but were correlated positively and significantly with age. Information on the accuracy with which the elderly perceive body position is scant. There is limited evidence, however, that their perception of their position in space (in the sagittal plane) is sometimes compromised. The results of studies using force plates to investigate the standing posture of the elderly suggest a perceptual problem. Elderly subjects tend to have a center of pressure relative to their feet that is posterior compared to that of younger individuals.[33] The standing posture of some elderly individuals who have been hospitalized and bed-bound for a short time also suggests a perceptual problem. They stand leaning backward, require assistance to prevent falling in that direction, and voice concern about falling forward when pulled to an upright position.[34]

Logic suggests that perceptual problems accompanying aging might be deemed problematic. Particularly disconcerting are misjudgments of verticality, whether allocentric or egocentric. Tobis and associates[31,32] found a relationship between errors in visual perception of rod position and falling status. They reported visual variables to be more important than other physical characteristics as predictors of falls.[32] The retropulsive behavior of the patients described by Bohannon[34] seems to be a consequence of a misperception by them of their position in space.

Balance Performance

Balance is defined herein as the ability to sustain or recover postural stability by maintaining or returning the center of gravity within the base of support. Balance depends on an adequate level of sensory, perceptual, and motor performance.

There is extensive evidence that standing balance decreases with age. Two measurements in particular show age effects. The maximum duration of unilateral stance has been shown in numerous studies to decline with age.[35-37] Sway during static standing has also been shown to increase as people age.[38,39]

The need for balance, if not self-evident, is easily verified through the observation of men and women as they go through everyday activities. Balance is necessary during bilateral stance if the upper extremities are to be freed for activities such as dressing or grooming. Similarly, balance is required whenever an individual assumes unilateral stance. Unilateral stance is assumed twice during each gait cycle, once by each lower extremity. Although the duration of single-limb stance during gait is not long (about 0.6 second at 50 cm/sec and 0.3 second at 200 cm/sec),[40] it does require a degree of balance. Other activities entailing balanced unilateral standing are climbing curbs or stairs, stepping over obstacles, and lower-body dressing (if standing). Without sufficient balance during bilateral or unilateral stance, an individual will fall unless support is gained by using the upper extremities or obtained by assistance from another individual.

Studies of the elderly have verified the importance of balance. MacRae and associates[41] found unilateral standing time to correlate positively with self-assessed health. Balance, whether described by unilateral stance time,[41-42] forward reach,[43] or sway,[44] has been shown to correlate with fall status. That is, as balance decreases, the likelihood of a fall increases.

FURTHER DETERIORATION OF NEUROLOGIC AND FUNCTIONAL PERFORMANCE AFTER STROKE

Stroke is one of several neurologic pathologies affecting primarily the elderly. As stroke is one of the most common diagnostic groups treated by those working with the elderly,[45] it provides a useful context for the discussion of deficits in neurologic and functional performance encountered in clinical practice. Consistent with the first section of this chapter, the neurologic impairments addressed will be those of muscle, perceptual, and balance performance. Each is likely to deteriorate further after stroke.

Muscle Performance

Muscle weakness (paresis) is probably the most obvious and is definitely the most common impairment that accompanies stroke.[46] Although noted primarily in the limb muscles contralateral to the side of the brain lesion, a lesser weakness of the ipsilateral muscles is also present.[47,48] In addition, nonlimb muscles such as those of the trunk[49] and neck,[50] and those of mastication[51] and respiration[52] can also be affected. At the trunk, the strength of forward flexion appears to be particularly impaired.[49] Fortunately, muscle strength tends to be recovered after stroke. The greatest recovery occurs during the first several weeks and months.[53] The ultimate strength realized by a patient is determined largely by the initial degree of paresis following stroke.[54] Thus, a patient who is totally hemiplegic 1 week after stroke is not likely to reach an ultimate state of mild hemiparesis 6 months later. The greater percentage increase in strength demonstrated by patients with more extensive weakness does not compensate for their initial degree of impairment.[55] They will remain, as a rule, weaker than patients who were stronger initially after stroke.

The muscle performance of patients with stroke is related to function for the same reasons that it is related to function in elderly individuals. The strength required for most functional activities, however, is not great. Consequently, it is when the elderly experience the cumulative weakness accompanying aging and neurologic disorders such as stroke that the importance of muscle strength to function becomes particularly apparent. In studies of patients with stroke, muscle strength has been shown to correlate significantly with measures of general[56,57] and specific function. Included among such specific functions are dressing,[58] stand-pivot-sit transfer,[59] level ground ambulation,[60–62] and stair climbing.[63]

Perceptual Performance

Impairments in perceptual performance are commonplace in patients with stroke. Visuoperceptual impairments have been most widely documented. Deficits in auditory[64] and tactile perception[65] also occur after stroke but will not be addressed directly hereafter. Some mention will be made of misperception of position in space.

Visuoperceptual Performance

The visuoperceptual impairment most frequently studied in patients with stroke is visual neglect. Although visual neglect can exist along any of three orthogonal axes (horizontal, vertical, or radial),[66] it is most often noted along the horizontal axis and in such cases is referred to as *unilateral neglect.* Mattingly and associates[67] have defined unilateral neglect as a "multicomponent attentional disorder consisting of an initial automatic orienting of attention toward the ipsilateral side and a subsequent impairment in contralesionally reorienting attention, both of which are superimposed on a generalized reduction in attentional resources" (p. 597). Unilateral neglect, which is identified most often through drawing,[68] bisection,[69] or cancellation tests,[70] is present in 12 to 85 percent of patients with stroke.[71] Unilateral neglect is more common among, but not limited to, patients with right-brain lesions.[72] The unilateral neglect demonstrated by patients with stroke decreases with time.[67,70,73] For patients with the more common left neglect, a residual rightward bias may persist 12 months poststroke after an apparent recovery.[67]

The implications of unilateral neglect are readily apparent when severe. A patient with the disorder may shave only one side of the face, eat from only one side of a plate, or continually collide with objects on the left side while propelling a wheelchair or ambulating. Research supports the relationship between neglect and function. Marsh and Kersel[70] found measurements of unilateral neglect to correlate significantly with scores of overall function (that is, Barthel). Nogaki[74] reported that severe or moderate unilateral spatial neglect is one of the critical determinants of standing balance and activities of daily living. Nouri and Lincoln[75] found neglect scores to correlate significantly with road driving test grades.

Another visuospatial disorder apparent among some patients with stroke is an error in the judgment of visual vertical.[76] Dieterich and Brandt[77] reported errors in excess of 20 degrees among patients with stroke who demonstrated lateropulsion. The errors in judgment of visual vertical demonstrated by the patients was related to their balance (lateropulsion) scores. Fortunately, the patients improved over time in both their perception of visual vertical and their standing balance.

Perception of Position in Space

After stroke, perception of position in space can be disrupted. Many patients show a tendency to stand with their center of pressure posterior[33] and their bodies to one side of their base of support. The latter behavior is particularly apparent among patients with left hemiparesis who demonstrate a pusher (lateropulsion) syndrome. Observation of their behavior indicates that their perception of an appropriate standing posture is often posterior and/or to the left of true vertical or upright. Although there is little published evidence of this fact, it does have major consequences for standing balance and function.

Balance Performance

The balance of patients with stroke is impaired far beyond that of individuals who are merely old.[78–84] As might be expected, standing balance is more likely than sitting balance to be impaired after stroke.[78] Patients with left hemiparesis are more likely to show impairments in sitting balance than patients with right hemiparesis.[79] The balance of patients with stroke tends to improve with time,[78] which is fortunate given the relationship between balance and function. Sitting balance has been shown to correlate with overall function[80] and with specific functional activities such as dressing.[58] Standing balance is associated positively with transfer capacity,[59] level-ground walking performance,[61,81,85,86] and stair-climbing ability.[63]

TREATMENT OF NEUROLOGIC AND FUNCTIONAL LIMITATIONS RESULTING FROM AGE AND STROKE

Functional limitations, whether resulting from age or stroke, are an appropriate primary focus of therapeutic interventions. Interventions aimed at muscle performance, perception, and balance can also be appropriate given their relationship to function. Such interventions, whether corrective or compensatory, will be the focus of the following.

Muscle Performance

Exercise Programs

Exercise programs, including those that use body weight or external loads for resistance, appear to be safe and effective for increasing muscle performance and function among the elderly. Faigenbaum and associates[87] claimed that even cardiac patients who are clinically stable and aerobically trained can perform "moderate to heavy resistance exercise without experiencing complications" (p. 108).

To be effective, exercise programs for the elderly must be of sufficient intensity, frequency, and duration. The programs should also take into account the concept of specificity of training. For many individuals, body mass may provide a sufficient stimulus to provide strengthening when segment masses are accelerated or decelerated during the performance of functional activities such as sit-to-stand or stair climbing. Both of these activities demand considerable voluntary torque production by the body.[9–11, 13, 88–91] The torque production demands of the former activity can be modified by altering seat height or employing arm rests.[13,14,90,91] The requirements of the latter activity can be changed similarly by altering step height or by use of handrails. The resistance inherent in stair climbing can be supplemented by carrying extra weight.[10] External strengthening loads most often take the form of weights but can be provided by springs, elastics, water, pistons, dynamometers, or manual resistance. Whether employing body weight or external resistance, exercise programs have been shown to be adequate to strengthen elderly men and women who live independently or in institutional settings.[22,23,92–98] Advanced age, even over 80 years, does not prevent an individual from gaining strength after participation in an appropriately designed program.[22,23,92–94] In addition to increases in strength, the programs can lead to improvements in function as well. Both Judge and associates[22] and Fiatarone and associates[23], have reported increases in gait speed among elderly individuals participating in exercise programs with an emphasis on strengthening exercises. The elderly trained by Binder and associates[93] showed increases in gait speed and the average number of city blocks they could walk. Their subjects also improved in stand-up performance and balance.

For patients with stroke, the prerequisites for effective exercise programs are consistent to a degree with those for the elderly. Functional activities that challenge their neuromuscular system appear to be of value for increasing strength and function. Patients with whom Åsberg[99] initiated regular sit-to-stands within 1 to 2 days of admission and with whom she continued the resistance exercise for 1 to 2 weeks were less disabled 5 to 7 days after stroke than patients in a control group. Inaba and associates[100] showed more than 20 years ago that patients with stroke who performed progressive resistance exercise with a weight machine realized greater increases in lower-extremity muscle strength and functional ability than patients in a control group or active exercise group. Although not performed on patients with stroke, research on patients with spastic paresis from other pathologies shows that the strength of eccentric actions is not as impaired as the strength of concentric actions[101–103] and that eccentric training may result in greater strength increases than concentric training.[103] These findings probably warrant greater application to be the patient with stroke.

Other Treatments

For patients with stroke, exercise programs focused on reducing paresis and associated functional deficits can be supplemented by other treatments (modalities). Primary among such modalities are functional electrical stimulation, biofeedback, and acupuncture. Considerable evidence exists for the effectiveness of functional electrical stimulation. Substantial increases in strength[104–106] and volitional movement[106–108] have been reported in patients with stroke who have been treated with functional electrical stimulation for limited periods of time. In some studies the increases realized over the course of treatment have exceeded several hundred percent. Biofeedback, alone or in combination with functional electrical stimulation,[109–111] has been shown to be of some value in restoring muscle performance in patients with stroke. Kraft and associates[112] found a treatment combining electromyography and electrical stimulation to yield significantly better motor outcomes than either low-intensity electrical stimulation or proprioceptive neuromuscular facilitation exercises. Naeser and associates[113] described acupuncture as a "beneficial treatment modality for stroke patients with hand paresis" (p. 127). Significant increases in tip pinch and three-jaw chuck strengths were demonstrated by eight chronic patients who received 20 or 40 treatments over a 2- or 3-month period. Patient responsiveness to treatment was noted to be dependent on the preservation of at least half of the motor pathway areas.[113,114] Other researchers have found accupuncture to affect function as well.[115]

Perceptual Performance

Conceivably, training might be provided for any individual with a perceptual deficit. Given the incidence and severity of perceptual problems among patients with stroke, such patients are probably the individuals most often treated for perceptual problems. Interventions aimed at assuaging the unilateral neglect that sometimes accompanies stroke have been described in the literature with some regularity. The interventions will be discussed hereafter under the categories of ameliorating impositions or training regimens.

Ameliorating Impositions

Several types of impositions have been described for ameliorating unilateral neglect. They include various types of cues or anchors, stimulations and body orientations, and the use of an eye patch.

Numerous investigations have examined the effects of cues or anchors in the left hemispace on left neglect. Riddoch and Humphreys[116] found cues in the left hemispace to be useful but indicated that the patient had to cognitively acknowledge the cue for it to be effective. Weinberg and associates[117] reported that vertical anchoring improved reading performance. Several reports have discussed the use of the left upper extremity as an anchor at the margin of activity. Robertson and associates[118] reported three cases where anchoring with the left upper extremity was helpful. In another study, Robertson and North[119] did not find use of the left hand in the left to be an anchor to reduce left neglect. Finger movements of the left hand space, on the contrary, did decrease neglect during a letter cancellation task. Movement of the left fingers in the right space or of the right fingers in the left space did not help. The improved cancellation performance accompanying left-hand activation was found in yet another study to be eliminated by simultaneous right-hand activation, whether in the left or right hemispace.

A number of forms of stimulation have been found to affect neglect behavior. Vallar and associates[121] reported a reduction in left neglect among 17 adults with right-brain lesions who received vestibular (caloric) stimulation. Vallar and colleagues[122] also noted that optokinetic stimulation had an influence on perception of stimuli from the left hemispace. If patients with right-brain lesions and left neglect observed leftward-moving dots, their neglect was reduced. If, however, they observed rightward-moving dots, their left neglect was exacerbated. Karnath and coworkers[123] documented a small but significant reduction in left neglect with vibration of the upper trapezius muscles of the left side.

Orientation of the head seems unimportant to the manifestation of neglect. Since neglect is a perceptual rather than a sensory disorder, turning the head toward the neglected side has no salutary effect. Turning the trunk toward the neglected side, on the other hand, can have a significant result regardless of whether the head is turned or not.[123,124]

Butter and Kirsch[125] placed a patch over the right eyes of patients with stroke in an attempt to reduce left neglect. Although 11 of 13 patients showed benefits while performing at least one of five tests, benefits appeared to be limited to the time during which the patch was worn.

Training

The extent to which training assists in the recovery of visuospatial perception cannot be determined unequivocally from the research published to date. Edmans and Lincoln[126] found that training by figure copying, sequencing, and scanning had little effect. Although Towle and associates[127] found that 7 weeks of group treatment resulted in some minimal changes among a sample of patients with stroke, there were no obvious changes in daily life skills. Weinberg[128] reported some benefits from training in spatial orientation and sensory awareness. Gordon[129] found treatment to result not only in increased scores on a composite psychometric index but in time spent reading also. Gouvier and associates[130] described some quite favorable responses to visual-scanning training. Their subjects were trained progressively using a lightboard: first while sitting stationary in a chair, next while being pushed in a chair toward the board, and finally while propelling themselves in a chair toward the board. Following training, they made fewer obstacle contacts during a wheelchair propulsion task. Neither Webster and colleagues[131] nor Wagenaar and colleagues,[132] however, noted as favorable a response to visual-scanning training.

Compared to the results briefly summarized heretofore, those of Soderback and coworkers[133] appear to have considerable potential in the treatment of neglect. They used video feedback of functional performance at three kitchen tasks. Specifically, they showed each patient a video of his or her performance, stopping the presentation at illustrative points to highlight neglect behaviors. The patients' perception and behavior were discussed with them. Clear changes in behavior at the kitchen tasks was noted, leading the authors to conclude that the program was effective for "remediation and relearning."

Balance Performance

Research focused on the treatment of balance has increased conspicuously over the past decade. Writings on the topic have included information relevant to the elderly and to patients with stroke or other neurologic diagnoses. Treatment options described in the literature have focused on balance directly, on impairments that influence balance, or on both.

Treatment of the Elderly

In cases where the imbalance of the elderly can be traced with some confidence to a particular impairment, treatment should focus directly on that impairment. For example, in cases of retropulsion where a misperception of sagittal plane vertical appears to be an issue, a motor relearning program based on the inculcation of a correct perception of vertical is in order.[34] Similarly, where balance is compromised by positional vertigo, vestibular habituation is in order.[134]

In most elderly individuals, the factors contributing to balance problems are multifactorial. It should not be surprising, then, that interventions shown to be effective at increasing balance of such individuals also possess multiple components. Activities aimed at strength, flexibility, aerobic capacity, speed, and balance are among the more common components of effective treatment programs described in the literature.[93,135-138]

Treatment of Patients with Stroke

The standing balance of patients with stroke can be treated directly or indirectly. As with other elderly individuals, the first step in reestablishing independent standing for some patients with stroke is their recognition of true vertical. Once they have acknowledged that they have a retropulsion or lateropulsion problem, motor relearning can begin. After the ability to balance has been restored under static conditions, a progression of more difficult static and dynamic challenges can be introduced. Although the goal of some interventions at this stage is a reduction in weight-bearing asymmetry,[139–142] such a goal is not easily justified. As long as an individual's center of gravity is controlled within his or her base of support, a state of balance exists regardless of the extent of asymmetry. Moreover, weight-bearing asymmetry is only weakly correlated with function, and improvements in symmetry that accompany training are not necessarily reflected in better functional performance.[139] A specific type of dynamic training that has been studied in some detail involves perturbations on a movable platform.[143,144] Such training has been shown to increase the magnitude of anterior-posterior displacement to which patients can respond without a loss of balance.

Indirect treatments of balance can be either compensatory or corrective. Assistive devices such as walkers or canes[145] and orthotics such as ankle-foot orthoses[146] can compensate effectively for imbalance or its underlying impairments (for example, weakness). They allow some patients to balance who would otherwise be dependent on help from others. They also alter the mechanics of stance. Because devices reduce the challenge to a patient's own internal balance mechanism, they must be withdrawn as soon as possible if independence in balance is to be restored expeditiously.[147] Electrical stimulation may be of value in treating balance dysfunction after stroke. Fuller and Davies[148] described the case of a patient with sitting and standing difficulties who had "immediate and astonishing changes" in body posture with electrical stimulation over the third and seventh spinal processes. Maležič and associates[149] reported a 50.8 percent improvement in the rate of weight shift during stimulation of pelvic and knee muscles. Two different papers have described a normalization of postural control after a course of acupuncture.[115,150]

SUMMARY

The neurologic impairments that so often accompany aging and result in functional performance deficits are exacerbated in patients with frank neurologic pathology such as stroke. Through exercise and other interventions directed at neurologic impairments, deficits in physiologic and functional performance can be reduced. Many of the interventions described heretofore remain underused in the elderly in general and patients with stroke in particular.

REFERENCES

1. Bassey, EJ and Harries, UJ: Normal values for handgrip strength in 920 men and women aged over 65 years, and longitudinal changes over 4 years in 620 survivors. Clin Science 84:331–337, 1993.
2. Christ, CB, Boilean, RA, Slaughter, MH, Stillman, RJ, Cameron, JA, and Massey, BH: Maximal voluntary isometric force production characteristics of six muscle groups in women aged 25 to 74 years. Am J Human Biol 4:537–545, 1992.

3. Rice, CL: Strength in an elderly population. Arch Phys Med Rehabil 70:391–397, 1989.
4. Shephard, RJ, Montelpare, W, Plyley, M, McCracken, D, and Goode RC: Handgrip dynamometry, Cybex measurements and lean mass as markers of the ageing of muscle function. Br J Sp Med 25:204–208, 1991.
5. Gross, MT, McGrain, P, Demilio, N, and Plyler, L: Relationship between multiple predictor variables and normal knee torque production. Phys Ther 69:54–62, 1989.
6. Bemben, MG, Massey, BH, Bemben, DA, Misner, JE, and Boilean, RA: Isometric muscle force production as a function of age in healthy 20- to 74-yr-old men. Med Sci Sports Exerc 23:1302–1310, 1991.
7. Phillips, SK, Rook, RM, Siddle, NC, Bruce, SA, and Woledge, RC: Muscle weakness in women occurs at an earlier age than in men, but strength is preserved by hormone replacement therapy. Clin Science 84:95–98, 1993.
8. Lundgre-Lindquist, B and Rundgren, A: Functional capacity among the elderly in Sweden. Int Disabil Studies 10:6–9, 1988.
9. Andriacchi, TP, Andersson, GBJ, Fermier, RW, Stern, D, and Galante, JO: A study of lower-limb mechanics during stair-climbing. J Bone Joint Surg 62(A):749–757, 1980.
10. Moffet, H, Richards, CL, Malouin, F, and Bravo, G: Load-carrying during stair ascent: A demanding functional task. Gait Posture 1:35–44, 1993.
11. Richards, CL: EMG activity level comparisons in quadriceps and hamstrings in five dynamic activities. In Winter, DA, Norman, RW, Wells, RP, Hayes, KC, and Patla, AE (eds): Biomechanics IX-A. Human Kinetics, Champaign, IL, 1985, pp 313–317.
12. Gooptu, C, and Mulley, GP: Survey of elderly people who get stuck in the bath. Brit Med J 308:762, 1994.
13. Arborelius, UP, Wertenberg, P, and Lindberg, F: The effects of arm rests and high seat heights on lower-limb joint load and muscular activity during sitting and rising. Ergonomics 35:1377–1391, 1992.
14. Tenetti, ME, Liu, W-L, and Claus, EB: Predictors and prognosis of inability to get up after falls among elderly persons. J Amer Med Assoc 269:65–70, 1993.
15. Weiner, DK, Long, R, Hughes, MA, Chandler, J, and Studenski, S: When older adults face the chair-rise challenge. J Am Geriatr Soc 41:6–10, 1993.
16. Alexander, NB, Schultz, A, and Warwick, DN: Rising from a chair: Effects of age and functional ability on performance biomechanics. J Gerontol 46M:91–98, 1991.
17. Wheeler, J, Woodward, C, Ucovich, RL, Perry, J, and Walker, JM: Rising from a chair. Influence of age and chair design. Phys Ther 65:22–26, 1985.
18. Himann, JE, Cunningham, DA, Rechnitzer, PA, and Patersen, DH: Age-related changes in speed of walking. Med Sci Sports Exerc 20:161–166, 1988.
19. Dobbs, RJ, Lubel, DD, Charlett, A, Bowes, SG, O'Neill, CJA, Weller, C, and Dobbs, SM: Hypothesis: Age-associated changes in gait represent, in part, a tendency toward Parkinsonism. Age Ageing 21:221–225, 1992.
20. Bowes, SG, Charlett, A, Dobbs, J, Lubel, DD, Mehta, R, O'Neill,CJA, Weller, C, Hughes, J, and Dobbs, SM: Gait in relation to aging and idiopathic Parkinsonism. Scand J Rehabil Med 24:181–186, 1992.
21. Bassey, EJ, Bendall, MJ, and Pearson, M: Muscle strength in the tricepts surae and objectively measured customary walking activity in men and women over 65 years of age. Clin Science 74:85–89, 1988.
22. Judge, JO, Underwood, M, and Gennosa, T: Exercise to improve gait velocity in older persons. Arch Phys Med Rehabil 704:400–406, 1993.
23. Fiatarone, MA, Marks, EC, Ryan, ND, Meredith, CN, Lipsitz, LA, and Evans, WJ: High-intensity strength training in nonagenarians. J Amer Med Assoc 263:3029–3034, 1990.
24. Cohen, JJ, Sveen, JD, Walker, JM, and Brummel-Smith, K: Established criteria for community ambulation. Top Geriatr Rehabil 3:71–77, 1987.
25. Robinett, CS and Vondran, MA: Functional ambulation velocity and distance requirements in rural and urban communities. Phys Ther 68:1371–1373, 1988.

26. Hoxie,RE and Rubenstein, LZ: Are older pedestrians allowed enough time to cross intersections safely? J Am Geriatr Soc 42:241–244, 1994.
27. Wilson, B: The measurement of perceptual impairment. Clin Rehabil 1:169–173, 1987.
28. Lincoln, NB: The recognition and treatment of visual perceptual disorders. Topics Geriatr Rehabil 7(1):25–34, 1991.
29. Freedman, M, Leach, L, Kaplan, E, Winocur, G, Shulman, KI, and Delis, DC: Clock Drawing. A Neuropsychological Analysis. Oxford University Press, New York, 1994.
30. Huntzinger, JA, Rosse, RB, Schwartz, BL, Ross, LA, and Deutsch, SI: Clock drawing in the screening assessment of cognitive impairment in an ambulatory care setting: A preliminary report. Gen Hosp Psychiatry 14:142–144, 1992.
31. Tobis, JS, Reinsch, S, Swanson, JM, Byrd, M, and Scharf, T: Visual perception dominance of fallers among community-dwelling older adults. J Am Geriatr Soc 33:330–333, 1985.
32. Tobis, JS, Nayak, L, and Hoehler, F: Visual perception of verticality and horizontality among elderly fallers. Arch Phys Med Rehabil 62:619–622, 1981.
33. Yoshida, K, Iwakura, H, and Inoue, F: Motion analysis in the movements of standing up from and sitting down on a chair. Scand J Rehabil Med 15:133–140, 1983.
34. Bohannon, RW: Idiopathic retropulsion: Response to a motor relearning program. Physical Therapy Forum March 19, 20–21, 1993.
35. Briggs, RC, Gossman, MR, Birch, R, Drews, JE, and Shaddeau, SA: Balance performance among noninstitutionalized elderly women. Phys Ther 69:748–756, 1989.
36. Bohannon, RW, Larkin, PA, Cook, AC, Gear, J, and Singer, J: Decrease in timed balance test scores with aging. Phys Ther 64:1067–1070, 1984.
37. Jedrychowski, W, Mroz, E, Tobiasz-Adamczyk, B, and Jedrycnowksa, I: Functional status of the lower extremities in elderly males; A community study. Arch Gerontol Geriatr 10:117–122, 1990.
38. Overstall, PW, Johnson, AL, and Exton-Smith, AN: Instability and falls in the elderly. Age Ageing 7:92–96, 1978.
39. Kollegger, H, Baumgartner, C, Wöber, C, Oder, W, and Deecke L: Spontaneous body sway as a function of sex, age, and vision: Posturographic study in 30 healthy adults. Eur Neurol 32:253–259, 1992.
40. Hirokama, S: Normal gait characteristics under temporal and distance constraints. J Biomed Eng 11:449–456, 1989.
41. McRae, PG, LaCourse, M, and Moldavon, R: Physical performance measures that predict faller status in community-dwelling older adults. J Orthop Sports Phys Ther 16:123–128, 1992.
42. Gehlsen, GM, and Whaley, WH: Falls in the elderly: Part II. Balance, strength and flexibility. Arch Phys Med Rehabil 71:739–741, 1990.
43. Duncan, PW, Studenski, S, Chandler, J, and Prescott, B: Functional reach: Predictive validity in a sample of elderly male veterans. J Gerontol 47M:93–98, 1992.
44. Maki, BE, Holliday, PJ, and Topper, AK: A prospective study of postural balance and risk of falling in an ambulatory and independent elderly population. J Gerontol 49M:72–84, 1994.
45. Kauffman, T, and Jackson, O: Defining the geriatric population. Clin Manage 10(6):18–22, 1990.
46. Wade, DT, Langton Hewer, R, Skilbeck, ED, and David, RM: Stroke. A Critical Approach to Diagnosis, Treatment, and Management. Year Book Medical Pub, Chicago, IL, 1985.
47. Hamrin, E, Eklund, G, Hillgren, A-K, Borges, O, Hall, J, and Hellström, O: Muscle strength and balance in post-stroke patients. Upsala J Med Sci 87:11–26, 1982.
48. Colebatch, JG and Gandevia, SC: The distribution of muscular weakness in upper motor neuron lesions affecting the arm. Brain 112:749–763, 1989.
49. Bohannon, RW: Trunk muscle strength is impaired multidirectionally after stroke. Clin Rehabil 9:47–51, 1995.
50. Mastaglia, FL, Knezevic, W, and Thompson, PD: Weakness of head turning in hemiplegia: A quantitative study. J Neurol Neurosurg Psychiatry 49:195–197, 1986.

51. Cruccu, G, Fornarelli, M, and Manfredi, M: Impairment of masticatory function in hemiplegia. Neurology 38:301–306, 1988.
52. Annoni, JM, Ackerman, D, and Kesselring, J: Respiratory function in chronic hemiplegia. Int Disabil Studies 12:78–80, 1990.
53. Sunderland, A, Tinson, D, Bradley, L, and Langton Hewer, R: Arm function after stroke. An evaluation of grip strength as a measure of recovery and a prognostic indicator. J Neurol Neurosurg Pyschiatry 52:1267–1272, 1989.
54. Bohannon, RW and Smith, MB: Upper extremity strength deficits in hemiplegic stroke patients: Relationship between admission and discharge and time since onset. Arch Phys Med Rehabil 68:155–157, 1987.
55. Bohannon, RW: Muscle strength changes in hemiparetic stroke patients during inpatient rehabilitation. J Neuro Rehabil 2:163–166, 1988.
56. Friedman, PJ: The star cancellation test in acute stroke. Clin Rehabil 6:23–30, 1992.
57. Olsen, TS: Arm and leg paresis as outcome predictors in stroke rehabilitation. Stroke 21:247–251, 1990.
58. Bohannon, RW. Determinants of gown donning performance soon after stroke. Eur J Phys Med Rehabil 2:70–73, 1992.
59. Bohannon, RW: Determinants of transfer capacity in patients with hemiplegia. Physiother Can 40:236–239, 1988.
60. Nakamura, R, Hosokawa, T, and Tsuji, I: Relationship of muscle strength for knee extension to walking capacity in patients with spastic hemiparesis. Tohoku J Exp Med 145:335–340, 1985.
61. Bohannon, RW: Selected determinants of ambulatory capacity in patients with hemiplegia. Clin Rehabil 3:47–53, 1989.
62. Bohannon, RW: Knee extension power, velocity, and torque: Relative deficits and relation to walking performance in stroke patients. Clin Rehabil 6:125–131, 1992.
63. Bohannon, RW and Walsh, S: Association of paretic lower extremity muscle strength and standing balance with stair-climbing ability in patients with stroke. J Stroke Cerebrovasc Dis 1:129–133, 1991.
64. DeRenzi, E, Gentilini, M, and Barbieri, C: Auditory neglect. J Neurol Neurosurg Psychiatry 52:613–617, 1989.
65. Lakshmi, MV, Tallis, R, Ribbands, M, and Hollis, S: Device for quantifying tactile neglect in stroke patients. J Biomed Eng 13:516–519, 1991.
66. Kageyama, S, Imagase, M, Okubo, M, and Takayama, Y: Neglect in three dimensions. Am J Occup Ther 48:206–210, 1994.
67. Mattingly, JB, Bradshaw, JL, Bradshaw, JA, and Nettleton, NC: Residual rightward attentional bias after apparent recovery from right hemisphere damage: Implications for a multicomponent model of neglect. J Neurol Neurosurg Psychiatry 57:597–604, 1994.
68. Andrews, K, Brocklehurst, JC, Richards, B, and Laycock, PJ: The prognostic value of picture drawings by stroke patients. Rheumatol Rehabil 19:180–188, 1980.
69. Friedman, PJ: Spatial neglect in acute stroke: Line bisection test. Scand J Rehab Med 22:101–106, 1990.
70. Marsh, NV and Kersel, DA: Screening tests for visual neglect following stroke. Neuropsychol Rehabil 3:245–257, 1993.
71. Halligan, PW and Cockburn, JM: Cognitive sequelae of stroke: Visuospatial and memory disorders. CRC Rev Phys Rehabil Med 5:57–82, 1993.
72. Edmans, JA, and Lincoln, NB: The frequency of perceptual deficits after stroke. Clin Rehabil 1:273–281, 1987.
73. Stone, SP, Patel, P, Greenwood, RJ, and Halligan, PW: Measuring visual neglect in acute stroke and predicting its recovery: The visual neglect recovery index. J Neurol Neurosurg Psychiatry 55:431–436, 1992.
74. Nogaki, H, Ohba, Y, Matusmoto, K, Morimatsu, M, and Fukuoka Y: Statistical analysis of post-stroke patients in rehabilitation institution. Jap J Geriatr 28:678–682, 1991.

75. Nouri, FM and Lincoln, NB: Predicting driving performance after stroke. Clin Rehabil 6:275–281, 1992.

76. Bruell, JH, Peszcznski, JH, and Volke, D: Disturbance of perception of verticality in patients with hemiplegia: Second report. Arch Phys Med Rehabil 38:776–780, 1957.

77. Dieterich, DM and Brandt, T: Wallenberg's syndrome: Lateropulsion, cyclorotation, and subjective vertical in thirty-six patients. Ann Neurol 31:399–408, 1992.

78. Ray, R and Nair, A: The elderly reach independence through a community stroke rehabilitation programme. Ann Acad Med 20:314–323, 1991.

79. Bohannon, RW, Smith, MB, and Larkin, PA: Relationship between independent sitting balance and side of hemiparesis. Phys Ther 66:944–945, 1986.

80. Sandin, KJ, and Smith, BS: The measure of balance in sitting in stroke rehabilitation prognosis. Stroke 21:82–86, 1990.

81. Bohannon, RW, Walsh, S, and Joseph, MC: Ordinal and timed balance measurements: Reliability and validity in patients with stroke. Clin Rehabil 7:9–13, 1992.

82. Mizrahi, J, Groswasser, Z, Susak, Z, and Reider-Groswasser, I: Standing posture of craniocerebral injured patients: Bilateral active force patterns. Clin Phys Physiol Meas 10:25–37, 1989.

83. Lee, WA, Deming, L, and Sahgal, V: Quantitative and clinical measures of static standing balance in hemiparetic and normal subjects. Phys Ther 68:970–976, 1988.

84. Wing, AM, Goodrich, S, Virji-Babul, N, Jenner, JR, and Clapp, S: Balance evaluation in hemiparetic stroke patients using lateral forces applied to the hip. Arch Phys Med Rehabil 74:292–299, 1993.

85. Morita, H: Rehabilitation of post-stroke hemiplegic patients. I. Gravity-center-swaying and walking ability. J UOEH 11:261–273, 1989.

86. Keenan, MA, Perry, J, and Jordon, C: Factors affecting balance and ambulation following stroke. Clin Orthop 182:165–171, 1984.

87. Faigenbaum, AD, Shriner, GS, Cesare, WF, Kraemer, WJ, and Thomas, HE: Physiologic and symptomatic responses of cardiac patients to resistance exercise. Arch Phys Med Rehabil 71:395–398, 1990.

88. Lyons, K, Perry, J, Gronley, JK, Barnes, L, and Antonelli, D: Timing and relative intensity of hip extensor and abductor muscle action during level and stair ambulation. Phys Ther 63:1597–1605, 1983.

89. Wretenberg, P and Arborelius, UP: Power and work produced in different leg muscle groups when rising from a chair. Eur J Appl Physiol 68:413–417, 1994.

90. Wretenberg, P, Lindberg, F, and Arborelius, UP: Effect of arm rests and different ways of using them on hip and knee load during rising. Clin Biomech 8:95–101, 1983.

91. Rodosky, MW, Andriacchi, TP, and Andersson, BJ: The influence of chair height on lower limb mechanics during rising. J Orthop Res 7:266–271, 1989.

92. Fisher, NM, Pendergast, DR, and Calkins, E: Muscle rehabilitation in impaired elderly nursing home residents. Arch Phys Med Rehabil 72:181–185, 1991.

93. Binder, EF, Brown, M, Craft, S, Schechtman, KB, and Birge,SJ: Effects of a group exercise program on risk factors for falls in frail older adults. J Aging Phys Activity 2:25–37, 1994.

94. Grimby, G, Aniansson, A, Hedberg, M, Henning, GB, Grangard, U, and Kvist, H: Training can improve muscle strength and endurance in 78- to 84-year-old-men. J Appl Physiol 73:2517–2523, 1992.

95. Roman, WJ, Fleckenstein, J, Stray-Gundersen, J, Alway, SE, Peshock, R, and Gonyea, WJ: Adaptations in the elbow flexors of elderly males after heavy-resistance training. J Appl Physiol 74:750–754, 1993.

96. Nichols, JF, Omizo, DK, Peterson, KK, and Nelson, KP: Efficacy of heavy-resistance training for active women over sixty: muscular strength, body composition, and program adherence. J Am Geraitr Soc 41:205–210, 1993.

97. Jones, CJ, Rikili, RE, Benedict, J, and Williams, P: Effects of a resistance training program on leg strength and muscular endurance of older women. J Aging Phys Act 2:182–195, 1994.

98. Charette, SL, McEvoy, L, Pyka, G, Snow-Harter, C, Guido, D, Wiswell, RA, and Marcus, R: Muscle hypertrophy response to resistance training in older women. J Appl Physiol 70:1912–1916, 1991.

99. Åsberg, KH: Orthostatic tolerance training of stroke patients in general medical wards. Scand J Rehabil Med 21:179–185, 1989.

100. Inaba, M, Edberg, E, Montgomery, J, and Gillis, MK: Effectiveness of functional training, active exercise, and resistance exercise for patients with hemiplegia. Phys Ther 53:28–35, 1973.

101. Griffin, JW, Tooms, RE, Veander-Zwaag, R, O'Toole, ML, and Bertorini, TE: Eccentric and concentric muscle performance in patients with spastic paresis secondary to motor neuron disease. A preliminary report. Neuromusc Disord 4:131–138, 1994.

102. Knutsson, E, Gransberg, L, and Mårtensson, A: Faciliation and inhibition of maximal voluntary contractions by activation of muscle stretch reflexes in patients with spastic paresis. Electroenceph Clin Nuerophysio 70:37P–38P, 1988.

103. Knutsson, E, Mårtensson, A, and Gransberg, L: The effects of concentric and eccentric training in spastic paresis. Scand J Rehab Med 24 (Suppl 27):31–32, 1992.

104. Levin, MF and Hui-Chan, CWY: Relief of hemiparetic spasticity by TENS is associated with improvement in reflex and voluntary motor functions. Electroenceph Clin Neurophysiol 85:131–142, 1992.

105. Merletti, R, Zelaschi, F, Latella, D, Galli, M, Angeli, S, and Sessa, MB: A control study of muscle force recovery in hemiparetic patients during treatment with functional electrical stimulation. Scand J Rehabil Med 10:147–154, 1978.

106. Baker, LL, Yeh, C, Wilson, D, and Waters, RL: Electrical stimulation of wrist and fingers for hemiplegic patients. Phys Ther 59:1495–1499, 1979.

107. Smith, LE: Restoration of volitional limb movement of hemiplegics following patterned functional electrical stimulation. Percept Mot Skills 71:851–861, 1990.

108. Lagassé, PP, and Roy MA: Functional electrical stimulation and the reduction of co-contraction in spastic biceps brachii. Clin Rehabil 3:111–116, 1989.

109. Intiso, D, Santilli, V, Grasso, MG, Rossi, R, and Caruso, I: Rehabilitation of walking with electromyographic biofeedback in foot-drop after stroke. Stroke 25:1189–1192, 1994.

110. Winchester, P, Montgomery, J, Bowman, B, and Hislop, H: Effects of feedback stimulation training and cyclical electrical stimulation on knee extension in hemiparetic patients. Phys Ther 63:1096–1103, 1983.

111. Fields, RW: Electromyographically triggered electrical muscle stimulation for chronic hemiplegia. Arch Phys Med Rehabil 68:407–414, 1987.

112. Kraft, GH, Fitts, SS, and Hammond, MC: Techniques to improve function of the arm and hand in chronic hemiplegia. Arch Phys Med Rehabil 73:220–227, 1992.

113. Naeser, MA, Alexander, MP, Stiassny-Eder, D, Lannin, LN, and Bachman,D: Acupuncture in the treatment of hand paresis in chronic and acute stroke patients: Improvement observed in all cases. Clin Rehabil 8:127–141, 1994.

114. Naeser, MA, Alexander, MP, Stiassny-Eder, D, Galler, V, Hobbs, J, and Backman, D: Real versus sham acupuncture in the treatment of paralysis in acute stroke patients: A CT scan lesion site study. J Neuro Rehab 6:163–173, 1992.

115. Johansson, K, Lindgren, I, Widmer, H, Wiklund, I, and Johansson, BB: Can sensory stimulation improve the functional outcome in stroke patients? Neurology 43:2189–2192, 1993.

116. Riddoch, MJ, and Humphreys, GW: The effect of cueing on unilateral neglect. Neuropsychologia 21:589–599, 1983.

117. Weinberg, J, Diller, L, Gordon, WA, Gertfman, LJ, Lieverman, A, Lakin, P, Hodges, G, and Ezrachi, O: Visual scanning training effect on reading related tasks in acquired right brain damage. Arch Phys Med Rehabil 58:479–486, 1977.

118. Robertson, IH, North NT, and Geggie, C: Spatiomotor cueing in unilatral left neglect: Three cases studies of its therapeutic effects. J Neuro Neurosurg Psychiatry 55:799–805, 1992.

119. Robertson, IH and North, NT: Spatio-motor cueing in unilateral neglect: The role of hemisphere, hand and motor activation. Neuropsychologia 30:553–563, 1992.

120. Robertson, IH and North, NT: One hand is better than two: Motor extinction of left hand advantage in neglect. Neuropsychologia 32:1–11, 1994.

121. Vallar, G, Bottini, G, Rusconi, ML, and Sterzi, R: Exploring somatosensory hemineglect by vestibular stimulation. Brain 116:71–86, 1993.

122. Vallar, G, Antonucci, G, Guariglia, C, Pizzamiglio, L: Deficits in position sense, unilateral neglect and optokinetic stimulation. Neuropsychologia 31:1191–1200, 1993.

123. Karnath, HO, Christ, K, and Hartje, W: Decrease of contralateral neglect by neck muscle vibration and spastical orientation of trunk midline. Brain 116:383–396, 1993.

124. Karnath, HO, Schenkel, P, and Fischer, B: Trunk orientation as the determining factor of the "contralateral" deficit in the neglect syndrome and as the physical anchor of the internal representation of body orientation in space. Brain 114:1997–2014, 1991.

125. Butter, CM, and Kirsch, N: Combined and separate effects of eye patching and visual stimulation on unilateral neglect following stroke. Arch Phys Med Rehabil 73:1133–1139, 1992.

126. Edmans, JA and Lincoln, NB: Treatment of visual perceptual deficits after stroke: four single case studies. Int Disabil Studies 11:25–33. 1989.

127. Towle, D, Edmans, JA, and Lincoln, NB: An evaluation of a group programme for stroke patients with perceptual deficits. Int J Rehabil Research 13:328–335, 1990.

128. Weinberg, J, Diller, L. Gordon, WA, Gerstman, LJ, Lieberman, A, Lakin, P, Hodges, G, and Ezrachi, O: Training sensory awareness and spatial organization in people with right brain damage. Arch Phys Med Rehabil 60:491–496, 1979.

129. Gordon, WA, Hibbard, MR, Egelko, S, Diller, L, Shaver, MS, Lieberman, A, and Ragarsson, K: Perceptual remediation in patients with right brain damage: A comprehensive program. Arch Phys Med Rehabil 66:353–359, 1985.

130. Gouvier, WD, Cottaum, G, Webster, JS, Beissel,GF, and Wofford, JD: Behavioral interventions with stroke patients for improving wheelchair navigation. Int J Clin Neuropsychol 11:295–310, 1989.

131. Webster, JS, Cottaum,G, Gouvier, WD, et al: Wheelchair obstacle course performance in right cerebrovascular accident victims. J Clin Exp Neuropsychol 11:295–310, 1989.

132. Wagenaar, RC, Van Wieringer, PCW, Netelebas, JB, Meiger, OG, and Kuik, DJ: The transfer of scanning training effects in visual inattention after stroke: Five single-case studies. Disabil Rehabil 14:51–60, 1992.

133. Söderback, I, Bengtsson, I, Ginsburg, E, and Ekholm, J: Video feedback in occupational therapy: Its effect in patients with neglect syndrome. Arch Phys Med Rehabil 73:1140–1146, 1992.

134. Norré, ME and Beckers, A: Vestibular habituation training for positional vertigo in elderly patients. Arch Gerontol Geriatr 8:117–122, 1989.

135. Lichtenstein, MJ, Shields, SL, Shiavi, RG, and Burger, C: Exercise and balance in aged women: A pilot controlled clinical trial. Arch Phys Med Rehabil 70:138–143, 1989.

136. Topp, R, Mikesky, A, Wigglesworth, J, Holt, W, and Edwards, JE: The effect of a 12-week dynamic resistance strength training program on gait velocity and balance of older adults. Gerontologist 33:501–506, 1993.

137. Lord, SR, Caplan, GA, and Ward, JA: Balance, reaction time, and muscle strength in exercising and nonexercising older women: A pilot study. Arch Phys Med Rehabil 74:837–839, 1993.

138. Lord, SR and Castell, S: Physical activity program for older persons: Effect on balance, strength, neuromuscular control, and reaction time. Arch Phys Med Rehabil 75:648–652, 1994.

139. Winstein, CJ, Gardner, ER, McNeal, DR. Barto, PS, and Nichoson, DE: Standing balance training: Effects on balance and locomotion in hemiparetic adults. Arch Phys Med Rehabil 70:755–762, 1989.

140. Sackley, CM: The relationships between weight-bearing asymmetry after stroke, motor function and activities of daily living. Physiother Theory Pract 6:179–185, 1990.
141. Sackley, CM, Baguley, BI, Gent, S, and Hodgson, P: The use of a balance performance monitor in the treatment of weight-bearing and weight-tranference problems after stroke. Physiotherapy 78:907–913, 1992.
142. deWeerdt, W, Brossley, SM, Lincon, NB, and Harrison, MA: Restoration of balance in stroke patients: A single case design study. Clin Rehabil 3:139–147, 1989.
143. Hocherman, S, Dickstein, R, and Pillar, T: Platform training and postural stability in hemiplegia. Arch Phys Med Rehabil 65:588–592, 1984.
144. Dickstein, R, Hocherman, S, Dannenbaum, E, Shina, N, and Pillar, T: Stance stability and EMG changes in the ankle musculature of hemiparetic patients trained on a moveable platform. J Neuro Rehab 5:201–209, 1991.
145. Milczarek, JJ, Kirby, RL, Harrison, ER, and Macleod, DA: Standard and four-footed canes: their effect on the standing balance of patients with hemiparesis. Arch Phys Med Rehabil 74:281–285, 1993.
146. Majica, JAP, Nakamura, R, Kobayashi, T, Handa, T, Morohashi, I, and Watanabe, S: Effect of ankle foot orthosis (AFO) on body sway and walking capacity of hemiparetic stroke patients.Tohoku J Exp Med 156:395–401, 1988.
147. Balliet, R, Harbst, KB, Kim, D, and Stewart, RV: Retraining of functional gait through reduction of upper extremity weight-bearing in chronic cerebellar atexia. Int J Rehabil Med 8:148–153, 1987.
148. Fuller, FF and Davies, JM: The effect of vibration and transcutaneous electrical stimulation on postural control in a patient with stroke. Can J Rehabil 2:79–86, 1988.
149. Maležič, M, Hesse, S, Schewe, H, and Mauritz, K-H: Restoration of stranding, weight-shift and gait by multichannel electrical stimulation in hemiparetic patients. Int J Rehabil Res 17:169–179, 1994.
150. Magnusson, M, Johansson, K, and Johansson, BB: Sensory stimulation promotes normalization of postural control after stroke. Stroke 25:1176–1180, 1994.

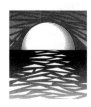

CHAPTER 9

Cardiopulmonary Rehabilitation of the Geriatric Patient

Cynthia Coffin Zadai, MS, PT, CCS
Scot C. Irwin, MS, PT, CCS

BEHAVIORAL OBJECTIVES

Upon completion of this chapter, the reader will be able to:

1 Define and identify the cardiopulmonary adaptations that accompany the aging process.
2 Specify the pathologic changes that accompany cardiopulmonary disease.
3 Describe how pathologic changes that accompany cardiopulmonary disease differ from the normal process.
4 Describe the response of the cardiopulmonary system to exercise.
5 Examine and evaluate the cardiopulmonary system of the geriatric patient.
6 Set goals and prescribe a treatment or training program for the geriatric patient with cardiopulmonary complications.

Anatomic and Physiologic Changes in Oxygen Transport with Age
Oxygen Uptake
Tissue Changes of Age
Structural and Physiologic Changes
Pathologic Changes in the Pulmonary System
Pathologic Changes in the Cardiac System
Cardiopulmonary Response to Exercise: Alterations with Age

Patient Examination
Observation
Palpation
Auscultation
Exercise Testing and Functional Assessment
Protocol and Modality Selection
Monitoring Parameters
Patient Preparation
Beginning an Exercise Test
During the Exercise Test
Stopping the Test
Setting Goals
Training Program

The elderly segment of the population is a complex and challenging group of individuals. The combination of old age and disease produces systemic changes that inhibit the cardiopulmonary responses to increased oxygen demand. Aerobic production of energy is a basic foundation of every individual's ability to meet increased exertional demands. Exercise training can be performed safely and effectively by deconditioned or diseased older individuals when the adequacy and appropriateness of their cardiopulmonary responses have been assessed, the purpose and practicality of their goals reviewed, and the safety and efficacy of the exercise prescription assured. Geriatric clients who are deconditioned or limited by cardiopulmonary disease have demonstrated increases in strength, endurance, overall functional abilities, and well-being when individualized exercise programs have been implemented.[1] The purpose of this chapter is to delineate methods for assessing cardiopulmonary responses to exercise in the elderly and to make suggestions for exercise programming.

The pulmonary system has not heretofore been considered a limiting factor in the performance of exercise for the healthy adult or child;[2] consequently, the respiratory response to exercise was simply observed and recorded but did not generally receive specific attention during functional evaluations or exercise program planning. Recently, however, there is evidence to suggest that well-trained athletes are in fact more limited at maximal exercise by their pulmonary mechanics than by their cardiac output.[3] The concept of the respiratory system as a limiting factor in low-level exercise is also relatively recent. Diseased individuals with respiratory limitation are difficult to assess and to prescribe exercise for. The clinical research procedures that document the ventilatory mechanics, gas exchange efficacy, and pathophysiologic responses to exercise have been difficult for this symptomatic and functionally impaired patient group to perform. Exercise was often considered to be contraindicated for dyspneic individuals prior to the gradual reversal in thinking that has occurred over the last two decades.

Conversely, the cardiovascular system's response to exercise has been extensively investigated, especially over the last two decades. The cardiovascular effects of deconditioning were well-documented in the early 1960s, and exercise programs have progressively become more accepted as a therapeutic modality.[4] The one exception to this extensive study has been in the area of geriatrics: only recently has there been in-depth study of "normal" cardiovascular responses in the elderly.

The recent increased interest in research about the older cardiac patient may be the result of changing demographic and sociologic patterns, creating a growing interest in the subjects of exercise and care for the elderly. Not only has there been a progressive increase in the number of individuals living well beyond the demarcation line of old age,[5] but the expectations or definitions of acceptable levels of function for that segment of the population have also changed. With society's increased focus on exercise and the positive expectation for an active elderly population has come a willingness and eagerness of older individuals to participate in physical activity programs. This new service demand has mandated development of clinical procedures for safe and effective exercise assessment and prescription for older clients. Concomitantly, research studies have demonstrated not only that exercise is beneficial for maintaining a functional baseline condition in the unimpaired older individual, but that it can be therapeutic for reversing the effects of impairment and improving the baseline condition of diseased individuals who have become deconditioned as a result of their symptom limitations (i.e., dyspnea and angina).[6–8] Therapeutic evaluation and program planning have now reached the point where the older individual who was once confined to bed because of angina and dyspnea resulting from cardiopulmonary disease can be evaluated and treated with a total rehabilitation program, including an individualized exercise prescription that considers the severity of disease, attempts symptom reversal, and has functional improvement as its goal.

The purpose of this chapter is to describe the effects of aging and disease on the oxygen transport system. Guidelines are included for patient evaluation and treatment procedures to be considered for use with elderly individuals who demonstrate cardiopulmonary limitation.

ANATOMIC AND PHYSIOLOGIC CHANGES IN OXYGEN TRANSPORT WITH AGE

In view of society's increased awareness regarding our environment and the risk factors for cardiac and pulmonary disease, it is not surprising that research has been directed toward the effects of our atmosphere on the cardiopulmonary system and the effects of risk-factor reduction on cardiopulmonary disease incidence and progression.[9,10] However, researchers have found it difficult to separate the anatomic and physiologic changes of age and the effects of deconditioning from the pathologic response of the cardiopulmonary system to both the passive environment and the created environment (for example, smoking). The cardiopulmonary system is in constant contact with all components of the atmosphere. More than other organs, the heart and lungs are exposed to the noxious effects of the air that we breathe. Hence, physiologic changes in the cardiopulmonary system because of age, disease, or environmental impact are difficult at best to separate and to identify.

Oxygen Uptake

The participation of the cardiac and pulmonary systems in the uptake and distribution of oxygen includes several component steps. The musculoskeletal thoracic pump is responsible for initiating skeletal muscle contraction to increase thoracic volume and to lower intrathoracic pressure. The lower intrathoracic pressure creates gas flow from the higher-pressured atmosphere into the conducting tubules where the gas is warmed, filtered, humidified, and mixed with exiting gases to produce an alveolar oxygen tension of 90 to 100 mmHg. Alveolar oxygen is diffused across the 70-square-meter blood gas interface into pulmonary capillary blood via an approximate 40 mmHg pressure gradient where it combines with hemoglobin and drains into the left atrium. The heart delivers the oxygenated blood to itself and other tissues by a self-generated rhythmic contraction. The cardiac pump pressure overcomes systemic pressure and generates blood flow through the arterial vascular system to the tissues where oxygen is extracted and used in quantities related to oxygen demand. The basis of all functional activity is, therefore, dependent upon each link in the system for oxygen uptake, transport, and delivery described by the equation

$$V_{O_{2max}} = Q \times (a - V_{O_2})$$

$$\begin{aligned}
\text{Where } V_{O_{2max}} &= \text{maximum ventilation rate of oxygen} \\
Q &= \text{cardiac output} \\
a &= \text{arterial oxygen content} \\
v &= \text{central venous oxygen content}
\end{aligned}$$

This formula represents all of the complexities of oxygen uptake in a simple form. Oxygen consumption at a maximal level ($V_{O_{2max}}$) is the best single measure of an individual's cardiopulmonary fitness. An impairment at any step or link in this system of oxygen delivery through aging, deconditioning, or disease will be reflected in a decrease in maximum oxygen consumption and eventually an impairment in functional capability.

Tissue Changes of Age

The anatomic structures of the cardiopulmonary system are functionally specific. The musculoskeletal pump is responsible for ventilation through the coordinated contraction of the diaphragm and associated ventilatory muscles, the displacement of the rib cage, and the expansion of the underlying lung. The force generation required to accomplish ventilatory pump motion, intrathoracic pressure change, and gas flow depends on the resting length and strength of the ventilatory muscles, the compliance of the thoracic cage, and the compliance and recoil of lung tissue. Aging produces a progressive decrease in chest wall and bronchiolar compliance, beginning at approximately 24 years of age.[11] This stiffening results from a structural change in the bones, cartilage, and elastic structures; there is an increase in cross-linking of collagen fibers, a decrease in resiliency of elastic and cartilaginous tissue, and a decrease in collagen of the annulus fibrosis.[1,12,13] Concurrently, there is an alteration in the location and structure of the elastic fibers within the lung, increasing the lung's compliance and decreasing its elastic recoil.[14,15] Because the decrease in rib cage and supporting structure compliance is relatively greater than the increase in lung compliance, there is a resultant overall decrease in the thoracic system or total lung compliance by age 60.[11,15] Change in elastic structures at the alveolar level is also accompanied by loss of tissue from the alveolar walls and septra, increasing the size and number of alveolar fenestra[16,17] and thereby decreasing surface area available for gas exchange. Increased rigidity of the conducting tubules, changes in the structure of smooth muscles, and an increase in the thickness of the mucosal bed combine to decrease the radius of the conducting tubules and increase resistance to gas flow.[12,18] These changes summarily result in decreased efficiency of gas exchange and increased work of breathing for a mechanically disadvantaged pump.

Vascular changes of age affect each tissue layer differently and vary in their degree and distribution throughout the body.[19] There is increased irregularity of cells in the intima, and they are no longer uniform in their orientation to the longitudinal axis of the vessel.[20] There is thickening of the subendothelial layer with increased connective tissue, calcification, and lipid deposition. The media layer also demonstrates increased calcification with fraying of the elastic fibers. These changes produce regional differences in vascular diameter and can create increased resistance and turbulence in the blood flow. The heart itself demonstrates little change in chamber size, but there is a slight increase in wall thickness of the left ventricle.[21,22] The valves may show signs of thickening or nodular ridges along the attachments of the aortic cusps.[21,23] The conduction system displays relatively little change in the atrioventricular (AV) node or the bundle of His, but the number of proximal bundle fascicles connecting the left (L) ventricle to the main bundle may be less.[20] An increase in small foci of fibrosis has been shown on the myocardium itself.

Structural and Physiologic Changes

Total lung compliance changes of age alter pulmonary function both statically and dynamically. Although the total lung capacity does not appear to change significantly with age, vital capacity (VC) is reduced while the functional residual capacity (FRC) and residual volume (RV) are increased (Table 9–1). This retention of volume results in several changes of physiologic significance. The functional resting position of the chest is changed to that of partial inspiration, which places the inspiratory muscles in a relatively shorter position on their length and tension curve. This resting position also produces a relatively higher intrathoracic pressure at end expiration, resulting in increased airway resistance and a greater ventilatory requirement to create an adequate pressure or volume change for inspiratory flow. The added retained volume in an overly compliant lung will also produce regional areas of collapse and hyperinflation, which alter ventilation-perfusion (V/Q) ratios and decrease the efficiency of gas exchange.[24] By way of comparison, a 20-year-old person would use 40 percent of the total elastic work of breathing at rest to expand the chest wall, whereas an older individual could expend 70 percent or more.[15] The ability of the ventilatory muscles to generate or to sustain such power output decreases with age.[25] The V/Q variations result in a gradual progressive decline in resting partial pressure of arterial oxygen (Pa_{O_2}) throughout life (see Table 9–1).[26] Given all these changes, an increase in the work of breathing and oxygen demand results in relatively less oxygen delivered to fuel the work.

Physiologic changes in the cardiovascular system primarily involve the determinants of cardiac output. The progressive decline in maximal heart rate associated with aging has been well documented. Although resting heart rate and the heart rates achieved with submaximal levels of exercise may not be directly related to age, they do vary in response to the individual's degrees of conditioning and impairment. Heart-rate responses and

Table 9–1. **Normal Changes Seen with Aging**

Parameter		Change with Increased Age	
Vital capacity (VC)	Decreased*		
Functional residual capacity (FRC)	Increased†		
Residual volume (RV)	Increased†	change dependent on size and sex	
Forced expiratory volume (FEV$_{1.0}$ liter)	Decreased*		
Forced expiratory flow (FEF$_{25-75\%}$ liter/sec)	Decreased*		
		Standard Values/Age-related change	
Partial pressure of arterial oxygen (Pa_{O_2})	Decreased	80–100 mmHG: 104 − (.42 × age) ‡	
Partial pressure of arterial carbon dioxide (Pa_{CO_2})	Unchanged	35–45 mmHG	
pH	Unchanged	7.35–7.45	

*From Morris, et al: Prediction nomogram: Spirometric values. Am Rev Resp Dis 108:57, 1971, with permission.
†From Kenney, RA: Physiology of Aging. Yearbook Medical Publishers, Chicago, 1982, with permission.
‡From Murray,[26] with permission.

physiologic stimuli such as postural change and cough have also been shown to decrease as age increases.[23,29] The stroke volume component of cardiac output is also affected by preload and afterload conditions, which are altered by aging. Early diastolic filling is decreased in the aging heart, possibly due to mitral valve thickening or decreased ventricular (L) compliance.[20] There is an increase in afterload with aging, possibly produced by a stiffened ascending aorta and a decreased cross-section of the peripheral vascular bed. This collective increased load is most likely to be responsible for the age-associated decrease in stroke volume and cardiac output.[19,23,30] Neurohumeral regulatory changes also affect the physiologic response of the elderly individual. Although there may be an increase in the plasma-catecholamine levels with advancing age,[31] there is a decrease in the end-organ responsiveness to beta-adrenergic stimulation.[19,20] This variation in circulating catecholamines or decreased neuroresponsiveness may partially account for the decreased heart rate and blood pressure response to activities such as a cough or Valsalva's maneuver. This attenuated responsiveness is also partly attributed to decreased baroreceptor sensitivity.[31]

Blood pressure changes in aged individuals are dependent on many factors, including extracellular fluid volume, vascular tone and reactivity, the autonomic nervous system, and the arterial baroreceptor reflex. Each component factor can affect responsiveness in the aged individual somewhat differently. Resting systolic and diastolic BPs tend to rise with advancing age. However, the range is quite variable, and whether this reflects genetic or environmental influences is not yet known.[20]

PATHOLOGIC CHANGES IN THE PULMONARY SYSTEM

The pulmonary anatomic and functional changes of aging previously described are not dissimiliar to the pathologic changes seen in patients with chronic lung disease. It is difficult and may be impossible to separate aging from disease in the early stages of chronic obstructive pulmonary disease (COPD) because both are characterized by small changes that occur over time and neither interferes with resting or low-level ventilatory function. The pathologic tissue changes seen with both emphysema and chronic bronchitis are similar to the tissue changes of advancing age. Distinguishing between normal and pathologic change requires documentation of the degree, type, and extent of impairment and compromise.[14,25] Cumming and Semple[32] note that emphysema is a condition characterized by abnormal enlargement of the terminal airspaces and is partly an expression of normal senescence, a loss of elastic tissue from the lung that leads to expiratory collapse of the larger air passages, difficulty in expiration, and dilatation of the terminal airways. The American Thoracic Society[33] defines chronic bronchitis on the basis of its symptoms. A subject who has a chronic or recurrent productive cough on most days for a minimum of 3 months per year in not less than 2 successive years is considered to have chronic bronchitis. Although emphysema and chronic bronchitis are described separately, their clinical coexistence is common. An older individual who has both problems complains of coughing, sputum production, frequent upper respiratory infections, and dyspnea on exertion. Objective functional measures will demonstrate a reduction in vital capacity due to an increased residual volume, decreased forced expiratory volume in 1 second (FEV_1) and a reduced arterial oxygen tension (Pa_{O_2}) with increased carbon dioxide tension (Pa_{CO_2}) (see Table 9–1 for comparison). The pulmonary systemic changes produced by disease further increase the work of breathing and decrease the energy supply available to perform work. Progressive retention of volume demonstrated with COPD places the ventilatory pump at a mechanical disadvantage. The ribs are held more horizontally, and the shorter inspiratory muscles are at an increasingly less effective point on the optimum length-tension curve. Simultaneously, the increasing stiffness of connective tissue, the progressive narrowing of airways increasing resistance to gas flow, and the declining ventilation/perfusion ratio combine to increase the ventilatory muscles' workload and decrease the system's ability to supply oxygen even at rest.[34,35] The problem intensifies during activity, wherein a larger percentage of the oxygen uptake is consumed by the ventilatory muscles. The result may be fatigue and failure of the ventilatory pump in addition to depletion of the oxygen available to other tissues.

PATHOLOGIC CHANGES IN THE CARDIAC SYSTEM

Coronary artery or ischemic heart disease (CAD or IHD) is the most common disease in individuals over age 60 in the United States. The disease process begins in youth and is intimately associated with specific risk factors, including age. In 90 to 95 percent of the cases, the reduction of blood flow to the heart muscle is a result of atherosclerotic narrowing of the coronary lumen.[36] This reduction in flow creates the three major disease manifestations of ischemic pain (angina), infarction, and sudden death. Angina and infarction impair function by decreasing maximum cardiac output and maximum oxygen consumption. Additionally, infarction or death of heart muscle will limit the distensibility of the heart and reduce stroke volume. Collectively, these pathologic changes produce a self-limiting impediment to cardiac pump function. Increased systemic demands for oxygen necessitate an increase in CO or myocardial pump work. Increased work requires an increased oxygen supply to the myocardium. The restricted coronary blood flow produces ischemia, which increases left end-diastolic pressure, prolongs systole as the heart is unable to relax, and stiffens the ventricle wall. These physiologic changes reduce perfusion of the myocardium and worsen the ischemia.[37,38] The outcome of this vicious circle for patients with CAD is a failing pump due to a self-limiting disease process that impairs exercise capacity by producing the primary symptoms of angina and dyspnea.

CARDIOPULMONARY RESPONSE TO EXERCISE: ALTERATIONS WITH AGE

The cardiopulmonary system's response to exercise in the normal healthy adult includes efficient function of five major components: chest wall and lung mechanics; alveolar ventilation; alveolar to arterial gas exchange and transport; adequate cardiac acceleratory and pump mechanics; and adequate perfusion to the tissues. With the onset of exercise, each component steps up its contribution relative to the stress experienced. Initially, the ventilatory pump and cardiac pump respond to an increased oxygen demand with an increase in their respective volumes. This increase in volume is progressively greater than the increase in rate up to approximately 50 percent of VC and $V_{O_{2max}}$.[2] At that point, in both the ventilatory and cardiac systems, there is a relatively greater increase in rate as tidal volume (V_t) and SV level off to produce progressively a larger minute ventilation (VE) and CO, respectively.[2,34] The increased lung volume enhances alveolar ventilation, thereby improving V/Q matching over a greater alveolar surface and increasing the oxygen available from external respiration. The increased CO transports the oxygenated blood more rapidly to the exercising muscle, enhancing internal respiration and returning the carbon dioxide produced to the lung. The cardiopulmonary response generated will be in direct ratio to the oxygen demand. Once the oxygen supply successfully meets the demand, that level of exercise is termed steady state, and cardiopulmonary component functions plateau. Demands that require energy supply beyond the maximum capacity of the aerobic system require reliance on additional anaerobic metabolism.

Each of the described cardiopulmonary component responses are slowed or decreased by age. The elderly individual will have a greater oxygen uptake response for any given submaximal metabolic demand.[38] Lower levels of work demand relatively larger increases in tidal and stroke volumes initially. A 50 percent level of maximum exercise capacity is reached sooner because of the decreased maximum capacity. Therefore, larger increases in the contribution from ventilatory rate and heart rate will be seen at lower levels of exercise. Because the system's responses to stress are slowed, lower workload levels will require a longer amount of time to reach steady state and to return to the resting level after exercise.

Once an individual is exercising, the ability to sustain a high V_t or to increase the ejection fraction is limited by both the strength and endurance of the ventilatory and cardiac muscles. Strength and endurance properties of muscle decrease with age, thereby limiting both the amount and duration of work an older person can perform. When the normal aging changes combine with a loss of fitness and deconditioning, there is a significant reduction in cardiopulmonary reserve capacity. The impact of this reduction may become noticeable during normal activities of daily living (ADL) if the total capacity is also reduced by disease (Fig. 9–1). For example, most individuals use approximately 40 percent of $\dot{V}_{O_2}$ to walk at a normal pace.[39] Individuals appear to alter their pace to accommodate any limitation in $\dot{V}_{O_2}$. As $\dot{V}_{O_{2max}}$ is reduced, a person's pace will be slowed to keep the oxygen consumption at a 40 percent level.[40] Eventually, as aging or deconditioning progresses and the maximum value decreases, any pace will require the utilization of anaerobic as well as aerobic energy sources because the individual will have to exceed 50 to 60 percent of the $\dot{V}_{O_{2max}}$ to walk. This process produces the symptom of dyspnea and is analogous to exercise-induced dyspnea produced in normal younger adults when jogging or running. Differentiation of shortness of breath or dyspnea produced by exercise versus aging versus pathology is critical in elderly individuals who are symptomatic at rest or with activity prior to institution of and progression through an exercise program.

PATIENT EXAMINATION

The key to success in treating the geriatric patient who may or may not have cardiopulmonary complications is an accurate and comprehensive ex-

CARDIAC RESERVE: EFFECTS OF AGE AND DISEASE

Normal Athlete 18–20 years old	Rest 4–6 L/min	Required for ADL	RESERVE CAPACITY			
						24 L/min maximum
Effects of Age > 60 years old	Rest 4–6 L/min	Required for ADL	RESERVE CAPACITY			Aging loss
						18 L/min maximum
Effects of Age and Deconditioning > 60 years old	Rest 4–6 L/min	Required for ADL	RESERVE CAPACITY		Deconditioning loss	Aging loss
						14 L/min maximum
Effects of Age, Deconditioning and Disease	Rest 4–6 L/min	Required for ADL	RESERVE CAPACITY	Ischemia/ infarction loss	Deconditioning loss	Aging loss

FIGURE 9–1. Effects of aging, deconditioning, and disease on cardiac output.

amination. The physical examination includes observation, palpation, auscultation, and exercise testing (Fig. 9–2).

Observation

The patient interview and chart review are the initial steps of patient examination and precede any hands-on examination. They are included in the observation phase and can be noted during the interview.

Careful scrutiny of a patient's chart or family and patient interviews can provide answers to pertinent questions that will be valuable for program planning. An accurate medical history can specify whether the patient is chronically ill with an acute exacerbation, recently aware of the symptoms associated with exercise, or unable to easily perform the ADL. Answers to all the interview questions (Fig. 9–3) provide information not only about the patient's physical condition but also about his or her mental attitude. For example, did the patient seek medical attention voluntarily or was there coercion? Is the patient aware that a problem exists? Is the patient eager to participate in a rehabilitation program?

A social history can be enlightening regarding the patient's support system. The family and friends of an individual can either support or detract from a patient's progress throughout the program. Knowledge of the pa-

I. Observation

  A. Patient position
    1. use of upper extremities
    2. use of musculature

  B. Thoracic cage
    1. symmetry
    2. ratio of AP to Lat diameter

  C. Breathing
    1. rate and depth
    2. rhythm
    3. pattern

II. Palpation

  A. subcostal angle/AP to Lat diameter
  B. localized expansion/symmetry
  C. excursion/mobility
  D. locate painful areas

III. Auscultation

  A. Normal breath sounds
  B. Abnormal breath sounds
  C. Adventitious breath sounds

FIGURE 9–2. A physical examination is part of the patient evaluation.

I. Patient interview

  A. Patient perception of problem/disease process

    1. specific didactic knowledge

    2. emotional reaction

      a. embarrassment

      b. anxiety

      c. preoccupation

      d. denial

  B. Family perception of problem/disease process

  C. Patient description of disease progress and physical performance ability

  D. Patient history of dyspnea/orthopnea

II. Chart review

  A. Medical history

    1. previous admissions and diagnosis

    2. present medical problems: active/inactive

      a. present medications

      b. admitting diagnosis/objectives/care plan

  B. Laboratory studies

    1. pulmonary function tests/ABGs

    2. metabolic studies/blood work

    3. recent ECG

    4. significant radiographic findings

III. Work/social history

  A. Present and past jobs/working environment

  B. Present and past living locations

  C. Social habits

    1. smoking

    2. alcohol

    3. physical activity

FIGURE 9–3. Answers to pertinent questions will inform the therapist not only of the patient's physical condition but also of the patient's mental attitude.

tient's financial circumstances will guide practical planning regarding the rehabilitation setting and potential equipment needs.

    If the patient is appropriately draped and positioned during the interview, his or her posture, use of musculature, rate, rhythm, and pattern of breathing, and some degree of jugular venous distention (JVD) may be obvious. Figure 9–4 view *(a)* illustrates a common positional adaption of emphysematous patients; view *(b)* shows an increased anterior-posterior (AP) diameter observed in the lateral view; and view *(c)* shows the appropriate anatomic area to note for supraclavicular retraction and use of accessory muscles in COPD and where to look when assessing JVD as the patient reclines to 45 degrees

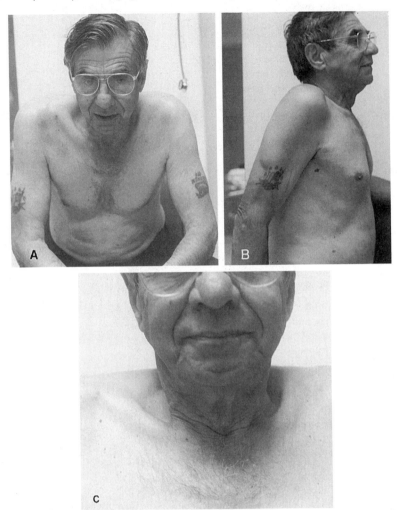

FIGURE 9–4. Signs of musculoskeletal adaptation to pulmonary disease. *(A)* Use of upper extremities to fix shoulder girdle. *(B)* Increased AP diameter, retraction above clavicles. *(C)* Visible accessor musculature.

supine. Observation also includes examination of the trunk and extremities for other signs of disease and chronic change. Cardiopulmonary disease is often accompanied by chronic musculoskeletal changes or peripheral adaptions such as clubbed fingers or swelling of the feet and ankles.

Palpation

The palpation step of the examination can be used to confirm normalities and/or abnormalities noted during observation and discriminate among or clarify symptoms described by the patient during the interview. Elderly patients often experience a myriad of musculoskeletal pains, particularly when they begin even a low-level exercise program, because dormant problems may become more apparent with activity.

Palpation is used on the anterior chest surface to assess the width of the subcostal angle, effective contraction of the abdominals, and coordinated motion of the diaphragm (Fig. 9–5). A gentle pressure and rotary fingertip motion over the sternum, along the rib borders, and over the posterior thoracic surfaces including the vertebral column is used to assess chest wall pain (Fig. 9–6). Many patients who describe chest wall discomfort during the interview have been unable to distinguish between musculoskeletal pain and angina. During palpation, it is useful for the examiner to refer to the described *chest pain* symptoms by using the same descriptions of pain or discomfort used by the patient during the interview. If you have asked the patient to describe in his or her own words any discomfort experienced above the waist, personal descriptors such as "burning," "tightness," "pressure," "squeezing," or "heaviness" can help distinguish between chest wall pain elicited during palpation and angina. Palpation of a tender area at rest or reproduction of pain through range-of-motion movement categorizes that pain as musculoskeletal. Angina, on the other hand, can be reproduced through activity that increases myocardial oxygen demand—such as exercise, eating, or emotional stress—and is relieved by medication or rest.

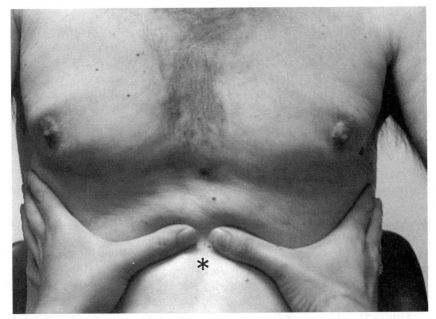

FIGURE 9–5. Palpation of the subcostal angle with thumbs at the xiphoid process and fingers along the ribs and intercostal spaces. Move fingertips centrally to subxiphoid space (*) to assess the abdominal contraction-coordinated diaphragmatic motion.

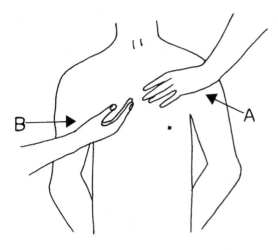

FIGURE 9–6. Palpation instructions: *(A)* Use the palmar surface and fingers to locate deformities and areas of pain. Continue palpation along the sternal and vertebral borders and along the intercostal spaces. *(B)* Use the ulnar border to palpate vocal fremitus: transmission of breath sounds through the chest wall.

Posteriorly, palpation at the lower costal borders is useful to determine symmetry of rib cage motion as well as overall thoracic motion. Elderly and COPD patients commonly have reduced excursion due to an increase in RV (Fig. 9–7).

Auscultation

Use of a stethoscope to auscultate breath and heart sounds establishes the normal character of sound that is baseline for each individual. This baseline is useful throughout treatment or intervention to identify acute changes and gradual decline or improvement in chronic conditions. Auscultation and classification of breath sounds are somewhat dependent upon the clinician's work setting because terminology varies among facilities. The gross classification categories of normal, abnormal, and adventitious breath sounds are consistent in the literature.[41] Normal breath sounds vary in intensity with the size of an individual. However, by using each patient as his or her own control, a norm can be established. There will be a gradual decrease in intensity and character of sound from central to peripheral lung surfaces and a shortening of the audible expiratory portion of the breathing cycle as the listener moves the stethoscope away from the trachea (Fig. 9–8). Abnormal breath sounds may be either a decrease in or the absence of normal breath sounds, or the auscultation of normal breath sounds in an inappropriate location (for example, bronchial breath sounds auscultated over the lower lobes). Adventitious breath sounds are additional breath sounds auscultated simultaneously with normal and abnormal breath sounds. They are generally thought to be caused by airway narrowing, collapse, consolidation, fluid, or secretions. Change in adventitious or abnormal breath sounds can be rapid, as in the onset of bronchospasm; be gradual over time, as in the development of a pleural effusion or tumor; or improve dramatically with

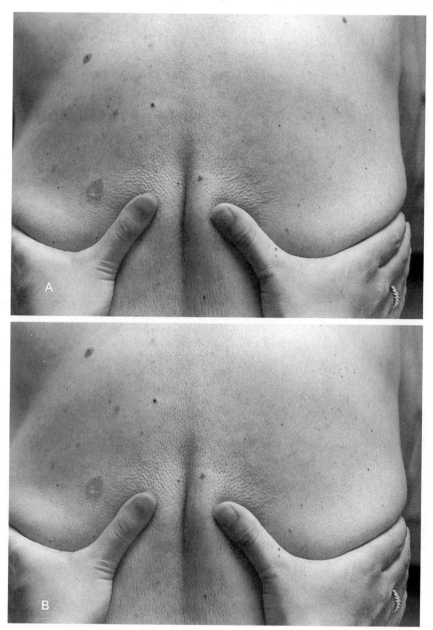

Figure 9–7. Minimal motion is observed *(A)* before inspiration and *(B)* after inspiration.

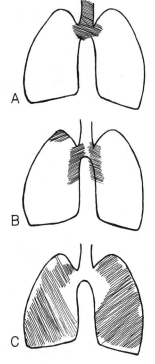

FIGURE 9–8. Auscultation. *(A)* Location of bronchial or tracheal breath sounds (loud, coarse, and audible equally during inspiratory and expiratory phase). *(B)* Location of bronchovesicular breath sounds (softer and audible slightly longer during the inspiratory phase). *(C)* Location of vesicular breath sounds (distant with expiration audible during one-half to one-third of the expiratory phase).

treatment, as in removal of secretions. Often breath sounds are useful clinical correlates to objective findings such as pulmonary function tests (PFTs) or chest radiography. Adventitious breath sounds are generally grouped under headings of rales, rhonchi, and wheezes and are described in terms such as "fine," "coarse," "wet," "dry," "continuous," and "crackling." Because of the variety and range of terms available to describe adventitious breath sounds, they are not specifically covered here. Although this examination technique is still considered somewhat subjective, clinical study has demonstrated the reliability of this assessment technique when used by a group of individuals who learn and employ a common terminology.[42]

Auscultation of heart sounds and the classification of these sounds into normal, abnormal, and additional sounds are also useful. The three clinically significant heart sound changes from normal are S_3 heart sounds or gallops, pericardial friction rubs, and murmurs. The S_3 sound is a low-frequency sound distinctly separated from the first and second sounds. The third heart sound is heard during diastole after the second sound and is commonly heard at the point of maximal impulse in patients with heart failure. S_3 heart sounds are normal in children under 5 years of age and can be heard in well-trained athletes, but they are usually pathologic in people over 40 years of age. S_3 heart sounds can develop after exercise and are an indication that the exercise has been excessive. S_3 gallops are associated with poor ventricular compliance, large areas of infarction or ischemia, and enlarged hearts.[43]

Pericardial friction rubs are usually easy to hear. They are often described as squeaky or snoring sounds. Rubs are associated with pericarditis or pericardial effusions. Both conditions described are contraindications to exercise, and the patient with these sounds should be referred for additional medical evaluation.

Finally, murmurs are heart sounds that result from stenosis or incompetent valves. The variety and causes of murmurs are quite numerous and can be studied elsewhere. The development of new murmurs is of greater clinical importance. Patients who develop a new murmur have had a change in their cardiac function either because of a recent infarction or the progression of chronic disease. When a new murmur is discovered, the patient should discontinue his or her exercise program and be referred for medical evaluation.

EXERCISE TESTING AND FUNCTIONAL ASSESSMENT

Indications for exercise testing of elderly individuals are many and varied. The major goals are to assess functional impairment or disability and to objectify the symptoms of dyspnea and angina. Older individuals who have been relatively inactive prior to evaluation may be intimidated or fearful of exercise testing, so the preliminary steps to testing should include explanation, demonstration, and practice to aid the examiner in selecting the proper setting and modality as well as to gain the client's trust and cooperation. Results of the exercise test provide an objective baseline by defining the oxygen requirements for exercise, assessing the adequacy of the cardiopulmonary response to stress, exposing pathologic cardiopulmonary, conditions, analyzing the musculoskeletal response to functional activity, and determining the factors limiting exercise performance. These parameters provide the basis for treatment design and exercise prescription.

Protocol and Modality Selection

The appropriate protocol and method for exercise-testing the geriatric patient depend on the individual's past medical history and present functional condition. Because dyspnea is a relatively subjective symptom, a patient's perception of his or her limitation varies widely. Healthy, regularly exercising older individuals require a vigorous protocol such as the Bruce or Balke (Fig. 9–9), to elicit symptoms and to measure the limits of exercise performance. Geriatric patients with the severe pulmonary impairments of bronchoconstriction and airway obstruction require modified protocols to elicit a safe exercise response that still produces an actual exercise limit and enables accurate measurement of maximal values (Fig. 9–10).

PROTOCOL

12-Minute Walk*	Level walking for 12 min. distance recorded.	No equipment necessary yet correlates well with study results of more complex tests; can be used for patients who cannot accomplish either treadmill, walking or bike riding because of dyspnea.
Low Level Functional	See Figure 9-10.	Intermittent walk test for use with moderate to severely impaired patients. Allows flexibility of workload assignment and establishes an accurate baseline.
Balke Test*	Treadmill: speed constant at 3.0 mph; grade initially 0 percent increased by 3.5 percent every 2 min.	Slight increase in speed for patient with less impairment allows pulmonary and cardiovascular stress to come before leg fatigue.
Bruce †	Treadmill: speed initially 1.7 mph; grade initially 10 percent; both are increased every 3 min in a specified manner.	Can be used with relatively fit individuals to stress accurately all systems' response to exercise. Good to assess exercise-induced bronchospasm in fit individuals.
Bicycle Test ‡	Specific workload, i.e., watts or Kgm/min. patient rides for a preset time, next workload determined by patient response.	Intermittent subjective test based on patient response. Requires lower extremity strength and endurance to reach high metabolic response level.

* McGavin, CR, Cupta, SP, McHardy, GJR: Twelve minute walking test for assessing disability in chronic bronchitis. Br Med J 1:822, 1976.
† From Physician's Handbook for Evaluation of Cardiovascular and Physical Fitness, Tennessee Heart Association, 1972.
‡ Ellestad, NH: Stress Testing: Principles and Practice. FA Davis, Philadelphia, 1979.

FIGURE 9–9. Exercise-testing protocols.

Consideration should be given to the potential method of exercise as well as the best protocol for testing each patient. A patient's baseline and maximum capacity are determined with the training modality he or she will be using during exercise conditioning to reliably and validly demonstrate improvement after training. If available, bicycle ergometry and treadmill walking provide the simplest exercise equipment modalities for aerobic exercise assessment and conditioning. Timed distance walking can also be used if no equipment is available. Simple questions to the patient regarding his or her walking or bike-riding ability prior to protocol selection can aid decision making. Individuals who have not bicycled either recently or regularly are

Collect resting data: Supine and sitting	ECG, BP, RR, HR, O$_2$sat, PFT's
Stage I:	Objective assessment of dyspnea/1.5–2 mph, 0% grade Walk 6 min = 4 min stabilization + 2 min gas collection Rest: Patient returns to baseline HR, RR, and O$_2$ sat
Stage II:	Functional ambulation assessment/treadmill set at speed and incline equal to functional work capacity based on physiologic and symptomatic response to Stage I Walk 6 min = 4 min stabilization + 2 min gas collection Rest: Patient returns to baseline HR, RR and ABG's
Stage III:	Maximum exercise tolerance/treadmill set to produce HR of 70–85% max or predicted ventilatory max (35 x FeV$_1$) Walk 6 min = 4 min stabilization + 2 min gas collection Rest: Patient returns to baseline HR, RR, and ABG's
Criteria to terminate test:	85% predicted or HR$_{max}$, desaturation to 85% or lower SaO$_2$, reaching a ventilatory maximum (35 x FEV$_1$), development of significant cardiac arrhythmias, or development of significant symptoms

FIGURE 9–10. Low-level functional protocol.

most likely to be limited by their leg musculature prior to either cardiac or pulmonary limitation. Included here are several test protocols and their potential advantages, given the condition of the individual to be tested and the goal of the exercise test (Fig. 9–11).

Monitoring Parameters

After protocol selection, monitoring requirements are assessed to determine cardiopulmonary response measures that will indicate a patient's functional exercise level most accurately and safely. Elderly individuals with stable, uncomplicated histories who complain of fatigue on exertion may require monitoring of heart rate (HR), blood pressure (BP), electrocardiogram (ECG), respiratory rate (RR), and symptoms to demonstrate their functional level and ability to participate in an exercise program. The geriatric client whose medical history includes frequent upper respiratory tract infections, two-pillow orthopnea, and dyspnea on exertion of walking one block or less requires additional monitoring to include resting and exercise pulmonary function, oxygen saturation, and analysis of expired gas at maximum exercise. The client with symptoms of chest tightness during stair climbing and paroxysmal nocturnal dyspnea will require continuous 12-lead ECG monitoring and assessment of heart sounds before and after maximal exercise.

Monitoring can be accomplished with a variety of equipment combinations. HR, RR, BP, breath sounds, and heart sounds require only a stetho-

TREADMILL TEST WORKSHEET

Institution:_____

Name_____ Patient No._____ Date_____ Age_____

Sex_____ Weight_____ Height_____ Diagnosis_____

Reason for test_____ Protocol_____

12 Lead ECG Interp._____

Time_____ Medications_____

Time last dose_____ Time last cigarette_____ Time last meal_____

Physician:_____ Activity Status:_____

TEST RESULTS

Minutes Completed_____ Limiting Factors_____

Resting Heart rate_____ Max. Heart rate_____ Resting BP_____/_____

Max. BP_____/_____ BP Response_____

Chest Pain_____

Summary ST Segment Changes_____

Heart Sounds_____ Arrhythmias_____

Physical Work Capacity_____

_____ Remarks/Recommendations_____

Interpreted by_____ M.D._____

FIGURE 9–11. Cardiac treadmill test worksheet. Copyright, Blessey, Huhn, Ice, Irwin, Oschrin, Physical Therapy, Inc., 1977, with permission.

scope, an aneroid sphygmomanometer, and clinical skill. ECG tracings assessed via telemetry will reveal only rhythm disturbances, whereas a hardwired 12-lead ECG unit with a printout strip-chart recorder is required for accurate ST segment evaluation. Oxygen saturation (Sa_{O_2}) can be monitored noninvasively with an oximeter. This accurately reflects saturation with a correlation coefficient of 0.9 between oximeter Sa_{O_2} and arterial blood Sa_{O_2}.[44] Spirometry measures can be taken to assess static volume and flow at rest, with spirometers ranging from water seal to electronic calculator models. Exercise ventilation measures and analyses of expired gases require more equipment than is generally found in a routine clinical setting; however, this equipment is generally available in an exercise laboratory setting. The severity of the patient's condition will dictate the monitoring parameters necessary to ensure a safe and clinically useful exercise test. Figures 9–11 and 9–12 provide examples of worksheets for recording monitor values.

Patient Preparation

The entire process of the exercise test, including the preparation, monitoring, effort necessary, and expected results, is explained to the patient well

Date			Name				Age				
	Pre-Exercise	HR	BP	RR	O_2 Sat		Target Heart Rate:				
	Supine						Barometric Pressure:				
	Sitting						Comment:				
	Standing										
		HR	BP	RR	O_2 Sat		O_2	CO_2	N	Tissot	
Stage I	2 min									Temp	
	4 min									Time	
	6 min						Comment:				
	1 min										
	5 min						O_2	CO_2	N	Tissot	
Stage II	2 min									Temp	
	4 min									Time	
	6 min						Comment:				
	1 min										
	5 min						O_2	CO_2	N	Tissot	
Stage III	2 min									Temp	
	4 min									Time	
	6 min						Comment:				
	1 min						Limiting Factor:				

FIGURE 9–12. Sample low-level exercise test worksheet.

ahead of time. Informed consent is required for use of invasive procedures. We have found that step-by-step reminders throughout the process and supportive conversational encouragement can make a great difference in patient cooperation and achievement.

Beginning an Exercise Test

Once a patient is set up with monitoring equipment, a review of the step-by-step process is useful. If the patient has never walked on a treadmill, demonstration will be necessary. Any hand signs or signals that the patient will need to indicate stress should be reviewed because patients using a mouthpiece for expired gas collection will be unable to speak. When the first stage is begun and the patient is exercising, one team member is directly responsible for monitoring the patient's response and giving the patient feedback and encouragement. Other team members can collect data from the monitoring devices and record the results.

During the Exercise Test

Observation of and interaction with the patient during the test provide the examiner with additional information. Patients may develop symptoms such as pursed-lip breathing, use of accessory muscles, or a discoordinated breathing pattern prior to an actual complaint of dyspnea. Conversely, there are individuals who develop an increased RR, shortness of breath (SOB), and clammy skin with no abnormal change in BP, HR, Sa_{O_2}, and breath sounds. Those RR, SOB, and skin symptoms may relate simply to anxiety resulting from fear such as loss of control with treadmill walking. It is essential to remain in constant visual and verbal communication with the patient during testing to integrate the subjective and objective responses observed. Subjective symptoms and observable clinical signs that may be useful indicators in conjunction with objective measures include facial expressions, breathing pattern, walking or riding pattern (musculoskeletal response), color/pallor, diaphoresis, and subjective complaints.

Stopping the Test

Criteria for stopping an exercise test in geriatric and pulmonary-impaired patients are often more subjective or patient-oriented than for the younger adult or strictly cardiac-impaired patient.[45] Elderly and severely impaired pulmonary patients may not have exercised for years, and the test activity itself may elicit previously unrecognized symptoms. Knee or hip pain and muscle cramps are common complaints that stop the test. The test completion point for a healthy, active older individual can be achievement of a predicted maximum HR and simple exhaustion. Most commonly during testing in our clinic, the test for the older person is stopped at the patient's request, and symptom limitations of deconditioning are usually the reason. The deconditioned older individual will exhibit a higher HR response at lower levels of exercise accompanied by an appropriate BP and RR. That limitation would be categorized as the patient having reached *symptom-limited* maximum and the subjective complaint such as leg fatigue or dyspnea recorded. The testing of individuals in our clinics who have a positive diagnostic test for cardiac or pulmonary disease will be stopped if they demonstrate significant ST depression (2 mm or more), serious arrhythmias, inappropriate BP response to an increase in workload (10 to 20 mmHg drop in systolic pressure, 20 to 30 mmHg increase above 90 diastolic pressure), decrease in Sa_{O_2} below 85 percent, increase in Pa_{CO_2} of 20 torr above resting level, or development of a discoordinated breathing pattern.

SETTING GOALS

The geriatric individual whose dyspnea is related to cardiopulmonary disease in addition to advanced age is evaluated and considered for treatment in a context different from that of the essentially healthy geriatric patient who is simply limited by deconditioning. Each of these individuals has lost a portion of his or her reserve capacity and will have limitation in the potential to improve $\dot{V}_{O_{2max}}$ that is dependent on the degree of impairment.

Short-term goals for disease are related to stabilization of the medical condition and patient education to gain an understanding of disease process. The educational component related to disease is essential in this population because the disease processes are progressive. Risk factor reduction has been shown effective in reducing incidence of recurrence. Acceptance of the need for risk-factor reduction and self-managed maintenance aids patients in setting and meeting their individually appropriate goals and maintaining positive gains. Long-term goals focus on a decrease in frequency or exacerbation of symptoms, an increase in exercise tolerance, an improved feeling of well-being, and prevention of further functional loss.[48-50] Short-term goals in the less impaired patient may focus on initiation of a training program and adapting that program into a life schedule. Long-term goals may relate to increases in and maintenance of ADL, exercise capacity, and endurance.

Other important factors to consider when setting goals with older persons relate to patient motivation, education, and compliance. If a patient does not feel safe in either the exercise environment or with the instructor, that individual will be reluctant to begin or to continue with the program. Patient education is integrated into all phases of the program and delivered at the appropriate level for each individual. A basic comprehension of anatomy and physiology related to the aging process can provide patients with an understanding of the changes they have observed in their own abilities. Education can provide motivation to decrease the risk factors for disease or reverse the effects of their deconditioning once they understand the process for change. Consideration is given to the patient's comprehension level and retention ability. Frequent review of the material that has been taught and reminders about the goals to be achieved are beneficial. Goals must therefore be individual, realistic, and attainable. In our clinic, we found that patients who understand their needs and capabilities feel safer in the setting, enjoy the process, and are more likely to comply with the program and attain their goals.

TRAINING PROGRAM

Exercise prescription for the geriatric patient with cardiopulmonary disease includes all the components utilized for programs that train young, healthy individuals, yet the parameters, environment, and goals are vastly different. Whether the patient is an elderly individual with the simple cardiopulmonary change of age or an elderly patient with long-standing COPD or CAD, the same elements should be considered. These elements include appropriate environment; proper exercise modality, intensity, duration, and frequency; and realistic overall goals. Guidelines for each element of the program are determined by the patient's personal preference and performance during the examination and testing period.

Setting/Environment

The most appropriate setting for patient training is determined by the geographic area of the country as well as by the facilities available. Warm, sunny, stable climates are conducive to outdoor walking, cycling, or swimming programs. Cold, wet, and unpredictable climates require the frequent, continual use of an indoor facility. Cardiopulmonary-impaired patients should be educated to note their responses to temperature, humidity, and pollution index during exercise. Because patient tolerance to both temperature and humidity is individualized, no specific number guidelines are recommended. Patients who note changes in HR or dyspnea owing to humidity should be encouraged to exercise indoors in controlled environments or in drier climates. Patients should be instructed to exercise in moderate temperatures rather than in extreme temperatures. Studies have shown that ozone levels of greater than 0.37 ppm create significant adverse health effects.[46] This level is usually broadcast as part of the air quality index on radio stations, so patients can choose whether or not to exercise indoors on particularly bad days. Additionally, each patient should be assessed for group participation or individual work. Some elderly individuals respond well in a setting where other people are equally "out of shape" by using the group for support; other older persons may be intimidated or embarrassed in a group and may not participate unless they receive individual attention. Last, but no less important, a safe environment is a major consideration for the elderly segment of the population. Adequate supervision, appropriately trained medical personnel, and accessibility are three major factors to consider whether you are beginning a program or referring a patient to a program.

Exercise Mode

Selecting the appropriate exercise modality also depends on personal preference and equipment or facility availability. Patients who have familiarity with and love for cycling can be set up on indoor stationary bike programs or with outdoor cycling groups if their baseline condition and the environment permit. Patients who enjoy swimming and hate jogging are obvious candidates for swim programs. The inner-city individual who prefers the protected indoor environment to the outdoors can participate in hallway or indoor-mall walking. Patient familiarity and comfort with the type of activity can be a useful motivational tool and an aid in compliance with any program. Any exercise mode chosen should be easily accessible on a 7-day-per-week basis to increase the likelihood of compliance.

Exercise Prescription

The three elements to be considered in exercise prescription are intensity, duration, and frequency. Based on the results of the exercise test, an individual prescription is formulated incorporating all three aspects. For a central cardiovascular training effect to occur, minimal criteria must be met in all categories; that is, it must have an intensity of ≥ 60 percent of HR_{max}, for a duration of 20 minutes or more, with a frequency of three times a week or more.[45,47]

Elderly patients without cardiopulmonary impairment may be able to meet these criteria, exercise aerobically, and achieve a cardiovascular training effect. Because of their advanced age, geriatric individuals can achieve training effects at lower HRs than those of younger individuals, owing to the decline in the HR_{max} with age.[38] Geriatric patients with cardiopulmonary impairment, however, may be restricted from aerobic training by symptoms of dyspnea or angina. At the present time, the question remains whether patients with COPD ever achieve the hallmark "anaerobic threshold" even at the higher HRs they demonstrate with lower levels of exercise.[34,35] These individuals are more likely to rely on a large component of anaerobic metabolism even at low levels of exercise or at rest. The improvements seen in COPD patients after exercise training are not consistent with the changes demonstrated by exercising normals (central cardiovascular training effect).[48–50] Their exercise training improvements are measured by increased exercise capacity and ADL performance.

Intensity

The intensity component of exercise prescription has been cited as most significant to ensure the achievement of improved aerobic capacity changes that have been demonstrated in normals.[51] Common prescriptions use HR as an indicator of intensity by selecting a target value that is a percentage of the maximum predicted HR or the HR_{max} achieved during testing. This method attempts to prescribe exercise intensity as a percentage of V_{O2max}. The older individual limited by cardiopulmonary disease cannot use heart rate as a calculated reflection of predicted oxygen consumption to ensure an effective intensity of exercise. Often this measure does not correlate well with actual oxygen consumption levels achieved by either pulmonary or cardiac patients. The oxygen cost of breathing can dramatically alter the V_{O_2} response curve, and HRs are often modified by medications taken by cardiac patients. Instead, the intensity of exercise is calculated for this group by the amount of work performed over a given period of time. Workload is then prescribed in terms of endurance. The intensity component of the prescription is given in the distance to be covered per unit of time. This time-and-distance prescription is especially useful for individuals incapable of palpating a peripheral pulse and for whom HR does not equate with intensity. HR can be a useful clinical indicator for geriatric individuals who can palpate a peripheral pulse. Once an exercise prescription has been calculated considering the time and distance necessary to increase endurance, the HR level achieved during that exercise is recorded. Patients are instructed to maintain that HR level throughout the exercise session. Additionally, the HR can also be correlated to the level of oxygen demand that produced significant symptoms during the patient's exercise test. The patient is given that HR value as a number *not to exceed* during the exercise session. Frequently the HR as an indicator of intensity is superseded in significance for the older individual by the component of duration.

Duration

The major goal of exercise training in older individuals is to improve the exercise capacity, thereby increasing the patient's ability to perform ADL. That improvement requires increased endurance. Consequently, the concept of endurance is elevated in importance. Individuals who cannot complete 6 minutes of a low-level protocol during exercise testing cannot receive an exercise prescription aimed at some intensity percentage of maximum HR to be performed for 20 minutes three times per week. Common exercise prescriptions begin at the lowest possible intensity level (for example, 1.5 mph, 0 percent grade, or 0.25 kpm $\times$ 30 rpm). The initial prescription has a total duration time that equals the eventual goal, but exercise is initially performed intermittently (for example, four 5-minute segments with 2-minute rest periods between segments). The total duration time progresses as rapidly as is feasible toward a minimum of 20 minutes of continuous exercise. Initially, this may be accomplished in two or more intermittent exercise sessions per day. For example, 14 minutes in the morning breaks into five 2-minute walks with three 1-minute rests that are repeated in the afternoon. The prescription is based on the exercise test results. For example, a patient who walked for 6 minutes at 1.5 mph, 0 percent grade at his or her maximum could begin at 1.5 mph, 0 percent grade and walk 3 minutes, rest 1 minute, walk 3 minutes, rest 1 minute during seven cycles for a total of 21 minutes of walking. The initial exercise session would be monitored similarly to the exercise test to assess the patient's response. The program could be progressed to 5 minutes of walking, 1 minute of rest for four walking sessions, then 8 minutes of walking, 1 minute rest for three sessions. Gradual increases in duration would occur before an increase in the intensity component of the prescription because the goal remains a duration of at least 25 minutes. We have found that 25 minutes of continuous exercise afford enough endurance capacity to perform most ADL at home. Prescriptions are also focused predominantly on duration because increases in grade and speed can produce unnecessary pain or injury in older individuals.

Frequency

Training should be performed by elderly persons four to five times per week once the duration has reached 20 to 30 minutes of continuous exercise. Individuals who are working on intermittent programs building up to constant exercise may attempt daily training unless they are limited by symptoms or the environment on any given day. Patients are taught to assess their baseline condition (that is, degree of bronchospasm, change due to humidity, general fatigue level) and to be responsible for selecting the days and times when they feel best able to perform their training activity.

Exercise Performance

Because the aging process itself slows the response to increased oxygen demand and prolongs the recovery time, periods of warm-up and cool-down are essential. The warm-up exercises we recommend are low-level, slow stretching and rhythmic bending through small ranges. An initial posture evaluation and general muscle-strength assessment provide the basis for the design of warm-up exercises. Patients are given an individual warm-up exercise program designed in response to their posture, strength, and range-of-motion (ROM) findings to address such things as increasing kyphosis, limited hip ROM, weak abdominals, or forward head. These exercises are performed in conjunction with breathing exercises to mobilize the thorax and to increase ventilation prior to starting the training program. Cool-down exercises focus on slow stretching of the skeletal muscles involved during training. Rhythmic bend-and-stretch coordinated with breathing can also aid in controlling the RR postexercise.

ADDITIONAL THERAPEUTIC MEASURES

Cardiac Medications

There is a wide array of cardiac medications commonly prescribed for geriatric patients. The medications include beta-adrenergic blocking agents, calcium channel blockers, nitrates, antiarrhythmics, diuretics, antihypertensives, and digitalis derivatives. All of these drugs can influence a patient's HR, BP, symptoms, and ECG responses to exercise. The beta blockers, such as Inderal, Tenormin, Sectral, and Lopressor, have a rather marked depressive effect on resting and exercise cardiac hemodynamics. A careful review of the normal effects and side effects of each patient's medications is essential prior to starting an exercise program.

Pulmonary Medications

The common medication groups used for patients with pulmonary disease include oxygen, systemic and inhaled bronchodilators, steroids, and antibiotics. The goals of therapy include increasing oxygen supply and decreasing oxygen demand through a decrease in the work of breathing.

Antibiotics are used to combat the effects of infection. The use of long-term oxygen therapy has been shown to decrease morbidity and mortality in COPD patients as well as improve functional capacity.[52,53] Bronchodilators are operative through the autonomic nervous system to produce primarily smooth muscle relaxation in the tracheobronchial tree; side effects can include increased HR and skeletal muscle tremor, which can be significant in the exercising patient. Chronic steroid use produces a complex array of side effects. Of primary consequence are the musculoskeletal changes that weaken muscles and bones, mandating careful assessment and exercise prescription for patients on steroids. Medication therapy in this patient group is complex and requires careful review for each patient on an individual basis.

Bronchopulmonary Hygiene

COPD patients, as previously described, have complicated symptomatology that often includes chronic cough and sputum production. Many treatment modalities are available to assist in airway clearance, including inhaled mucolytics, inhaled and oral bronchodilators, humidity and physical therapy techniques of postural drainage, percussion, shaking/vibration, breathing exercises, and cough. Patients who improve with the therapeutic use of these techniques may increase air flow, decrease flow resistance, improve Sa_{O_2}, and decrease the work of breathing. Many individuals therefore benefit from a course of therapy prior to or in conjunction with exercise training.

SUMMARY

Exercise prescription and cardiopulmonary assessment are key components in keeping older individuals physically active and healthy. The combination of disease and age invariably works to reduce the cardiopulmonary system's ability to adequately deliver oxygen. Without an appropriate system for aerobic energy production, ambulation and higher levels of activity can be impaired or eliminated. Loss of the ability to perform activities of daily living in the elderly will continue to burden health care funds, families, and society. The concepts presented in this chapter provide safe and effective models for implementing individualized exercise programs for older clients, resulting in healthier, more physically active and productive individuals.

REFERENCES

1. Shephard, RJ: Physical Activity and Aging. Croom-Helm, London, 1978.
2. Astrand, PO and Rodahl, K: Textbook of Work Physiology. McGraw-Hill, New York, 1977.
3. Dempsey, JA: Is the lung built for exercise? Med Sci Sports Exerc 18:143, 1986.

4. Saltin, B, Blomquist, CG, Mitchell, JH, et al: Response to exercise after bedrest and after training. Circ 37(Suppl III): VII–1, 1968.

5. Rowe, JW and Besdine, RW: Health and Disease in Old Age. Little, Brown, Boston, 1982.

6. DeVries, HA: Physiological effects of an exercise training regimen upon men aged 52–88. J Gerontol 25:325, 1970.

7. Irwin, SC: Cardiac rehabilitation for the geriatric patient. Top Geriatric Rehab 2:44, 1986.

8. Patrick, DF: Pulmonary rehabilitation of the geriatric patient. Top Geriatric Rehab 2:55, 1986.

9. ATS: Cigarette Smoking and Health. Official ATS statement, 1740 Broadway, New York, November 1984.

10. Blessey, RL: Atherosclerosis: An overview of the basic mechanism of atherogenesis, pathophysiology and natural history. In Irwin, SC and Tecklin, J (eds): Cardiopulmonary Physical Therapy. CV Mosby, St Louis, 1985.

11. Mittman, C, et al: Relationship between chest wall and pulmonary compliance and age. J Appl Physiol 10:1211, 1965.

12. Smith, E and Serfass, R (eds): Exercise and Aging: The Scientific Basis. Enslow, Hillside, NJ, 1981.

13. Hall, DA: The Aging of Connective Tissue. Academic Press, New York, 1976.

14. Wright, RR: Elastic tissue of normal and emphysematous lungs: A tridimensional histologic study. Am J Pathol 39:355, 1961.

15. Turner, JM, Mead, J, and Wohl, ME: Elasticity of human lungs in relation to age. J Appl Physiol 25(6):664, 1968.

16. John, R and Thomas J: Chemical compositions of elastins isolated from aortas and pulmonary tissues of humans of different ages. Biochem J 127:261, 1972.

17. Pump, KK: Fenestrae in the alveolar membrane of the human lung. Chest 65:431, 1974.

18. Hernandez, JA, et al: The bronchial glands in aging. J Am Geriatr Soc 13:799, 1965.

19. Yin, FCP: The aging vasculature and its effects on the heart. In Weisfeld, ML (ed): The Aging Heart. Raven Press, New York, 1980.

20. Wei, JW: Cardiovascular anatomic and physiologic changes with age. Top Geriatric Rehab 2(1):10, 1986.

21. Pomerance, A: Pathology of the myocardium and valves. In Caird, FI, Dalle, JC, and Kennedy, RD (eds): Cardiology in Old Age. Plenum Press, New York, 1976.

22. Gerstenblith, G, Frederiksen, J, Yin, FCP, et al: Echocardiographic assessment of a normal adult aging population. Circ 56:273, 1977.

23. Wei, JY: Heart disease in the elderly. Cardiovasc Med 9:971, 1984.

24. Holland, J: Regional distribution of pulmonary ventilation and perfusion in elderly subjects. J Clin Invest 47:81, 1968.

25. Zadai, CC: Pulmonary physiology of aging: The role of rehabilitation. Top Geriatric Rehab 1(1):49, 1985.

26. Murray, JF: The Normal Lung, WB Saunders, Philadelphia, 1976.

27. Muiesan, G, Sorbini, CA, and Grassi, V: Respiratory function in the aged. Bulletin de Physio-Pathologie Respiratoire 7:973, 1971.

28. Astrand, I, Astrand, PO, Hallback, I, et al: Reduction in maximal oxygen uptake with age. J Appl Physiol 35:649, 1973.

29. Wei, JY, Rowe, JW, Kestenbaum, AD, et al: Post-cough heart rate response: Influence of age, sex and basal blood pressure. Am J Physiol 245:R–18, 1983.

30. Nicols, WW, O'Rourke, MF, Avolio, AP, et al: Effects of age on ventricular-vascular coupling. Am J Cardiol 55:1179–1985.

31. Shimada, K, Kitazumi, T, Sadakne, N, et al: Age-related changes of baroreflex function, plasma, norepinephrine, and blood pressure. Hypertension 7:113, 1985.

32. Cumming, G and Semple, SG: Disorders of the Respiratory System. Blackwell Scientific Publications, Oxford, 1973.

33. American Thoracic Society: Chronic bronchitis, asthma and pulmonary emphysema. Am Rev Respir Dis 85:762, 1962.

34. Pardy, RL, Hussain, SNA, and Macklem, PT: The ventilatory pump in exercise. In Symposium on Exercise: Physiology and Clinical Applications. Clinics in Chest Medicine 5(1):35, 1984.

35. Loke, J, Mahler, DA, Paul-Man, SF, et al: Exercise impairment in chronic obstructive pulmonary disease. In Symposium on Exercise: Physiology and Clinical Applications. Clinics in Chest Medicine 5(1):121, 1984.

36. Robbins, SL, Cotran, RS, Kumar, V: Pathologic Basis of Disease. WB Saunders, Philadelphia, 1984.

37. Epstein, SE, Cannon, R, Talbot, TL: Hemodynamic principles in the control of coronary blood flow. Am J Cardiol 56:4E, 1985.

38. Shephard, RJ: Physical Activity and Aging, ed 2. Aspen, Rockville, MD, 1987.

39. Blessey, RL, Hislop, HJ, Waters, RI, et al: Metabolic energy cost of unrestrained walking. Phys Ther 56:1019, 1976.

40. Hinman, JE, Cunningham, BA, Rechnitzer, TA, et al: Age-related changes in speed of walking. Med Sci Sports 20:161, 1988.

41. American College of Chest Physicians–American Thoracic Society: Joint Committee on Pulmonary Nomenclature: Pulmonary terms and symbols. Chest 67:583, 1975.

42. Luciano, DM and Lareau, MT: The auscultation and interpretation of breath sounds: An interrater reliability study. Unpublished study.

43. Stapleton, JF: The third sound of heart failure. Chest 91(6):801, 1987.

44. Cecil, WT, et al: A clinical evaluation of the accuracy of the Nellcor N–100 and Ohmeda 3700 pulse oximeter. J Clin Monit 4:31, 1988.

45. ACSM: Guidelines for graded exercise testing and exercise prescription. Lea & Febiger, Philadelphia, 1975.

46. Air Quality and Automobile Emission Control, vol. 2: Health Effects of Air Pollutants. Coordinating Committee on Air Quality Studies, National Academy of Sciences, National Academy of Engineering, National Research Council, Washington, DC, US Government Printing Office, September 1974.

47. Pollock, ML: The quantification of endurance training programs. In Wilmore, JH (ed): Exercise and Sports Sciences Reviews, vol 1. Academic Press, New York, 1973.

48. Alison, JA, Samios, R, and Anderson, SD: Evaluation of exercise training in patients with chronic airway obstruction. Phys Ther 61(9):1273, 1981.

49. Guthrie, AG and Petty, TL: Improved exercise tolerance in patients with chronic airway obstruction. Phys Ther 50(9):1333, 1970.

50. Belman, MJ and Kendregan, BA: Exercise training fails to increase skeletal muscle enzymes in patients with chronic obstructive pulmonary disease. Am Rev Respir Dis 123:256, 1981.

51. Hellerstein, HK, et al: Principles of exercise prescription for normals and cardiac subjects. In Naughton, J and Hellerstein, HH (eds): Exercise Testing and Exercise Training in Coronary Heart Disease. Academic Press, New York, 1973.

52. Nocturnal Oxygen Therapy Trial Group. Continuous or nocturnal oxygen therapy in hypoxemic chronic obstructive lung disease. A clinical trial. Ann Intern Med 93:391, 1980.

53. Sahn, SA, Nett, LM, and Petty, TL: Ten-year follow-up of a comprehensive rehabilitation program for severe COPD. Chest 77:2 (Suppl):311, 1980.

54. Boyer, JL and Kasch, FW: Exercise therapy in hypertensive men. JAMA 211:1668, 1970.

55. Bruce, RA: The benefits of physical training for patients with coronary heart disease. In Ingelfinger, FJ, et al (eds): Controversy in Internal Medicine, vol 2. WB Saunders, Philadelphia, 1974.

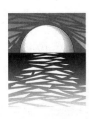

CHAPTER 10

Implications of Oncology in the Aged

Stephen A. Gudas, PT, PhD

BEHAVIORAL OBJECTIVES

Upon completion of this chapter, the reader will be able to:

1 List the major types of cancer that commonly occur in the elderly population.
2 Explain why detection of cancer in the elderly is often delayed.
3 Modify rehabilitation treatment goals in the geriatric cancer patient in light of the physiologic changes that accompany aging.
4 Outline a palliative and supportive program for the terminal geriatric cancer patient.
5 List the various members of the cancer rehabilitation team and state their roles in the management of geriatric cancer.
6 Identify clinical symptomatology and physical rehabilitation interventions in the elderly patient with myeloma, colon cancer, skin cancer, breast cancer, lymphoma, head and neck cancer, complications caused by metastatic disease, and lung cancer.

Among the older population, cancer is a significant health problem.[1] Cancer incidence and death rates rise continuously with age and are highest among the elderly.[2] Although cancer occurs at any age, the disease most commonly affects middle-aged and older adults. In the latter age group, cancer ranks second only to heart disease as a cause of death in the United States.[3,4]

Each specific type of cancer tends to have a peak incidence regarding age, although there is wide variability. The carcinoma family of tumors, such as those of the lung, skin, gastrointestinal (GI) tract, breast, and prostate, occur almost exclusively in older individuals. In men 75 years of age and older, prostatic cancer accounts for 25 percent of all cancer, and GI cancer comprises an additional 25 percent. In women in this same age group, breast cancer is responsible for 20 percent of malignant tumor incidence, and GI cancer comprises an additional 25 percent.[2]

The probability that a given individual will develop a malignant tumor within a 5-year period rises from 1 in 700 at the age of 25 to 1 in 14 at the age of 65.[4] This fact alone demands that the elderly population be well educated in the warning signs and symptoms of cancer and that physicians and other health professionals become more knowledgeable in the manner of presentation of neoplastic disease, in screening for cancer in the elderly, and in the general principles of therapeutic management and treatment of malignant disease in the elderly. One consideration is that 50 percent of all cancers occur in patients over 65 years of age.[5] Current direction in cancer management targets the elderly population as a special group requiring new emphasis regarding the detection and treatment of cancer.

Because the incidence of malignancy increases with age, we can expect a geriatric cancer epidemic by the year 2030, when 20 percent of the population of the United States will be age 65 or older. Practitioners should become knowledgeable about current issues in geriatric oncology, including appropriate treatment selection for geriatric patients with malignancies (surgical, radiotherapeutic, or medical); age bias in treatment selection; modification of toxicities from therapy in the elderly; cancer screening and prevention; and the special issues of informed consent and pain control in the geriatric cancer patient.[6] For example, geriatric patients are less likely to use a cancer information service.[7]

CANCER IN THE ELDERLY

From the standpoint of therapeutic intervention, some authors recommend that cancer be regarded similarly in all age groups.[8] Although this may well be an oversimplification of the cancer problem in the aged, no patient should be denied full comprehensive treatment on the grounds of age alone. Also, it should be remembered that malignant disease in the elderly may be only one of several life-threatening diseases present, and frailty and disability may coexist with the occurrence of malignancy, thus complicating the clinical picture.[4] For example, many elderly patients may not experience early detection of their disease, owing to the fact that warning symptoms are often unheeded or attributed to or masked by another disease already progressing. This delay, caused by insufficient vigilance on the part of the patient or family, is believed to be a significant factor in the development of tumors in the elderly population.[2] Statistics imply that older patients must be particularly alert for symptoms of cancer at high-risk sites.

The continuing development of new, more elaborate scanning techniques, such as radionuclide imaging, computerized axial tomography (CAT), and magnetic resonance imaging (MRI), has enhanced the detection and recognition of cancer.[9] Conventional diagnostic procedures are still used and have wide clinical usage; the importance of breast self-examination and mammograms to detect early breast cancer and of periodic chest radiographs to detect lung cancer is fairly well established for the older person. Indeed, screening techniques may be more urgent and applicable in the geriatric population, in which patient delay in reporting symptoms is common, leading to later detection and lessened chance of cure. The inverse relationship of age to clinical stage in bronchogenic carcinoma, for example, suggests that appropriate screening by periodic chest radiographs and cytologic sputum examinations may be more appropriate for the high-risk elderly population than for a younger age group in whom these screening methods have yielded fewer positive results.[10] However, one report concerning trends of cancer mortality did *not* support the hypothesis that recent increases in specific cancers in the elderly chiefly reflect improved diagnosis of cases that would formerly have been misrepresented or miscoded.[8] Cancer in the elderly is definitely on the rise.

Changes in the immune system may play a role in the development of cancer in the aged. A defect or decrease in T cell function and regulation with age has been reported, and there appears to be an association between immunodeficiency and increased cancer incidence.[11] Paradoxically, immune processes may also contribute to the geriatric cancer problem. A recent review suggested that T-cell dysfunction in the aged may permit the simultaneous development of autoimmunity and neoplasia.[12] Although results are inconclusive, further research in immunology will undoubtedly shed new light on the role of the immune system in the development of cancer in the elderly individual.

Multiple primary neoplasms, or the development of separate cancers in more than one organ system, are a common problem in old age; the longer a person lives, the more likely he or she is to develop primary malignant neoplasms at various sites.[13] During a prolonged follow-up period, up to 36 percent of elderly patients treated for cancer will eventually develop a second or third primary tumor.[14] In a series of 676 patients, 34 showed more than one site of malignancy, and 6 of these demonstrated three primary sites.[13] Because the likelihood of additional separate cancer occurrence increases with each year, clinicians should be aware of the possibility of a second primary tumor when reviewing patients who have enjoyed long survival periods following the initial appearance of cancer.

Many of the treatment procedures used in cancer management carry significant and pronounced cosmetic and functional morbidity. In general, the rehabilitation of the geriatric patient and alleviation or palliation of dysfunction and disfigurement are of the utmost importance.[15] Each type of cancer, and each individual, will present with specialized problems arising from the malignant process itself or iatrogenically from the effects of treatment. Geriatric oncology rehabilitation, therefore, requires a comprehensive knowledge of both disease process and treatment. Cancer rehabilitation in the elderly necessitates the involvement of a multidisciplinary team, members of which should have expertise in both gerontology and oncology.

Issues such as the quality of life are important and should be addressed.[16] The quality of life is characterized by an "individuality," including the person's integrity, independence, and autonomy. An acceptable physical status and well-being, adequate social interaction, and a comfortable or at least basic economic stability are all tantamount to the multidimensionality of the quality of life.[16] In assessing elderly people with cancer, physical therapy practitioners need to identify adaptive and ineffective behaviors that reflect the quality of life.[17] Adaptation can be reflected in the level of hope that is expressed. When it is not possible to improve physical health or socioeconomic well-being, the practitioner can become a resource to patients and families by emphasizing the development and achievement of short-term goals.

Too often rehabilitative efforts are directed toward employment-oriented goals or major physical achievements, which may be inappropriate for elderly persons.[18] In planning programs for geriatric cancer patients, the rehabilitative staff should modify goals according to the potential lifestyle and physical condition of the patient, keeping the physiologic changes of aging in mind. The geriatric cancer patient will gain from the rehabilitation procedure even if he or she does not meet the initial predetermined rehabilitative goal.[19] Rehabilitation that affords a degree of independence and increased function in daily living skills is of great importance; the value of coordinated rehabilitation services for the elderly person experiencing disabilities caused by cancer cannot be minimized. A comprehensive assessment of the patient, together with positive attitudes and frequent reevaluation, greatly enhances the likelihood of a successful treatment outcome.[19]

After it has been ascertained that additional radical medical or surgical treatment is unwarranted in the face of disease progression, the health-care professional can design a palliative and supportive care program for the terminally ill geriatric patient. At this stage, the health professional can intervene to alleviate pain, and proper positioning and supportive devices can assist in keeping the patient comfortable.

Both primary-care physicians and medical oncologists can provide, or ensure the provision of, effective cancer care and pain control in a home-based or inpatient hospice program.[20] The hospice interdisciplinary team can be a valuable resource for physicians who are supervising and rendering this care for the geriatric cancer patient.

Minority elderly should be carefully screened for cancer. Age-adjusted cancer mortality is 27 percent higher for African Americans than for the general U.S. population.[21] Social support seems to be associated with increased use of mammography and occult blood stool examinations among older African Americans. Interventions designed to increase utilization of social networks may be an effective way to increase use of cancer screening in this population. There is an urgent need to concentrate on problems unique to the elderly, particularly minority elderly, for early detection, diagnosis, and treatment.[22] Guidelines specific to older persons should be developed.[23]

Major areas related to psychosocial issues pertinent to the provision of cancer control services to older people include values and decision making; psychosocial barriers to screening and access to care and services; and quality of life, including rehabilitation.[24]

When the dying process becomes inevitable, every health practitioner must seek the answer to the basic question of how to provide the highest quality care for the terminally ill older person. Although dying is a physical process, cognitive and behavioral clues are often evident in the terminal patient. In an older individual dying from cancer, at times an abrupt change in thought and/or behavior may signal the beginning of the terminal phase of the disease.[25] Caregiver withdrawal is unfortunately common in terminal care and a shift by the patient toward anxiety or depression may receive less attention than in the younger age group. The elderly person, like all persons, approaches death from a distinctive and individualistic pathway and responds and reacts in a manner commensurate with his or her psychologic makeup. Patient's wishes and desires regarding care, disposition, and environment during the terminal phase of their disease should be respected within all possible and practical means. As an integral team member, the rehabilitation specialist can do much to facilitate meeting these specific patient requests.

Advances in detection and diagnosis and major breakthroughs in surgical, medical, and radiation oncology have afforded longer survival periods for many patients and, in some cases, complete cures, even in the face of systemic, metastatic disease. Admittedly, much success has been manifest in the pediatric tumor realm, but as research advances, more geriatric individuals with favorable cancers will experience longer survival periods during which the quality as well as the length of life will be emphasized. This chapter will explore some of the more common tumors that occur in the elderly and offer guidelines concerning the clinical presentation, treatment, and rehabilitation of cancer in this population.

PRIMARY AND SECONDARY LUNG CANCER

The average age of onset of primary lung cancer is 60 years. This disease is responsible for 33 percent of male cancer deaths and 11 percent of female cancer deaths and has demonstrated a marked increase in incidence in the last 50 years. Approximately 150,000 new cases will occur in the United States each year, with an incidence of 4 to 10 times higher in cigarette smokers than in nonsmokers.[26] Cromartie and his associates[27] reported that only 6.8 percent of a series of 702 patients were nonsmokers, which strongly suggests that tobacco is a contributory etiologic factor.

Lung cancer exhibits both hematogenous and lymphatic metastatic potential and often spreads widely before diagnosis.[28] Consequently, surgical resection may not be curative; this, combined with the low response rate of lung cancer to available chemotherapeutic modalities, makes treatment extremely difficult. In elderly patients, decreased survival is correlated with lymph node involvement and the extensiveness of the required surgical intervention—pneumonectomy versus lobectomy, for example.

Symptoms of the disease include dyspnea (20 percent), cough (75 percent), weight loss (40 percent), and occasional hemotysis.[28] These clinical manifestations may mimic other pulmonary conditions, an additional rationale for the elaborate diagnostic and staging procedures that are used.

Elderly patients, like others with primary lung cancer, undergo a sequential process of evaluation, which includes initial staging (liver, spleen, and bone scans and CAT scan of the brain) and final staging (histologic verification of lymph node or distant organ metastases).[29] This complex process significantly improves the accuracy of determining the extent of disease in older patients who do not have obvious clinical evidence of metastases at the time of diagnosis.

In one series, 123 elderly patients (over 70 years of age) with small-cell lung carcinoma (SCLC) were treated with chemotherapy, with good results. Chemotherapy should not be withheld from elderly patients with SCLC on the basis of age.[30] The survival period of patients who receive chemotherapy is significantly longer than that of untreated patients, even though frequent dose reductions for toxicity may be required. On the other hand, in some cases elderly patients with lung cancer have not benefited from the therapeutic improvements obtained during the 1980s with younger adults. Potentially operable non-small-cell lung cancers are more common in elderly patients, the disease is more likely to be localized at diagnosis, even though elderly patients are rarely treated with surgery.[31] Radiotherapy remains the most frequently used primary treatment in the elderly. Hematopoietic growth factors may be used to reduce bone marrow damage following cytotoxic chemotherapy, and may be a promising tool in elderly patients.[31]

One half of all cases of lung cancer occur in patients aged 65 and older.[32] Although adenocarcinoma is the predominant histologic subtype in the general population, squamous cell carcinoma has remained the most common type in the elderly. It is surprising that, although lung cancer presents at a less advanced stage with increasing age, the percentage of elderly patients undergoing treatment tends to decline despite the fact that they may well tolerate the aggressive therapy that may enhance survival.[32]

The progressivity and radioclinical features of lung cancer in the aged are not essentially different from those observed in younger patients.[33] Pretherapeutic evaluation must be thorough when surgery is possible, with special attention to the cardiovascular system. Studies that report postoperative mortality and morbidity rates paradoxically similar or lower in both younger and older patients probably are a result of patient selection.[33] Although age is not an absolute contraindication to surgical intervention, more rigorous selection and closer postoperative supervision are required for elderly lung cancer patients.

Both preoperative and postoperative physical therapy treatment will be required in the majority of elderly patients undergoing a thoracotomy for primary lung cancer. A complete chest evaluation is performed preoperatively. The therapist notes the rate and depth of respiration, use of accessory muscles of respiration, and any asymmetry of chest wall movement during breathing. The rehabilitation specialist also assesses the preoperative shoulder range of motion, general posture, and frequency and effectiveness of the patient's cough. The latter is particularly important, because postoperative sputum retention is a significant cause of morbidity in the lung cancer patient. Palpation is systematically carried out to determine whether structural abnormalities are present in the chest wall and thorax; vocal fremitus will be increased over the area of the tumor if the lesion is large and there is accompanying consolidation. Percussion over a tumor, used as an evaluative tool, often yields a dull, flat sound. Lastly, auscultation is performed by the therapist to determine the presence of abnormal or adventitious breath sounds. Normal breath sounds are frequently diminished over a large lung cancer. The postoperative program is explained to the patient, who is instructed in deep breathing, coughing, and splinting of the incision.[34]

Particularly in the geriatric patient, who might be frail, initially debilitated, and perhaps frightened of the surgical procedure, a preoperative visit by the rehabilitation specialist can allay some of the fears the patient may have, as well as familiarize him or her with the treatment procedures that will follow surgery. Especially in the elderly, postthoracotomy complications are common enough to warrant both preoperative and postoperative programs designed to give attention to areas such as weak or ineffective cough, heavy secretion production, oversplinting of the chest incision, and drying of the respiratory mucosa.

The postoperative physical therapy approach to these patients is multidimensional. Postural drainage techniques may be employed to assist in removal of secretions and to ensure adequate lung ventilation, but percussion and vibration are contraindicated directly over the tumor site if hemorrhage is present or if there is an ongoing course of radiation.[34] Modified drainage positions may be necessary; ultrasonic nebulization can be used to liquify secretions. The therapist should realize the potential dangers of aggressive physical therapy procedures performed on cachectic, elderly lung cancer patients.[35] Hemoptysis, atalectasis, and exhaustion of the patient may occur if vigorous percussion and vibration are employed. The postoperative program should include breathing exercises and instruction in coughing.

The incidence of postthoracotomy pneumonitis in patients over 65 is three times that of younger individuals. This suggests that the geriatric patient may need more attention in order to prevent this complication.[35] In the recumbent, semicomatose patient, positional rotation by the combined team may be necessary both to prevent secretion accumulation and to avoid skin breakdown, the latter being of special concern in the older patient, who may have poor skin nutrition. Lung cancer patients who do not undergo surgical resection will need modified postural drainage, instruction in coughing, and breathing exercises to ensure adequate lung expansion and secretion clearance and to prevent atelectasis and pneumonitis.

Following a lateral thoracotomy, range of motion to the ipsilateral upper extremity is indicated. Proprioceptive neuromuscular facilitation (PNF) diagonal patterns have been found beneficial in increasing functional shoulder range of motion and should be performed bilaterally for their coordinative beneficial effect. This ipsilateral shoulder may displace slightly downward, and the therapist should attempt to keep the shoulders level so that weight can be evenly distributed on the buttocks when the older person is in the seated position. A postural evaluation will assess the patient for shoulder displacement, which can be treated with appropriate exercise.

Stanley[36] reviewed the cases of over 5000 patients with lung cancer in which over 77 prognostic factors were considered. The three most important factors affecting survival were initial functional performance, defined as ability to carry out normal daily activities; extent of disease; and recent weight loss. The author substantiated the role of the rehabilitation team in ensuring adequate functional ability prior to surgery or other treatment.

Early hematogenous, or blood-borne, dissemination is distinctly common in lung carcinoma, and blood-borne metastases may involve the brain, liver, skeleton, and opposite lung. In men, lung and prostate cancer are responsible for most clinical metastatic bone disease. Secondary tumor deposits may be lytic or blastic. Osteolytic metastases may cause dissolution and resorption of extensive areas of bone and carry the threat of pathologic fracture, particularly in the long bones. Although metastatic disease may be less widespread in the older age group, the various organs involved by metastic tumor are similar to those seen in lung cancer in general.[38]

Lung carcinoma is the most common primary neoplasm to metastasize to the brain; the tumor cells embolize via the pulmonary veins and carotid artery, enjoying a fairly direct route to the central nervous system (CNS). In the elderly individual, neurologic signs may be the presenting symptoms of a silent lung tumor. In a review of 80 patients 65 years of age and older with a brain tumor, metastatic carcinoma was second in occurrence only to glioblastoma.[37] Solitary metastatic tumors may be surgically extirpated, but brain irradiation is more commonly used because the tumor foci are usually multiple.[37] The older patient who presents with a hemiparesis or other neurologic syndrome caused by brain metastases should be treated by the therapist much the same way as a patient whose nervous system has been compromised by trauma, vascular accident, or infection. The neurophysiologic facilitatitive approaches can be used in an attempt to regain motion, alleviate spasticity if present, and provide more normal motor patterns for the patient. Brain metastases formulate a dynamic process; with treatment with steroids and irradiation, the clinical neurologic picture is frequently marked by remissions and exacerbations. For this reason, it is often difficult to assess the efficacy of rehabilitation intervention on neurologic and functional improvement. Aggressive yet carefully coordinated physical therapy treatment techniques are necessary to give the benefit of the doubt in managing these patients.

Metastatic lesions in the lung will eventually occur in 20 to 30 percent of patients dying with malignant disease.[26] Almost any primary tumor can be responsible, and the lungs provide the first resting ground via the pulmonary arteries after cancer emboli are released into the systemic circulation. Parenchymal metastases are notoriously asymptomatic for long periods of time until sufficient pulmonary tissue has been compromised and the patient experiences progressive dyspnea. When severe shortness of breath ensues, deep-breathing exercises and supplementary oxygen inhalation can be of considerable benefit to these patients.

In contrast to parenchymal lung metastases, lymphangitic metastases— usually from breast, GI, or uterine cancer—cause an intense early pulmonary symptomatology consisting of severe dyspnea, tachypnea, and cough productive of large amounts of grayish sputum.[39] In these patients, the cancer cells are dispersed throughout the perivascular and periobronchiolar lymphatic channels, interfering with the normal cleansing action of the lung. Elderly patients exhibiting this type of metastatic lung disease may be acutely ill, and chest physical therapy procedures, particularly postural drainage to mobilize secretions, can be significantly beneficial in relieving their distress.

Another complication of lung carcinoma is metastic involvement of the vertebrae, which can result in epidural spinal cord compression, with resultant paraplegia or quadriplegia.[40] Metastatic spinal cord lesions are increasingly more common in the elderly patient suffering from cancer. Lung cancer is one of the most common primary tumors to cause this complication. Treatment is usually by radiation therapy, which may be combined with surgical compression and laminectomy in selected patients. The geriatric patient who presents with spinal cord symptomatology owing to metastatic epidural disease should be treated as any patient with spinal cord injury; although the survival period is usually short, the patient can benefit both physically and psychologically from proper positioning, maintenance of range of motion, mobilization of extremities, and strengthening programs to enhance whatever functional abilities are present.[41]

The paraneoplastic syndromes—such as polymyopathies, peripheral neuropathies, pulmonary hypertrophic osteoarthropathy, and hypercalcemia—occur more often in primary lung cancer than in any other type of cancer. Over 50 percent of elderly people who present with a polymyositis syndrome will be found to have an underlying carcinoma, usually in the lung, breast, large bowel, or prostate.[1] In polymyositis and its variants, the proximal muscles are swollen, tender, and weak. Patients with these syndromes may respond to a rehabilitation program of splinting, positioning, and judicious use of active assisted exercise. The latter is of use when the acute edema and inflammation begin to subside.

It is clear that either primary or secondary lung cancer results in clinical problems that go far beyond the realm of pulmonary symptomatology. The elderly lung cancer patient may present with a wide variety of complications that will require the intervention of a coordinated, well-disciplined cancer rehabilitation team. Throughout the course of the disease, the patient's physical comfort and mobility are of prime concern; many therapeutic modalities can be used to achieve this goal. In the future, newer methods of diagnosis, staging, and treatment, including polychemotherapy, will result in longer survivals and a more hopeful outlook—further evidence for the place of rehabilitation efforts as a contribution to optimal management in these patients.

HEAD AND NECK CANCER

Cancer of the head and neck region constitutes 5 percent of all malignancies in men and 2 percent of all cancer in women, collectively comprising 80,000 new cases annually and resulting in 25,000 deaths.[42] Head and neck cancer is largely a geriatric problem, most patients being over 60 at diagnosis.[45] The most common location is in the larynx, and the vast majority of tumors are of the squamous cell variety.

The head and neck area, with its areas and organs of special senses, has a special significance in one's body image. Surgical mutilation, which is frequently necessary to control or to eradicate neck and head cancer, has a much greater psychological impact than elsewhere in the body. In no other form of cancer is the team approach so greatly needed or appreciated. Cooperation of the entire team is mandatory in order for the full rehabilitation potential of the patient to be attained.

A summary of the major types of head and neck cancer is given in Table 10–1. Cancer of the oral cavity, anterior two-thirds of the tongue, and lip is relatively common. Alcohol and tobacco are major etiologic agents, associated with age, sex, and ethnicity. The vast majority of tumors occur in elderly men.[44] The increased cancer and precancer rates in older people may be due in part to age changes in the oral mucosa, making it more vulnerable to the action of carcinogens.[43] Survival rates with localized disease, particularly in cases involving only the lip, are excellent.[45]

Disabilities resulting from surgery—such as problems in speech, swallowing, facial and masticatory muscle control, and sensation—will necessitate the skills of various trained professionals. The speech pathologist evaluates and treats the patient who has undergone a laryngectomy or resection of structures used in speech, such as the tongue, lips, hard and soft palates, and buccal surfaces. The dietician is needed both preoperatively and postoperatively to assess nutritional problems, which are all too common when chewing and swallowing become painful or difficult following resection of head and neck structures. The rehabilitation specialist may prescribe assistive devices to aid the postoperative patient in achieving proper nutrition and motor control. Both physical and occupational therapists treat muscle dysfunction in the postsurgical head and neck patient and, by sensory stimulation and muscle reeducation and training, afford the patient maximum control and use of the muscles of expression and mastication.

Carcinoma of the paranasal sinuses is fortunately rare, comprising 3 percent or less of all head and neck cancer.[41] Over 90 percent of cases occur

Table 10–1. **Major Types of Head and Neck Cancer**

Location	Percentage Head and Neck Cancer	5-Year Survival	Comment
Oral cavity	10%–15%	50%–80%	80% occur in males, mean age of 60
Paranasal sinuses	3%	30%–60%	90% occur in maxillary sinus
Nasopharynx	<1%	30%–40%	Relative frequency of hematogenous spread is high
Oropharynx	10%–15%	20%–30%	In cancer of posterior ⅓ of tongue, 50%–70% will have positive cervical nodes
Larynx and hypopharynx	>50%	variable	Good prognosis if lesion detected early

Source: Adapted from Norante and Rubin,[42] p 163.

in the maxillary sinus, but only 10 percent in the ethmoid sinus. Sphenoid and frontal sinus cancers are extremely rare. The relative frequency is higher in women than most other head and neck cancers. Symptoms include bloody nasal discharge, pain in the teeth or face, nasal obstruction, and a palpable swelling in the area involved. The treatment of these cancers demands complex methods of radiation and surgery.[46] The radical surgery required may include orbital exenteration with en bloc dissection of the tumor mass, producing considerable cosmetic and functional defects. Maxillofacial prostheses are used as an adjunct or as a replacement for reconstructive surgery, because the defect may be too large or the blood supply too poor to allow surgical reconstruction. Also, the elderly person may not tolerate the multiple surgical procedures that may be required for adequate reconstruction. The use of maxillofacial prosthetic devices permits an early return of function for patients with severe deformities. Much research is needed in the area of muscle reeducation and training in the use of prosthetic devices to treat the defects resulting from surgery for head and neck cancer. The logical place to begin would be for health professionals to perform a *detailed* assessment of motor ability and sensation in the operative area so that the patient may make optimum use of remaining structures to provide acceptable use of the prosthesis.

In a review of 758 cases of head and neck cancer, a distinct prevalence in the elderly population was noted.[47] Although survival rates were similar to those of a younger age group, more patients were living longer with greater morbidity. Areas of concern in the elderly included anesthesia risk, reconstruction and wound healing, and response to chemotherapy and radiation therapy.

The ocular tissues can be the site of a number of malignant tumors in geriatric patients.[48] Secondary tumors, especially from lung primaries, are more common than primary ones if all patients are taken into consideration. These tumors can pose a serious threat to life and may result in visual loss or blindness as well. Primary-care physicians should be aware of the various malignant ocular tumors, including those of the eyelid, conjunctiva, intraocular structures, and orbit, and be prepared to refer the geriatric client for appropriate management.[48]

Thyroid carcinoma, although not a disease specific to the elderly, may occur in this population. In a series of differentiated thyroid carcinomas in a group of 268 patients over 60 several interesting findings were noted.[49] The follicular histologic type was more common than the papillary; the rate of cases with extrathyroid tumor and distant metastases was increased; bone metastases were increased; and the overall survival rate compared to younger patients was lower. A radical treatment approach, with total thyroidectomy, ^{131}I administration, and suppressive hormonal therapy, was recommended.[49]

Nasopharyngeal cancer is particularly common in Asians for reasons not completely understood. The majority of patients seek the aid of a physician because of cervical adenopathy; the incidence of nodal spread from these lesions is 70 to 90 percent. Symptoms include cranial nerve impairment, hearing loss, pain, and nasal obstruction.[42] Surgical resection is difficult because of the anatomic location. Recent research has examined the occupation of patients with this tumor, and a somewhat higher incidence was reported in persons who worked with wood or leather.[50]

The oropharynx may be defined anatomically to include the soft palate, tonsil, and posterior third of the tongue. Major symptoms of malignancy in these areas are sore throat, dysphagia, painful ulceration, or an exophytic growth that may be palpable by the patient.[42] A significant proportion (over 50 percent) of patients will have positive cervical nodes if the primary tumor is located at the base of the tongue. When cancer in this area or in any head and neck location becomes unresponsive to treatment, the irreversibility of the disease becomes a challenging problem to the cancer rehabilitation team. The health care professional and the patient's family should respond with appropriate supportive measures in order to assist the patient in remaining independent and productive.[51,52] Engaging the patient's cooperation in rehabilitative efforts may be difficult in light of so distressing a lesion and a seemingly hopeless situation.

The vast majority of head and neck cancers occur in the larynx and hypopharynx, and the majority of cases occur in the sixth and seventh decades of life.[47] The major symptoms are hoarseness, dysphagia, and, in advanced lesions, dyspnea and stridor caused by respiratory obstruction. Any geriatric patient presenting with acute or gradual onset of hoarseness should be considered to have or at least should be highly suspected to have laryngeal cancer until proven otherwise. The 5-year survival is quite variable, but the prognosis is favorable if lesions are detected early.[42] The multidisciplinary approach to treatment is stressed, and protocols employing surgery, radiation, chemotherapy, and immunotherapy in various combinations are becoming increasingly common.[53] In cases of early detection, conservative surgery, such as wide excision and subtotal laryngectomy, may be used, thus sparing the patient the considerable morbidity and dysfunction of total laryngectomy and the creation of a permanent stoma. In all cases, the judicious use of postoperative speech and physical and occupational therapies will afford the patient adequate communication techniques and acceptable physical function.

Most head and neck cancer patients require rehabilitation and treatment, not for the effects of the primary tumor or its metastases, but for the disabilities encountered after a radical neck dissection has been performed. This procedure usually requires the dissection of the cervical lymphatic chain, the internal and external jugular veins, the sternocleidomastoid muscle, and the spinal accessory nerve.[54] Because of the paralysis of the trapezius muscle, which is supplied by the spinal accessory nerve, there is a loss of ability to flex completely or to abduct the arm at the shoulder joint.[55] The degree of trapezius paralysis will depend on the amount of primary accessory innervation loss, because this muscle receives collateral innervation in some individuals from C-2, C-3, and C-4 spinal segments. The therapist employs active and active-assisted range-of-motion exercises and mobilization techniques to ensure adequate capsular mobility. Inferior displacement of the ipsilateral shoulder joint may also occur, along with protraction of the scapula—the latter caused by a combination of the loss of trapezius as a scapular stabilizer and an uneven or unopposed anterior shoulder muscle pull. An already chronically protracted scapula and kyphosis, which are commonly found in the geriatric age group, contribute significantly to the problem. Late scoliosis is possible.

Postural exercises emphasizing shoulder extension, external rotation, scapular retraction and adduction, and cervicothoracic extension are indicated. In one study of radical neck dissection patients, inferior shoulder displacement occurred in 50 percent, pain and discomfort in 42 percent, and reduction of active range of motion in the shoulder in 90 percent of the individuals studied.[54] Most often impaired are the complex acts involving the use of the arm over the head.

Recently a variation of the classical radical neck dissection has been tried successfully.[56] In this variant, the jugular vein, accessory nerve, and sternocleidomastoid muscle are dissected out during surgery and preserved. the cosmetic advantage as well as the lessened physical dysfunction in these patients undergoing a "functional" radical neck dissection is significant. The smaller degree of surgery involved reduces the metabolic stress in the patient, and this procedure may find applicability in the geriatric patient who for medical reasons cannot tolerate extensive surgical procedures. The number of patients undergoing this more conservative procedure has increased markedly. In practice, most neck dissections done today are functional. Patients still require postoperative exercise regimens to ensure full range of motion and adequate function of the ipsilateral upper extremity.

For all patients undergoing neck dissection, the therapist performs posture evaluation, sensory testing, specific manual testing, and goniometric evaluation. The therapeutic rehabilitation approach emphasizes maintaining or increasing the shoulder range of motion, strengthening the remaining musculature, and improving performance in activities of daily living (ADL). Strengthening the shoulder muscles is of great importance; no muscles can really substitute for the trapezius if the latter is completely paralyzed. The serratus anterior does help appreciably in stabilizing the scapula, and its strengthening should be emphasized. The geriatric patient may consider the cosmetic problems more significant than the functional ones. In these sedate patients, the shoulder disabilities may present seemingly little problem, and gentle ADL and functional activities may be all that is indicated. In all cases, goals should be mutually agreed upon by both therapist and patient.

Lastly, the importance of psychological counseling should be entertained in the treatment approach to the geriatric head and neck cancer patient. There is need for consideration of emotional factors during all phases of diagnosis and treatment of head and neck cancer.[57] Attention should be given also to the psychological needs of the staff and patient's family as well.

Head and neck cancer in the geriatric population will continue to be an engrossing clinical problem in the ensuing decades. The cosmetic, social, psychological, and physical ramifications are extensive, and older patients will present with complications requiring the services of various members of the cancer rehabilitation team. As with lung cancer, improved treatment regimens will afford longer survival periods; many patients with both localized and systemic disease will require these rehabilitative efforts to continue for longer periods. In response to this need, newer rehabilitation strategies may have to be developed to treat the clinical disability and dysfunction that will be observed.

BREAST CANCER

Breast cancer is the most common type of cancer in women; 1 in 9 women will develop a breast cancer at some time in her life. These tumors account for 27 percent of female cancer deaths.[58] There is a wide geographic variation, with incidence being highest in the United States and Western Europe and lowest in Japan.[59] The disease occurs at a median age of 50; 60 percent of cases occur in persons over 55 years of age;[60] and 13 percent occur in persons over 75 years of age. Another study reported that 36 percent of new breast cancer cases and 42 percent of deaths caused by breast carcinoma occurred in women 65 years of age and older.[61] The overall survival rate in breast cancer is approximately 50 percent, and despite advances in treatment, this figure has not changed appreciably in several decades. Herbsman and his associates[62] reported absolute 5- and 10-year survival rates of 54 percent and 41 percent, respectively, in 138 female patients over 70 years of age. The prognosis of breast cancer in elderly women is not better than that in other age groups, and it may be poorer, according to some reports.[59,60] One study reported a poor prognosis in patients over 75 years of age, this trend being present in all stages and periods of diagnosis.[59] The poor outcome among older patients may be related to the less aggressive treatment approaches that are taken in this patient population.

Comorbidity, impaired functional status, lack of social support, and differences in host physiology are all factors that can influence treatment efficacy and effectiveness, making extrapolation of study findings from younger to older women somewhat questionable.[63] Health-related quality of life may be more important to the elderly patient than risk of recurrence or death. Substantial variations in breast cancer diagnosis, treatment, and care exist, and these differences become greater with increasing age of the patient. Reasons for these variations and their relationship to subsequent outcomes is lacking. Physicians can best serve older patients with breast cancer by involving them carefully in decision making, taking into account available efficacy data, and individualizing care as much as possible.[63]

The typical presentation of breast cancer is a lump or nodule, which may be isolated, movable, and usually painless in the early stages. In geriatric women with large, pendulous, or atrophic breasts, the early signs may not be detected as often; an early detection depends on self-examination and annual examination by the physician. Over 50 percent of tumors occur in the upper outer quadrant of the breast.[58] Frequent breast self-examination and mammograms are as important for the geriatric woman as for her younger counterpart.

In determining the effect of age on treatment outcome in women with metastatic breast cancer treated with chemotherapy, age groups were compared in a recent study.[64] Women 70 years of age or older enrolled in clinical trials were similar to younger counterparts in response rates, time to disease progression, survival, and toxic effects of chemotherapy. They concluded that women should not be excluded from clinical trials of chemotherapy based on age alone.[64]

The treatment of primary breast cancer has become a complex process, combining the modalities of surgery, radiation therapy, hormonal manipulation, and chemotherapy. These combined approaches have offered significant prolongation of life in many patients, even those with disseminated disease. Survival periods of 5, 10, and even 15 years are becoming increasingly more common.

Kessler and Seton[65] stated that the management of operable breast carcinoma in women aged 70 years or older represents a unique problem. These patients often suffer from intercurrent diseases that reduce their life expectancy and increase their operative risk. Treatment of breast cancer should be based partially on the life expectancy of the woman at each age. A recent study outlined 94 patients over 65 years of age who were treated surgically.[66] The authors substantiated the contention that long-term survival was comparable with that found in the general population with breast cancer, despite a high percentage of deaths from intercurrent disease. Elderly patients may present with advanced disease when first seen clinically, but this finding does not generalize to all geriatric breast cancer patients.

Alberts and associates[67] compared 217 elderly and 209 middle-aged postmenopausal breast cancer patients and found that, when considered as a group, the elderly had a more favorable prognosis (median survival 20.3 months) than the middle-aged group (median survival 15.5 months). They felt that the more favorable prognosis in the elderly was due to effective nontoxic treatment. The chance of a breast tumor being malignant seems to increase with age.[68] The most evident risk factor for the tumor being malignant appears to be the influence of the estrogen hormone.

It is known that the relationship between aging and cancer is complex, because the intrication takes place at the cellular, organismal, and environmental levels.[69] Breast tumors in older patients may be slower growing and less aggressive. Plasma oxidants and antioxidants may play a role, based on the premise that breast cancer in the elderly is induced late in life. There is question as to whether the oxidant-antioxidant characteristics of a senescent organism can be causally related to the slow evolution of tumors in the aged patient.[69]

In one intriguing study, 381 women with breast cancer over age 70 were treated with either surgery plus tamoxifen or tamoxifen alone.[70] At a median follow-up of 34 months, there was no demonstrable difference in survival rate or quality of life in the two groups. Some patients treated with tamoxifen alone went on to surgical intervention for local treatment failure, and this did not appear to be disadvantageous to treatment outcome. This study has led to the opinion that operable breast cancer may be treated without surgical intervention in selected cases with small primary tumors. In a follow-up study along these lines, Horobin and associates[71] reported on 113 women with breast cancer over 70 years of age treated with tamoxifen alone. After 5 years, they concluded that tamoxifen provides an alternative treatment for operable breast cancer in older women in the short term and is particularly suitable for individuals with concurrent disease or who are unwilling to undergo surgery. In the long term, however, treatment by tamoxifen alone delays more definitive therapy. The authors concluded that further studies are warranted.

Other authors have found no significant difference between older and younger patients regarding detection and patterns of spread in breast cancer. It appears, then, that breast carcinoma in the elderly woman is not a disease significantly different from breast carcinoma in younger populations.

The radical mastectomy, which removes the breast, pectoralis major and minor muscles, and ipsilateral axillary lymphatics, was the mainstay in treatment for operable breast cancer for many decades. Extensive clinical trials have lent evidence to the observation that a modified radical mastectomy, in which the pectoral muscles are left intact, affords equal survival rates in breast carcinoma and produces less morbidity.[58] In most centers, the modified technique has replaced the standard Halsted radical mastectomy. Alternatives are lumpectomy, in which the tumor alone is excised, and simple mastectomy. Many clinical trials are under way in which these less radical procedures are employed in conjunction with radiotherapy and/or chemotherapy. More extensive disease, such as when the internal mammary lymph nodes are involved, will of necessity involve more extensive surgery.[72]

The removal of the pectoralis major and minor muscles during a radical mastectomy results in a moderate degree of dysfunction for varying periods of time after the surgery. It is the goal of the rehabilitation team, particularly the rehabilitation specialist and occupational therapist, to initiate and monitor exercises to ensure the return of range of motion and strength to the affected shoulder.

The usual disability encountered is an immediate postsurgical loss of abduction and forward flexion of the involved shoulder. This is mainly a result of the mastectomy incision extending up into the axilla; there is pulling on this incision when abduction and forward flexion are attempted. Edema in the operative area may also contribute to this loss of range of motion. The elderly patient may have a preexisting functional loss of range of motion in the operative shoulder, stressing the need for preoperative evaluation, if possible. Shoulder horizontal adduction, for which the pectoralis major is a prime mover, is seriously weakened if this muscle is resected. In time, the anterior deltoid and coracobrachialis muscle compensate for the loss of the pectoral muscles.[73]

Exercises performed postsurgically assist in increasing range of motion and strength and also in reducing edema. An exercise program should be performed three times daily, starting during the immediate postoperative period. Exercises are performed *slowly* and to the limit of endurance. This is extremely important because overexercising causes fatigue and pain. This fatigue may cause the patient to splint during movement or to develop substitution patterns that might be detrimental to further function. In all exercise programs, the therapist must be attentive to the cardiovascular and pulmonary changes, with resultant decreased endurance and decreased tolerance of exercise, that may occur in the elderly patient.

Shoulder internal rotation is frequently limited after a mastectomy and interferes with activities that involve the use of the hand on the upper back, such as bathing and hooking a bra. A manual muscle test is impractical during the first few weeks following a mastectomy; however, after this period the patient should be gently assessed for gross muscle weakness. Assessment of ADL and sensory testing are useful adjuncts to successful therapy.

Examples of exercises that are useful include ball squeeze with the elevated arm; pendulum exercises of the Codman's variety; wall climbing, which measures successive progress in shoulder range; exaggerated deep breathing to assist in chest expansion; bilateral external shoulder rotation; and pulley exercises.[74] An individualized program for the geriatric patient is essential; not all patients will be able to perform all exercises. The patient should aim for smooth, rhythmic motions when exercising; performing movements in front of a mirror helps tremendously. The rehabilitation professional should foster a positive, assured attitude in the patient, which is a necessary component for good recovery of function. The sensitive professional also will consider the psychologic and socioeconomic problems that may beset the breast cancer patient[75] and be prepared to refer the patient to team members who are trained to handle such problems.

Swelling of the ipsilateral arm occurs in one third to one half of mastectomy cases.[73,75] In 10 percent of cases, this edema may be severe, resulting in a grossly enlarged arm and loss of functional ability. The usual cause is surgical ablation of the lymphatic channels and nodes in the axillary region, but scarring, delayed wound healing, radiation fibrosis, venous obstruction, recurrent cancer, obesity, and infection may all be contributory. Elevation of the affected arm and frequent exercising will assist in lymphatic drainage and thereby reduce lymphedema. Intermittent compression with pneumatic devices and units is very effective in early or moderate lymphedema, but current research indicates that this treatment must be employed for several hours *daily* for any considerable or lasting benefit to be realized.[75] Newer equipment and techniques that allow sequential, graded application of pneumatic pressure have been found useful in treating lymphedema. Treatment may need to be carried out for several weeks before improvement is noted. Meticulous hand and arm precautions such as avoiding injections, cuts, and infections, especially in the elderly, should be followed to prevent or to reduce lymphedema. Fortunately, the overall incidence and degree of lymphedema in the postmastectomy breast cancer patient is decreasing, perhaps owing to early detection, improved surgical technique, newer radiation therapy modalities, and comprehensive and early therapeutic management. However, lymphedema may still be encountered in the elderly breast cancer patient, and the astute rehabilitation specialist should carefully observe the patient for its occurrence.

Breast cancer spreads both lymphatically and hematogenously; few cancers can result in as wide and varied a metastatic pattern. Metastases are common in bone, lung, pleura, liver, brain, and soft tissue. Skeletal involvement occurs clinically in over half of cases with disseminated breast carcinoma and can be found in up to 70 percent of cases coming to autopsy.[76] One theory states that older breast cancer patients tend to have a greater degree of soft tissue and bony metastases, as opposed to the visceral, liver, and lung metastases that are more common in the younger patient.[2]

Bone metastases may be of the osteolytic type, appearing as decorticated areas of decreased bone density, or osteoblastic, appearing as areas of scarring or increased bone density. In breast cancer, 70 percent of metastatic bone disease is osteolytic, 10 percent osteoblastic, and 20 percent mixed.[66] The axial skeleton is most frequently involved; metastases usually are found in the spine, pelvis, ribs, proximal femora, proximal humeri, and skull. Table 10–2 gives the frequency of metastases to specific bony sites in a sample of 25 patients with breast cancer metastatic to bone. This findings are comparable with larger series, in which metastases are most common in the vertebral column.[75]

In the elderly woman with disseminated bony disease, bone metastases may be asymptomatic. Pain usually heralds positive radiographs; it is usually deep and worsened by activity, particularly weight bearing. In geriatric patients, the clinician may dismiss bone pain as arthritis or muscle strain, and a careful clinical history of each patient is mandatory.[77] This point cannot be

Table 10–2. **Frequency of Metastases to Specific Bony Sites**[*]

Bony Site	Number of Patients	Percentage of Patients Having Bony Disease ($N = 25$)
Lumbar vertebrae	15	60
Throacic vertebrae	15	60
Ribs	13	52
Wing of ilium	10	40
Skull	9	36
Ischium	8	32
Femur—head and neck	8	32
Femur—intertrochanteric	7	28
Acetabulum	6	24
Pubic bone	6	24
Sacrum	4	16
Shoulder girdle (clavicle, scapula, upper humerus)	4	16
Femur—subtrochanteric	2	8
Cervical vertebrae	2	8
Sternum	1	4

[*]Detected by bone survey, bone scanning, or both.

stressed enough, because time is of the essence in this important, potentially treatable metastatic complication. Pathologic fractures occur in 50 percent of breast cancer patients with radiographic evidence of osteolytic metastases,[78] perhaps the greatest and most disabling complication in this disease. Fractures may rapidly incapacitate the elderly patient with decreased muscle mass and poor cardiac and pulmonary reserve. Femoral fractures are the most common and carry the greatest morbidity, chiefly because of the weight-bearing properties of this bone.

In the past, these patients rapidly became bedfast and had short survival periods. Little was done in the way of treatment because of the historically poor prognosis once a pathologic fracture occurred. However, the rationale for internal fixation of pathologic fractures of the long bones, followed by aggressive rehabilitative therapy, is now well established.[78–82] Surgery facilitates nursing, ambulation potential, radiotherapy, and transportation of the patient. The complications of the bedridden patient can be avoided.

Methyl methacrylate cement has recently been found to be a useful adjunct in fixation of malignant neoplastic fractures.[80] Radiation therapy is usually employed in addition to surgical fixation, and does not appear to alter fracture healing time.[79] The breast cancer patient with a hip nailing for metastatic fracture should be treated with the same rehabilitation efforts that would be used for any hip fracture patient. The rehabilitation specialist should employ early mobilization, early weight bearing (depending on the type of orthopedic device used), and graded exercises to restore strength and range of motion.

A fracture of a long bone is imminent if more than 50 percent of the cortex of the bone is destroyed by the metastatic deposit. Metastatic bone tumors are best treated *before* the extent of malignant invasion permits a fracture to occur.[82] The concept of prophylactic internal fixation has gained wide favor.[81,82] Internal stabilization of an imminent fracture eliminates pain, displacement of fragments, and an emergency situation created by the fracture. Ryan and his associates[81] reported on 18 prophylactic nailings in 14 patients (11 of 14 patients had breast cancer); all but 3 ambulated postsurgery and continued to do so until 1 to 2 weeks prior to death. In most patients, immediate or early weight bearing is allowed, thereby greatly increasing their mobility and functional ability.

Metastatic disease can lead to additional complications, such as hypercalcemia and quadriplegia or paraplegia from epidural spinal cord compression, as in metastatic lung cancer. Lastly, it is important to note that metastatic bone disease can be caused by primary tumors in the lung, kidney, prostate, and thyroid, among others. The same complications outlined above for breast cancer can ensue and will require similar treatment and rehabilitation management.

In summary, the rehabilitation effort for the breast cancer patient is multifaceted, begins with initial diagnosis, and continues throughout all phases of the disease. In the initial phase, the rehabilitation specialist treats respiratory problems, shoulder dysfunction, and lymphedema. Later, the management focuses on disabilities caused by metastatic deposits. The clinician may encounter neurologic deficit owing to brain metastases or generalized weakness owing to liver metastases, and these problems should respond to rehabilitation efforts. Lastly, the importance of supportive and palliative care for the terminally ill geriatric breast cancer patient cannot be underestimated, for it is integral to total cancer therapy and is most appreciated by the patients who seek it.

SARCOMAS COMMON TO THE GERIATRIC AGE GROUP

A wide variety of connective tissue tumors may affect the geriatric population. Although some of the primary soft tissue and bone tumors have peak incidences in childhood or early adulthood, many also have a high incidence in the elderly patient.

Adult pleomorphic rhabdomyosarcoma, a cancer of striated voluntary muscle origin, occurs in the sixth and seventh decades. At one time this cancer accounted for approximately 10 to 15 percent of malignant muscle tumors.[83] The tumors usually arise in the extremities; over half occur in the lower extremity.[84] The quadriceps, adductors, and biceps femoris are most commonly involved. The disease most often presents clinically as a hemorrhagic bruised area or soft tissue mass, which is characterized by nonencapsulation and local invasiveness. These tumors may metastasize both hematogenously and lymphatically; and even after wide surgical excision they recur in approximately 60 percent of cases.[85] At diagnosis, 30 percent of cases will already have pulmonary metastases, and metastases to regional lymph nodes will occur in 15 percent of patients.

In patients who undergo a wide surgical section, a considerable loss of muscle bulk may be expected. In order to obtain a wide surgical margin, the surgeon may resect an entire muscle or muscle group. Muscle reeducation performed by the rehabilitation specialist and occupational therapist will be important in restoring or increasing strength, mobility, and contour to the affected extremity. Ambulation training with appropriate assistive devices may be necessary, especially initially. Treatment should continue until the patient regains functional control of the limb or develops successful muscle substitution patterns to replace the function lost by muscle resection. The specific exercise approach will depend on the location and extent of surgery. In our cancer center, we have treated two geriatric patients with a quadriceps myectomy for malignant muscle tumors. After rehabilitation, both patients learned to ambulate successfully without assistive devices.

Because they often are located in the extremities and have shown a tendency to recur after local resection, these tumors may require amputation. The surgical procedure may include resection of regional lymphatics proximal to the stump. The site and level of amputation will depend upon the location, extent, and invasiveness of the primary tumor. The principles of management of the elderly cancer amputee are the same principles that would apply to any geriatric amputee. An adequate program of stump wrapping and exercise is instituted immediately after surgery. Dietz[73] claimed that preoperative training is of great value to the prospective amputee. During this period, the patient is not in any discomfort from a surgical wound, has not been immobilized, is not overmedicated for pain, and still has confidence in ambulation. Especially in geriatric cancer patients, the progress in rehabilitation can be facilitated by preoperative training in crutch or walker ambulation. This will be of great assistance in ambulation training in the postoperative recovery period. A diagnosis of malignancy should never in itself be a contraindication to prosthetic fitting. The overall 5-year survival rate for adult pleomorphic rhabdomyosarcoma is approximately 35 percent,[86] and many patients live for significant periods of time, even with disseminated disease. Many other sarcomas—fibrous histiocytoma and fibrosarcoma, for example—can also occur within muscles.[86]

Either upper- or lower-extremity prostheses should be used to ensure maximal patient function and mobility. Fitting of the prosthesis can be done early or sometimes immediately in the postoperative period in selected cases; this relatively new approach affords early ambulation. In all cases, adequate upper-extremity strength and balance are tantamount to a successful outcome. The therapist must instruct the patient in proper stump hygiene and correct stump wrapping, the latter to ensure a conical shape for optimal prosthetic fit. The prosthetist becomes an important member of the cancer rehabilitation team, joining the oncology nurse, social worker, rehabilitation specialist, occupational therapist, and physician in effecting good geriatric amputee care and rehabilitation.

Paget's disease is a disorder of unknown etiology, characterized by hyperactive destruction of bone and replacement of normal bone by expanded, soft, poorly mineralized osteoid tissue.[87] The disease rarely occurs in patients under 40 and usually involves the pelvis, skull, femur, spine, tibia, humerus, and scapula. Between 1 and 2 percent, and possibly as high as 7 percent, of cases will be complicated by the development of osteosarcoma. These tumors are most frequently located in the femur and humerus, occasionally in the pelvis and skull; occur at a mean age of 67.6 years; and carry a pathologic fracture rate of 33 percent.[87]

The prognosis in sarcomatous transformation of primary Paget's disease is unfavorable, with a mean survival of approximately 1 year following diagnosis. Nevertheless, the elderly patient with an orthopedic stabilization device for a fracture from osteosarcoma will respond well to therapy that is designed to increase functional range of motion, to maintain an increase in muscle strength, and to permit early ambulation. If an amputation is performed, the principles of geriatric amputee care and rehabilitation will apply. In an older patient, often prosthetic devices that are essentially more cosmetic than functional are prescribed, and this is acceptable from a rehabilitation standpoint if the patient's psychological status and physical comfort are improved. In the terminally ill patient, positioning, frequent turning, pain relief, and other measures of palliative care are important.

Liposarcoma, the malignant tumor of fat cells, represents approximately 18 percent of all soft-tissue sarcomas and occurs primarily after age 60.[86] Liposarcomas occur in the extremities—primarily the lower extremity—in over 60 percent of cases and in the retroperitoneum in an additional 15 percent of cases. Between 40 and 50 percent of tumors will metastasize to the lungs via the bloodstream.[88,89] Because the tumor frequently recurs after simple excision, radical soft-part resection is frequently necessary, and large surgical and functional defects are common.[88] An individualized assessment of each patient and muscle reeducation in treatment are the mainstays in ensuring as normal postoperative functioning as possible. Occasionally an amputation is performed to control an aggressive tumor. Research indicates that multimodality therapy employing radiation therapy, chemotherapy, and surgery may prolong life.[89] The overall 5-year survival rate is 35 to 40 percent.

Other soft-tissue sarcomas, such as leiomyosarcoma, fibrosarcoma, angiosarcomas, and other rare tumors, may be found in the geriatric population. Wide surgical excision and amputation are the primary treatment modalities for extremity tumors, and the resultant disabilities or amputations are managed similarly.

Other sarcomas, particularly lower-grade (I and II) and more differentiated tumors, tend to have relatively long survival periods even when pulmonary metastases eventually occur. Patients dying of metastatic sarcoma usually succumb to respiratory failure secondary to pulmonary disease, and it is uncommon to have disease elsewhere.

NON-HODGKIN'S LYMPHOMA AND CHRONIC LYMPHATIC LEUKEMIA

The maximum risk for the development of lymphoma occurs between 60 and 69 years, clearly making it a concern in the geriatric age group. It is somewhat more common than Hodgkin's disease, with an incidence of 9 per 100,000, and it has a male-to-female patient ratio of 1.7:1.[40] Older patients are more likely to present with advanced disease, and excessive symptomatology has been correlated with shorter survival.[91,92] The liver is involved in one third of cases, and 20 percent of patients have systemic symptoms of fever, chills, and weight loss.

Multiple involvement of systemic nodes is common on clinical presentation, and the involved nodes may lead to obstructive symptoms. The overall survival rate is approximately 20 to 30 percent at 5 years; aggressive treatment is recommended in many patients, especially those in poorer prognosis categories.[92] Elderly patients have a shorter survival rate than younger patients. Radiation therapy and chemotherapy are used extensively, and there are several clinical trials currently under way.

Chronic lymphatic leukemia (CLL) is a complex disease; it is the most commonly encountered leukemia (30 percent) and is clearly a disease of the aged.[93] Over 90 percent of the patients are over age 50 years of age, and 70 percent are over age 60 at diagnosis.[94] There is a 2:1 male-to-female patient predominance, and the median survival rate is between 3 to 5 years. Familial clustering, especially in siblings, has been demonstrated but has not been explained fully.

It is of interest that a large proportion of patients are asymptomatic when the disease is diagnosed. Symptoms do occur in most patients with time and include malaise and fatigue, weight loss, diaphoresis, enlarged lymph nodes, organomegaly, and general dysfunction.[94] In mild cases with few symptoms, patients may be quite functional and medical treatment may be electively withheld. In active disease, cyclic and/or combination chemotherapy produces encouraging responses.[95,96] Interestingly, the 5-year survival rate appears to be better determined by response to initial therapy than by clinical staging at diagnosis.[95] Bone marrow transplantation is used as a method of treatment for many leukemia patients. Bone marrow transplantation should not be withheld from patients over 50 years of age if the clinical condition is good and the disease is diagnosed at an early stage.

However, allogeneic marrow grafting cannot be considered as a first-line therapy in this age group.

Both lymphoma and leukemia in the aged can produce a clinical picture in the patient of generalized weakness; reduced tolerance for stress, activity, and exercise; and increased susceptibility to fatigue. The latter is also caused by the anemia that frequently accompanies these neoplastic processes. Cachexia, the syndrome of weight loss, anorexia, nitrogen and protein imbalance, and generalized wasting of body tissues—problems in any long-term disease—may ensue in these lymphoproliferative disorders, causing further loss of strength and making mobilization difficult.

For the aged patient who has become dysfunctional from the general effects of leukemia, lymphoma, or any metastatic cancer, a program consisting of gentle active exercise, positioning and turning, functional ambulation, and pain control may be beneficial. Treatment is based on the patient's willingness and ability to participate. Keeping the seriously weakened patient mobilized and ambulatory for as long as possible has pronounced effects on his or her functional level, physical comfort, psychological well-being, and overall condition. The patients then can become or remain active participants in the treatment of their disease. Exercise programs and ambulation schedules are determined individually, inasmuch as no two patients present with the same patterns of weakness or level of dysfunction.

CANCER OF THE PROSTATE

The median age for clinically overt prostatic cancer is 70 years. Prostate cancer exists in two forms: common localized tumors without clinical significance and less frequent, overt disease with metastases.[96] Only those tumors showing progression, with increased cell size and loss of differentiation, appear to acquire clinically aggressive behavior. Initial symptoms include cystitis, pain, dysuria, and polyuria.

A reliable assessment of prognosis can be expected by combined evaluation of histologic findings and clinical staging.[97] One group[98] found that patients over 70 who have early prostatic carcinoma will have a normal life expectancy if treated conservatively, but that patients under 70 live fewer years than expected.[76] Radical prostatectomy is widely employed; however, it fails to cure prostate cancer in many elderly patients because distant dissemination of the disease is often present at the time of diagnosis.[99]

Prostate cancer, like lung and breast carcinoma, spreads both hematogenously and lymphatically. The regional lymphatics are involved in 60 percent of cases, and early hematogenous spread through the paravertebral venous plexuses leads to early bone disease; the osseous involvement is most commonly osteoblastic (osteosclerotic).

Fully 70 percent of men with prostate cancer develop metastatic bone disease, occurring most commonly, in order of decreasing frequency, in the pelvis, sacrum, lumbar spine, femurs, dorsal spine, and ribs. These osseous lesions carry considerable pain and morbidity, making management a challenging clinical problem.[100,101]

Benign prostatic hyperplasia is probably the most common neoplasm in men, and carcinoma of the prostate now leads the list of newly diagnosed malignancies in males.[102] If a man lives long enough, he is likely to be affected by one or both diseases. The increasing size of the geriatric population and the frequency of these disorders result in a problem of impressive magnitude. Further investigation is required to determine the true value of screening and staging techniques. Controversy now exists regarding the relative propriety of transurethral and open surgical techniques for benign disease. Comparisons need to be made with newer, less invasive, and pharmacological approaches for prostate cancer.[102]

Although at present there is no cure for patients with widespread bone or visceral metastases, surgery, hormonal therapy, radiation therapy, and chemotherapy have all been used quite successfully in palliating this disease.[103] Prostate cancer, like breast cancer, is very commonly hormonally related, and for this reason orchiectomy and estrogens have been used in treatment. Preliminary reports indicate that chemotherapy can be palliative and give good symptomatic relief in many cases.[104] Most cell-mediated immunologic activity is depressed in many prostatic cancer patients.[105] Immunotherapy will undoubtedly play an as-yet undefined role in metastatic prostate cancer in the future. Withholding or reducing the intensity and aggressiveness of treatment for elderly prostate cancer patients is a widespread tenet lacking substantiation in the research literature. However, the benefit of wide local or radical surgery for less active, more typical prostate carcinoma has come into question. External beam radiation for prostate cancer can be given to elderly patients with acceptable morbidity and gratifying results.

Patients with widespread disease from prostate cancer are quite debilitated and appear older than their stated age. The lungs, liver, pleura, and other organs may be involved via the bloodstream, but it is the bone metastases that cause the most pain and distress in these patients. Severe spinal involvement may lead to restricted motion and a bedfast condition; the patient may need considerable assistance and encouragement in turning and positioning. Light range-of-motion exercises are frequently indicated to keep the extremities mobile. Ambulation, with a walker if necessary, should be encouraged in all patients. Although the lesions are mostly osteoblastic, careful monitoring of radiographs is important so that weight bearing may be adjusted accordingly. Orthotic devices for the low back may not be tolerated well, and the weight and pressure of the brace may actually aggravate symptoms. Transcutaneous electrical nerve stimulation (TENS) is sometimes useful as an adjunct for pain control and may lessen the amount of narcotic analgesic required for effective pain relief.

MYELOMA, COLON CANCER, AND SKIN CANCER

Multiple myeloma is a malignant tumor of plasma cells in the bone marrow, usually occurring during the sixth to eighth decades of life; 90 percent of cases occur after the age of 40.[106] It is the most common primary malignant bone tumor, per se, and is extremely difficult to treat.[107] Localized and indolent forms of the disease may also occur.[108]

The osseous lesions in myeloma are multicentric and characteristic; moth-eaten-like, lytic, and well-demarcated punched-out areas appear radiographically.[106] The most common presenting symptom is back pain that becomes increasingly unresponsive to treatment. Systemic abnormalities are common: 60 percent of patients will have hypercalcemia; renal impairment may be progressive; and repeated infections may occur owing to deficient antibody production. Exercise or ambulation tolerance may be low. Unfortunately, pathologic fractures caused by extensive bony destruction are all too common in this disease. Although the skeletal disease initially responds well to radiation, chemotherapy is eventually used in management. The elderly patient with advanced disease will need assistance in mobility, transfers, and general functional activity. Orthotic devices are sometimes employed in painful areas to restrict motion and also to provide support where the diseased skeleton may be unable to maintain stability. Tolerance of these devices is variable. Because of the high incidence of pathologic fracture, the orthopedic surgeon should be in close attendance.

Colon cancer is the second leading cause of death from cancer in the United States, with approximately 130,000 new cases per year resulting in 80,000 deaths. This represents 12 percent of male cancer deaths and 15 percent of female cancer deaths. The average age at diagnosis is between 60 and 70 years.[109] Although many factors may predispose an individual to the development of colon cancer, most cases have an unknown etiology. It is of interest that colon cancer has replaced stomach cancer as the leading gastrointestinal malignancy in the last 40 years.

One half of colon cancers occur in the rectum, but patients with lesions in the transverse colon tend to have the poorer survival rate: 28 percent after 5 years.[110] The most common surgery for colon cancer is resection of the distal colon and rectum and creation of a colostomy. A total colectomy and ileostomy construction may be performed for more extensive tumors. Chronologic age alone, in addition, should not be a deterrent to necessary surgical colectomy or colostomy.[109] Although diminished or weakened organ function is common in the elderly, the majority of patients appear to tolerate the surgery well.[111] Tumors may be more locally advanced and there is increased morbidity due to respiratory and urinary problems.[110] Colon cancer is more frequently found in the right and middle third of the colon in elderly patients; ileus and intestinal perforation are more common in the elderly. A hopeful attitude on the part of the patient, family, physician, and the cancer rehabilitation team is helpful in rehabilitation. Notwithstanding, more extensive surgical procedures, such as abdominoperitoneal resection, carry higher mortality and morbidity, especially in the elderly. Gingold[112] advocated electrocoagulation followed by radiation for small rectal adenocarcinomas in the aged.

Over one half of patients with gastrointestinal malignancy show malnutrition.[113] This is associated with greater postoperative complications and mortality. Prealbumin levels and weight loss percentages are the nutritional parameters most often altered. Preoperative nutritional support needs to be evaluated for effectiveness in reducing postoperative complications. A protocol of preoperative evaluation, intraoperative hemodynamic monitoring, and postoperative intensive care has been formulated for use in elderly or poor-risk patients undergoing abdominal surgery for cancer.[114]

In a recent study, it was found that patients over age 65 who underwent a curative resection of a colon carcinoma had a worse survival period (44 months versus 72 months) than a younger patient group.[115] However, other factors may be important, such as postsurgical stage of classification, degree of lymphocytic infiltration, and expression of immunological response.

Ileostomies and colostomies leave the patient without voluntary control of bowel elimination. Enterostomal therapy has become a specialized branch of nursing, and the diversification of collective devices, skin adhesives, and related appliances has been remarkable in the past few decades, offering a wide range of therapeutic approaches to individual problems. The enterostomal therapist begins intervention preoperatively with patient instruction. The immediate postoperative care is highly specialized, and the patient gradually learns to irrigate and to care for the stoma. Regular elimination schedules, protection of the skin, and the elimination of odors are but a few of the many facets of ostomy rehabilitation.

Colon cancer frequently metastasizes to the liver via the portal vein, and the lungs and other organs may be secondarily involved. Metastases to the regional retroperitoneal lymph nodes are extremely common in the disease. The patient with widespread metastases from colon cancer may be cachectic and weak and should benefit from a therapeutic program stressing exercise, ambulation, and pain control.

Skin cancer is the most common type of cancer in human beings.[116] An enormous variety of carcinogens—physical, chemical, and environmental—have proven to be important in its etiology. Repeated exposure of the skin to solar ultraviolet radiation is responsible for most skin cancers, and these tumors become progressively more common in older people.[117] Skin damage occurs with each prolonged exposure to the sun, leading to changes characteristic of aged skin.[118] These changes are believed to form the foundation for later development of malignant lesions. The use of magnifiers and skin microscopes to detect early lesions in the elderly population is strongly recommended.[119]

The majority of skin cancers are squamous (epidermoid) and basal cell carcinomas. The former is more aggressive and may metastasize beneath tissue planes and via the lymphatics. Basal cell carcinomas rarely metastasize but are locally destructive. In a series of 1271 cutaneous carcinomas, 496 were recurrent basal cell carcinomas.[120] Older patients, then, tend to be at risk for persistent or recurrent basal cell carcinoma. In malignant melanoma, advanced age is associated with deeper lesions and a poorer prognosis; this may be partially explained by a predominance of other unfavorable factors.[121] The frequent neglect of the lesion in elderly patients may be an important factor.

Patients who have undergone extensive facial surgery to eradicate skin cancer may need the services of the maxillofacial prosthodontist, speech pathologist, and physical therapist. In addition, because of the area involved and the considerable incidence of recurrence that may require additional surgery, psychological support is of great benefit to the patient.

SUMMARY

The cancer problem in the geriatric age group is multidimensional. Almost any cancer and its treatment will carry varying degrees of disability and dysfunction. Some tumors are more prevalent in the aged, and the local and systemic effects of cancer may be heightened in this age group.[122–124] In general, the elderly respond well to medical therapy and rehabilitation, and most endure the taxing treatment regimens without undue strain or morbidity.

Efforts should focus on the effects of cancer and cancer treatment on survival and quality of life, efficacy and toxicity of antineoplastic therapy, barriers to adequate treatment, alternative settings of cancer care, and special supportive-care needs in the elderly with cancer.[125] Also, longer-term efforts should focus on unique features of cancer in older patients, long-term effects of cancer and cancer treatment, and prevention and detection of new primary malignancies.

Challenging problems—such as pulmonary dysfunction, loss of range of motion, lymphedema, pathologic fractures from metastatic bone disease, epidural spinal cord compression, and loss of joint function and generalized weakness—can occur and will need the services of professionals who are highly trained and skilled in providing appropriate cancer rehabilitation procedures. Tumors like those outlined in this chapter are only a representative example of the array of malignancies that can affect the aged individual. With continued progress, research, and specialization in cancer rehabilitation, the elderly with cancer-related dysfunction will be able to reach maximal functional potential.

As we approach the 21st century, cancer rehabilitation will continue to exhibit a dynamic and evolving nature as a subspeciality. Rehabilitation specialists are challenged to meet with renewed vigor and sense of purpose the multitude of problems that are incurred so that more elderly patients will be restored to full health and function.

REFERENCES

1. Kurk, AE and Wardle, DF: Management of malignant disease in old age. In Denham, MJ (ed): The Treatment of Medical Problems in the Elderly. University Park Press, Baltimore, 1980.
2. Ratner, LH: Management of cancer in the elderly. Mt Sinai J Med 47:224, 1980.
3. Rubin, P (ed): Clinical Oncology for Medical Students and Physicians: A Multidisciplinary Approach, ed 5. American Cancer Society, 1978.
4. Hodkinson, HM: Cancer in the aged. In Brocklehurt, JC (ed): Textbook of Geriatric Medicine and Gerontology, ed 2. Chuchill Livingstone, New York, 1978.
5. Kerr, IG: Cancer chemotherapy in the elderly. Can Pharm J 118:289–290, 1985.
6. Guthrie, TH and Gaddis TG: Geriatric oncology. J Fla Med Assoc 80(2):112–116, 1993.
7. Rimer, BK, Catoe, KE, Graves, C, Burklow, S, and Anderson, DM: Older callers to the cancer information service. Monog Natl Cancer Inst 14:156–169, 1993.
8. Davis, DL and Schwartz, J: Trends in cancer mortality: US males and females, 1968–1983. Lancet 1/8586:633–636, 1988.
9. Horton, J and Daut, M: Detection and recognition of cancer. In Horton, J and Hill, G (ed): Clinical Oncology. WB Saunders, Philadelphia, 1977.
10. Holmes, FF and Hearne, E: Cancer stage to age relationship: Implication for cancer screening in the elderly. J Am Geriatr Soc 29(2):55, 1981.
11. Good, RA: Cancer and aging. Hosp Pract 15(11):10, 1980.
12. Lipsmeyer, EA: Simultaneous development of autoimmune disease and malignancy in two elderly patients. J Am Geriatr Soc 27:455, 1979.
13. Rao, DB, Batima, RR, Ray, M: Multiple primary malignancy in the aged. J Am Geriatr Soc 26:526, 1978.
14. Howell, TM: Multiple primary neoplasms in the elderly. J Am Geriatr Soc 28:65, 1980.
15. Payton, OD: Geriatric rehabilitation. In Teitelman, J and Yancey, K (ed): Modular Gerontology Curriculum Series. Health Sciences Consortium, High Point, NC, 1986.
16. Ishitani, K, Murakemi, S, and Kishi, A: Quality of life for older people under oncological treatment. Gan To Kagaku Rycho 19:1808–1816, 1992.
17. McGill, JS and Paul, PB: Functional status and hope in elderly people with and without cancer. Oncol Nur Forum 20:1207–1213, 1993.
18. Hunt, TE: Practical considerations in the rehabilitation of the aged. J Am Geriatr Soc 28:59, 1980.
19. Henriksen, JD: Problems in rehabilitation after age sixty-five. J Am Geriatr Soc 26:510, 1980.
20. Ramsey, A: Care of cancer patients in a home-based hospice program: A comparison of oncologists and primary care physicians. J Fam Prac 34(2):170–174, 1992.
21. Kang, SH and Bloom JR: Social support and cancer screening among older black Americans. J Natl Cancer Inst 85:737–742, 1993.
22. Yancik, R and Ries, LG: Cancer in the aged: An epidemiologic perspective on treatment issues. Cancer 68(11 suppl.):2502–2510, 1991.
23. Mettlin, C, Bonfligo, J, Berg, RL et al: Cancer control in the older person. Prevention and detection in older persons. Cancer 68(11 suppl.):2530–2533, 1991.
24. Vachon, ML, Robinovitch, A, Burkow, J et al: Cancer control and the older person: Psychosocial issues. Cancer 68(11 suppl.):2534–2539, 1991.

25. Kastenbaum, R: The physician and the terminally ill older person. In Rossman, I (ed): Clinical Geriatrics. JB Lippincott, Philadelphia, 1979.

26. Emerson, G, Philips, C, Rubin, P: Lung cancer. In Rubin, P (ed): Clinical Oncology for Medical Students and Physicians: A Multidisciplinary Approach, ed 5. American Cancer Society, 1978.

27. Cromartie, R, et al: Carcinoma of the lung: A clinical review. Ann Thorac Surg 30:30, 1980.

28. Deneffe, G, Lacquet, LM, Verbecken, E, and Vermaut, KG: Surgical treatment of bronchogenic carcinoma: A retrospective study of 720 thoracotomies. Ann Thorac Surg 45:380–383, 1988.

29. Mitz, V, et al: Sequential staging in bronchogenic carcinoma. Chest 76:653, 1979.

30. Shepherd, FA, Amdemichael, E, Evans, WK, Chalvardjian, P, Hogg-Johnson, S, Coates, R., and Paul, K: Treatment of small-cell lung cancer in the elderly. J Am Geriatr Soc 42(1):64–70, 1994.

31. Zagonel, V, Tirelli, U, Serraino, D, et al: The aged patient with lung cancer. Management recommendations. Drugs Aging 4(1):34–46, 1994.

32. Lee Chiong, TL and Matthay, RA: Lung cancer in the elderly patient. Clin Chest Med 14:453–478, 1993.

33. Bellamy, J: Surgery of bronchogenic cancer in elderly patients. Rev Pneumol Clin 48(5):225–229, 1992.

34. Hammon, L: Oncology. In Frownfeller, DL (ed): Chest Physical Therapy and Pulmonary Rehabilitation. Year Book Medical Publishers, Chicago, 1978.

35. Hammon, WE: Total pulmonary hemorrhage associated with chest physical therapy. Phys Ther 59:1247, 1979.

36. Stanley, KE: Prognostic factors for survival in patients with inoperable lung cancer. Journal National Cancer Institute 65:25, 1980.

37. Tomita, T and Raimondi, AJ: Brain tumors in the elderly. JAMA 246:53, 1981.

38. Sarma, DP: Lung cancer managed in patients 75 or older. J Surg Oncol 34(1):19–21, 1987.

39. Janower, ML and Stennerhasset, JB: Lymphangitic spread of metastatic cancer to the lung. Radiology 101:267, 1971.

40. Gilbert, RQ, Kim, JM, and Posner, JB: Epidural spinal cord compression from metastic tumor: Diagnosis and treatment. Ann Neurol 3:40, 1978.

41. Cox, ML, Ogle, SJ, and Hodkinson, DM: Paraplegia and quadriplegia in the elderly due to spinal cord lesions: Association with malignancy. J Am Geriatr Soc 29:126, 1981.

42. Norante, JD and Rubin, P: Head and neck tumors. In Rubin, P (ed): Clinical Oncology for Medical Students and Physicians: A Multidisciplinary Approach, ed 6. American Cancer Society, New York, 1983.

43. Pindborg, JJ: Oral cancer and precancer as diseases of the aged. Community Dent Oral Epidemiol 6:300, 1978.

44. Smith, EM: Epidemiology of oral and pharyngeal cancers in the United States: Review of recent literature. Journal of the National Cancer Institute 63:1189, 1979.

45. Love, JM, et al: Surgical management and epidemiology of lip cancer. Otolaryngol Clin North Am 12:81, 1979.

46. Robin, PE, Powell,DJ, and Starbie, JM: Carcinoma of the nasal cavity and paranasal sinuses: Incidence and presentation of different histological types. Clin Otolaryngol 4:431, 1979.

47. Lamp, HB, Lampe, KM, and Skillings, J: Head and neck cancer in the elderly. J Otolaryngol 15:235–238, 1986.

48. Shields, JA and Shields, CL. Malignant tumors of the eye in geriatric patients. Geriatrics 46(9):28–39, 1991.

49. Casara, D, Rubello, D, Saladini, G, DeBesi, P, Fassini, A, and Busnardo, B: Differentiated thyroid carcinoma in the elderly. Aging (Milano) 4:333–339, 1992.

50. Huygen, PL: Nasopharyngeal cancer: A clinical study with special reference to age and occupation. Clin Otolaryngol 5:37, 1980.

51. Pearson, PW: The dying patient with oral malignant disease. Otolaryngol Clin North Am 12:241, 1979.
52. Keith, CF: Wound management following head and neck surgery: The challenge of complex nursing intervention. Nurs Clin North Am 14:761, 1979.
53. Ferlito, A, et al: Therapeutic prospects in cancer of the larynx. J Laryngol Otol 94:405, 1980.
54. Ewing, M and Mayes M: Disability following radical neck dissection. An assessment based on the postoperative evaluation of 100 patients. Cancer 5:873, 1952.
55. Audgeon, BJ, DeLisa, JA, and Miller, RM: Head and neck cancer: A rehabilitation approach. Am J Occup Ther 34:243, 1980.
56. Ariyan, S: Functional radical neck dissection. Plast Reconstr Surg 65:16, 1980.
57. Breitbart, W and Holland, J: Psychosocial aspects of head and neck cancer. Semin Oncol 15:61–69, 1988.
58. Saulov, E: Breast cancer. In Rubin, P (ed): Clinical Oncology for Medical Students and Physicians: A Multidisciplinary Approach, ed 6. American Cancer Society, 1983.
59. Host, H and Lund, E: Age as a prognostic factor in breast cancer. Cancer 57:2217–2221, 1986.
60. Van Rosen, A, Gardelin, A, and Auer, G: Assessment of malignancy potential in mammary carcinoma in elderly patients. Am J Clin Oncol Cancer Clin Trials 10:61–64, 1987.
61. Schottenfield, D and Robbins, GF: Breast cancer in elderly women. Geriatrics 26:121, March, 1971.
62. Herbsman, H, et al: Survival following breast cancer surgery in the elderly. Cancer 47:235, 1981.
63. Silliman, RA, Balducci, L, Goodwin, JS, Holmer, FF, and Leventhal, E: Breast cancer in old age: What we know, don't know, and do. J Natl Cancer Inst 85(3):190–199, 1993.
64. Christman, K, Muss, HB, Case, LD, and Stanley, V: Chemotherapy of metastatic breast cancer in the elderly. The Piedmont Oncology Association epxerience. JAMA 268(1):96–97, 1992.
65. Kessler, HJ and Seton, JZ: The treatment of operable breast cancer in the elderly female. Am J Surg 135:664, 1978.
66. Hunt, EI, Fry, DE, and Bland, KI: Breast carcinoma in the elderly patient: An assessment of operative risk, morbodity, and mortality. Am J Surg 140:339, 1980.
67. Alberts, AS, Falkson, G, and van der Merwe, R: Metastatic breast cancer: Age has a significant effect on survival. S Afr Med J 79(5):239–241, 1991.
68. Pannella, A, Tibaldeschi, C, Prati, U, Roveda, L, Picchio, GL, Zambianchi, M, Cattaneo, G, and Pezza, A: Tumors of the breast in old age. Minerva Chir 48:443–452, 1993.
69. Gerber, M and Segala C: Aging and cancer: Plasma antioxidants and lipid peroxidation in young and aged breast cancer patients. EXS 62:235–246, 1992.
70. Bates, T, Riley, DL, Houghton, J, Fallowfield, L, and Baum, M: Breast cancer in elderly women: A cancer research campaign trial comparing treatment with tamoxifen and optimal surgery with tamoxifen alone. Br. J Surg 78:591–594, 1991.
71. Horobin, JM, Preece, PF, Dewar, JA, Wood, RA, and Cuschieri, A: Long-term follow-up of elderly patients with locoregional breast cancer treated with tamoxifen only. Br. J Surg 78:213–217, 1991.
72. Scatarige, JC, Fishman, EK, and Zinreich, ES: Internal mammary lymphadenopathy in breast carcinoma: CT appraisal of anatomic distribution. Radiology 167:89–91, 1988.
73. Dietz JH: Rehabilitation of the cancer patient. Med Clin North Am 53:607, 1969.
74. Healy, J: Role of rehabilitation medicine in the care of the patient with breast cancer. Cancer 28:1666, 1971.
75. Grabois, M: Rehabilitation of the postmastectomy patient with lymphedema. CA 26(2):75, 1976.
76. Viadana, M, Bross, L, and Pickren, B: An autopsy study of some routes of dissemination of cancer of the breast. Br J Cancer 27:336, 1973.
77. Galaski, CB: Skeletal metastases and mammary cancer. Ann R Coll Surg Engl 50:3, 1972.

78. Schumann, DJ and Amstute, H: Orthopedic management of patients with metastic carcinoma of the breast. Surg Gynecol Obstet 137:831, 1973.
79. Heisterberg, L and Johnsen, TS: Treatment of pathological fractures. Acta Orthop Scand 50:6, II:787, 1979.
80. Harrington, E, et al: The use of methylmethacrylate as an adjunct in fixation of malignant neoplastic fractures. Journal of Bone and Joint Surgery 54-A:1665, 1972.
81. Ryan, M, et al: Prophylactic internal fixation of the femur for neoplastic lesions. Journal of Bone and Joint Surgery 58-A:1071, 1976.
82. Wirth, CR: Metastatic bone cancer. Curr Probl Cancer 3:1, 1979.
83. Keyhani, A and Booker, RJ: Pleomorphic rhabdomyosarcoma. Cancer 22:956, 1968.
84. Lee, ES: Rhabdomyosarcoma in adults. Proceedings of the Royal Society of Medicine 59:414, 1966.
85. Bizel, LS: Rhabdomyosarcoma. Am J Surg 140:687, 1980.
86. Aust, JB: Soft tissue sarcomas. In Horton, J and Hill, GJ (eds): Clinical Oncology. WB Saunders, Philadelphia, 1977.
87. Schajowicz, F, Velan, O, and Arajo, EX: Metastases of carcinoma in the pagetic bone. A report of two cases. Clin Orthop Rel Res 220:290–296, 1988.
88. Campbell, DA, et al: Liposarcoma of the lower extremity. Surgery 88:453, 1980.
89. Evans, HL: Liposarcoma: A study of 55 cases with a reassessment of its classification. Am J Surg Pathol 3:507, 1979.
90. Solal-Celigny, P, Chastany, C, and Hersera, A: Age as the main prognostic factor in adult aggressive non-Hodgkin's lymphoma. Am J Med 83:1075–1079, 1987.
91. Elias, L: Differences in age and sex distributions among patients with non-Hodgkins lymphoma. Cancer 43:2540, 1970.
92. Ridders, RA, et al: Nodular non-Hodgkin's lymphoma (NHL): Factors influencing prognosis, and indications for aggressive treatment. Cancer 43:1643, 1979.
93. Paolino, W, Infelise, V, Rossi, M: Chronic lymphoid leukemia: Clinical observation about its natural progression. Acta Haematol 63:19, 1980.
94. Klingermana, HG, et al: Bone marrow transplantation in patients aged 45 years and older. Blood 67:770–776, 1986.
95. Keating, MJ, Scouros, M, and Murphy, S: Multiple agent chemotherapy (POAEH) in previously treated and untreated patients with CLL. Leukemia 2(3):157–164, 1988.
96. McNeal, JE: The origin and evolution of prostatic carcinoma. Cancer Detect Prev 2:565, 1979.
97. Kastendieck, H: Prostatic carcinoma: Aspects of pathology, prognosis, and therapy. J Cancer Res Clin Oncol 96:131, 1980.
98. Barnes, R, et al: Conservative treatment of early carcinoma of the prostate. Comparison of patients less than 70 with those over 70 years of age. Urology 14:359, 1979.
99. Walsh, PC: Radical prostatectomy for the treatment of localized prostatic carcinoma. Urol Clin North Am 7:583, 1980.
100. Forman, JD, Order, SE, and Zinreich, ES: Carcinoma of the prostate in the elderly: The therapeutic ratio of definitive radiotherapy. J Urol 136:1238–1241, 1986.
101. Pollen, JJ and Schmidt, JD: Bone pain in metastatic cancer of the prostate. Urology 13(2):129, 1979.
102. Van Arsdalen, KN: Prostate surgery. Clin Geriatric Med 6:609–631, 1990.
103. Barnes, RW: Endocrine therapy of prostatic carcinoma. Cancer Detect Prev 2:761, 1979.
104. Luckland, AT, et al: Sequential polychemotherapy for advanced prostatic carcinoma. A preliminary cooperative study on 30 patients. Eur Urol 5:250, 1979.
105. Catalona, WJ: Immunobiology of carcinoma of the prostate. Invest Urol 17:353, 1980.
106. Klos, JR and Burtz, JW: Multiple myeloma: An overview for the clinician. Journal of American Osteopathic Association 79:113, 1979.
107. Osby, E, Codmark, B, and Reizenstein, PL: Staging of myeloma. A preliminary study of staging factors and treatment in different stages. Recent Results Cancer Res 65:21, 1978.

108. Alexanian, R: Localized and indolent myeloma. Blood 56:521, 1980.
109. Bader, JF: Colorectal cancer in patients older than 75 years of age. Dis Colon Rectum 29:728–732, 1986.
110. Payne, SE, Chapuis, PH, and Pheils, MT: Surgery for large bowel cancer in people aged 75 years and older. Dis Colon Rectum 29:733–737, 1986.
111. Braun, L: Prognosis of colorectal carcinoma in persons aged over 80 years. Dtsch Med Wochernscher 111:1869–1873, 1986.
112. Gingold, BS: Local treatment (electrocoagulation) for carcinoma of the rectum in the elderly. J Am Geriatr Soc 29:10, 1981.
113. Beguiristain, GA, Medrano, GMA, Uriarte, ZC, and Alvarez, CJ: Preoperative nutritional status in geriatric patients with digestive neoplasm. Nutr Hosp 6:364–374, 1991.
114. Alexander, HR, Turnbull, AD, Salamone, J, Keefe, D, and Melendez, J: Upper abdominal cancer surgery in the very elderly. J Surg Oncol 47(2):82–86, 1991.
115. Digiorgio, A, Tocchi, A, Puntillo, G, Butti, C, Derone, G, Basso, L, alManour, M, Diegoli, L, and Flammia, M: Age as a prognostic factor following excisional surgery for colorectal cancer. Ann Ital Chir 61:647–650, 1990.
116. Bechtel, MA, Cullen, JP, and Owen, LG: Etiological agents in the development of skin cancer. Clin Plast Surg 7:265, 1980.
117. Fobres, PD, Davies, RE, and Urback, F: Aging, environmental influences, and photocarcinogenesis. J Invest Dermatol 73:131, 1979.
118. Willis, I: Sunlight, aging and skin cancer. Geriatrics 33:33, 1978.
119. Goldman, L: Direct skin microscopy as an aid in the early diagnosis of precancer and cancer of the skin in the elderly. J Am Geriatr Soc 28:337, 1980.
120. Levine, HL and Bailin, DL: Basal cell carcinoma of the head and neck: Identification of the high-risk patient. Laryngoscope 90:955, 1980.
121. Conen, HS, Cox, E, Manton, K, and Woodbury, M: Malignant melanoma in the elderly. J Clin Oncol 5(1):100–106, 1987.
122. Bharacha, NE, Raven, RH, and Schoenberg, BS: Primary malignant nervous system neoplasms: Birth cohort effect in the elderly. Arch Neurol 42:1061–1062, 1985.
123. Rossi Ferrini, P, Basi, A, and Casini, C: Hodgkin's disease in the elderly: A retrospective clinicopathologic study of 61 patients aged over 60 years. Acta Haematol 78:Suppl 1:163–170, 1987.
124. Edelam, DS, Russin, DS, and Wallack, MK: Gastric cancer in the elderly. Am J Surg 53(3):170–173, 1987.
125. Balducci, L, Ades, T, Carbone, PP, Friedman, M, Fulmer, T, Galakotos, A, and Yancik, R: Cancer control in the older person: Issues in treatment. Cancer 68(11 suppl.):2527–2529, 1991.

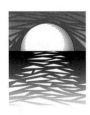

CHAPTER 11

Health Promotion for the Elderly

Mary Ferguson Livingstone Belmont, EdD, RN
Kristin N. Koehler, MA, RN
Alona Harris, EdD, RN

BEHAVIORAL OBJECTIVES

Upon completion of this chapter, the reader will be able to:

1 List three areas of health promotion that have particular relevance for the geriatric patient.
2 Discuss major barriers to participation in health-promotion activities.
3 Modify a health-promotion intervention plan according to different risk behaviors.
4 Analyze ethical issues involved in planning health promotion for the aged.

EVOLVING FORMS OF HEALTH PROMOTION

"What is health?" Pose this question to a dozen esteemed health professionals, and you will probably receive a dozen different, but acceptable, answers. The definition of health has changed over the centuries and continues to do so today.

In the past, being healthy meant not being sick; and being sick meant that you would probably die. Although cave drawings left by prehistoric humans suggest that people cared for the sick, it seems unlikely that great effort could be expended to protect the infirm in nomadic societies. Survival was partly determined by one's ability to move from a hostile environment.

In the classic essay *Mirage of Health*, René DuBois[1] writes that complete freedom from disease is almost incompatible with the process of living.

> Through the molding forces of biological and social evolution, and by altering the environment to his taste, man had made himself at home almost everywhere in the world—in the Arctic and in the tropics, as well as along the Mediterranean shores—in crowded apartment houses and desolated tundra, as well as the cozy villages of Somerset—in flimsy tents and in igloos, as well as in the chateaux of the Loire. And it seems to be his chosen fate that he will continue to search for new homes even though the adaptive changes made necessary by each move involve unforeseeable dangers. The Garden of Eden, the Promised Land that each generation imagines anew in its dreams, and all the Arcadias past and future could be sites of lasting health and happiness only if mankind were to remain static in a stable environment. But in the world of reality, places change and man also changes. Furthermore, his self-imposed striving for ever new distant goals makes his fate even more unpredictable than that of other living things. For this reason, health and happiness cannot be absolute and permanent values however careful the social and medical planning. (p. 2)

Biological fitness requires never-ending efforts of adaptation to the environment, which, because of our inquisitive nature, we are forever changing.

McKnight[2] provides an interesting perspective for understanding modern definitions of health by dividing health history into three phases: the engineering era, medical era, and postmedical era. These historical divisions apply only to industrial countries.

The *engineering era* occurred during the 18th and 19th centuries as the rural population poured into the urban areas in huge numbers, creating tremendous health threats associated with poverty and overcrowding, such as contagious diseases and starvation. It was during this era that the concept of organized public health efforts became evident for the first time. Three major strategies were used on a large scale to overcome social health problems: the pasteurization of food, the organization of efforts to produce and distribute food to starving populations, and the development of proper sewage systems and safe water supplies. Health advances of this era can be characterized as environmental improvements.

The *medical era* roughly spanned the period from 1920 to 1960. Again, three strategic developments had an impact on public health: wide-scale use of vaccines and antibiotics, extraordinary technological advances in medical machinery, and the establishment of comprehensive hospital complexes. Health care became available to the masses, and people no longer faced certain death from communicable diseases and infection. Major health advances of this era, characterized as preventive and curative medical treatment, enabled people to live significantly longer lives.

Problems confronting us now, in what might be called the *postmedical era*, flow directly from the health improvements of the two preceding eras and the resulting changes in lifestyle. We will consider several that are particularly evident in this decade: they are cost, poor planning for advanced years, and the increasing responsibility of individuals to moderate behavior that places health at risk.

COST OF HEALTH CARE

The cost of health care is staggering for those who do not have a comprehensive insurance plan. People survive catastrophic illness because of technology they cannot afford, thus placing enormous hardship on the individual and his or her family. Insurance programs of past decades were developed for a medical model that emphasized rapid cures for acute disorders.[3] It is imperative that we begin to focus economic concerns on the long-term management of chronic illness.

Although the life span has increased dramatically, the final years of many older people are without meaning. People may be isolated for many reasons. Physical and economic handicaps resulting from chronic disorders may prevent the person from engaging in activities with others. Often, retirement is approached without planning for activities that can enhance physical and psychological well-being.

Today, the leading causes of premature death and premature disability in industrialized countries are heart disease, cerebrovascular disease, cancer, and trauma—conditions largely influenced by lifestyle factors such as stress, diet, exercise, and smoking.[4] In other words, there has been a shift in the leading cause of death from disease that could be controlled only by public health and medical intervention to conditions that can be significantly influenced by making simple changes in behavior. The focus of health promotion and disease prevention, as well as of medical care, is to reduce the potential years of life lost (in premature mortality) and to ensure better quality of extended life. Contemporary health problems may be characterized as social concerns necessitating responses from multiple disciplines—political, legal, economic, religious, medical—to achieve resolution. Whereas the continuum of medical care once started with disease prevention and ended with cure, the end points have expanded to encompass rehabilitation in one direction, and a healthy lifestyle in the other. Thus, the medical field is maturing into the health field. No longer dominated by one discipline, the responsibilities for the health care of society are increasingly shared by many health practitioners.

DEFINITIONS OF INDIVIDUAL HEALTH

In 1974, the World Health Organization[5] defined health as a state of complete physical, mental, and social well-being, not merely the absence of disease and infirmity. This statement is, however, more a global goal for humanity than a working definition. By eliminating and curing many acute diseases and congenital disorders, we have created a situation whereby increasing numbers of people will complete a normal life span while suffering from unresolved long-term illnesses. Does this always mean that these people are unhealthy? Of course not: people have differing degrees of health. This may be clearer if you consider the person with controlled epilepsy who is in superb physical condition and emotional balance. Such a person could best be described as healthy, but with individualized health goals.

As important as the degrees of health one might attain is the multifaceted character of health; that is, the various components and indicators of health. Some of the most common terms used to describe a state of health, or process of being healthy, include holistic health, wellness, and self-care.

Holistic Health

Holism is a word derived from the Greek word *halos*, meaning "whole." Holistic health care encompasses the whole person, meaning the physical, psychological, and spiritual components of each individual. Spiritual considerations with respect to health care are rarely discussed in depth, but refer to a direction or feeling of purpose in life. Health in each area results in the health of the whole person, and conversely, illness in any area creates disharmony in the other areas. The concept of holistic health can be illustrated as a triangle whereby physical being, emotional well-being, and spirituality are each represented by a separate side. Disturbances in any side of the triangle will ultimately be evident in the remaining sides. Severe or prolonged emotional stress will eventually have physical manifestations, and vice versa. Even though a person may be physically and emotionally sound, life may be unfulfilling without spiritual purpose. Often, we see changes in the physical health of a person without giving sufficient consideration to the psychological and spiritual components of his or her illness, either as causes or potential complications.

Wellness

Health is a complex, dynamic state that changes constantly. Whereas we may consider ourselves well if we have no visible signs or symptoms of illness, the concept of wellness is really much more complex, involving our ability to adapt physically and psychologically to health threats. Wellness can be considered our current state of health plus all of our biological, psychological, and social reserves that contribute to our ability to maintain health equilibrium.

We can illustrate wellness as an iceberg, the visible tip representing the current state of our health.[6] Beneath the water lies the enormous base of the iceberg, representing additional layers that support our state of wellness: they are lifestyle behaviors, psychological properties, and philosophical beliefs. Lifestyle behaviors include nutrition, exercise, stress levels, and substance abuse. Psychological properties are what motivates our health-related behaviors. Philosophical areas refer to our spiritual interpretation of life, which ultimately shapes all of our behavior.

For example, someone can appear to be physically fit on the surface, but inside be lonely and isolated, thus diminishing his or her ability to maintain the equilibrium of this iceberg called wellness.

Self-Care

Common to the concepts of holism and wellness is the notion of self-care. According to Orem,[7] self-care is the practice of activities that individuals initiate and perform on their own behalf to maintain life, health, and well-being. In our society, people are expected to be responsible for their own well-being and to make life choices that will result in optimal health. Self-care has probably always been practiced by humans to some degree; currently it is evidenced by the proliferation of exercise, nutrition, and stress management programs. It is important to understand each person's unique definition of health in order to plan meaningful and effective health-promotion activities.

NATIONAL HEALTH GOALS FOR THE YEAR 2000

Because of the broad, organizational health accomplishments of this century, such as sanitation reform and widespread accessibility of medical care, more attention could be given to prevention, promotion, and protection in this country.[8] These efforts, however, were largely uncoordinated by professional or geographic location until the late 1970s. In 1979, the Public Health Service[9] published a landmark document, *Healthy People: The Surgeon General's Report on Health Promotion and Disease Prevention*, which presented general goals for reducing premature death and injury in different age categories by the year 2000. In the foreword to this document, Joseph A. Califano, Jr., then secretary of health, education, and welfare, wrote:

> We are killing ourselves by our own careless habits. We are killing ourselves by carelessly polluting the environment. We are killing ourselves by permitting harmful social conditions to persist—conditions like poverty, hunger and ignorance—which destroy health, especially for infants and children.

To know these things gives hope that we can devise new strategies for health. *1990 Health Objectives for the Nation,*[10] published in 1980 by the U.S. Public Health Services, was another landmark document that categorized, planned, and evaluated activities for systematically improving the nation's health. The document outlined fifteen sets of objectives concerning national goals for reducing most causes of premature death and disability in this country. The objectives were grouped into three categories: health promotion, health protection, and disease prevention (Fig. 11–1). Activities by disparate

1990 HEALTH OBJECTIVES FOR THE NATION

Health Promotion—any combination of health education and related organizational, environmental and economic interventions designed to promote health.

1. Smoking and Health
2. Misuse of Alcohol and Drugs
3. Nutrition
4. Physical Fitness and Exercise
5. Control of Stress and Violent Behavior

Health Protection—protective measures in the environment that can be used by government, private industries and communities, to protect people from harm.

6. Toxic Agent Control
7. Occupational Safety and Health
8. Accident Prevention and Injury Control
9. Fluoridation and Dental Health
10. Surveillance and Control of Infectious Diseases

Preventive Health Services—key preventive services that can be delivered by health providers to individuals.

11. High Blood Pressure Control
12. Family Planning
13. Pregnancy and Infant Health
14. Immunization
15. Sexually Transmitted Diseases

FIGURE 11–1. The U.S. Public Health Service's 1990 health objectives for the nation.

professional groups and local communities were finally unified by the strategies and goals embodied in these documents. Major reductions in the amount of illness and premature death for all age categories were evident in 1990, confirming the usefulness of forming national goals. Groups of health professionals and government officials repeatedly met to evaluate effectiveness of strategies used to meet the original objectives and to decide on new, attainable goals for the year 2000. Additional areas of concern focused on improvement of mental health, maintaining health and quality of life in older people, control of HIV infection and AIDS, cancer screening, and cholesterol screening.

Whereas a century ago Americans struggled to avoid life-threatening work conditions and contagious diseases, today we have come to enjoy and expect health in all aspects of our lives. At the same time, we pursue lifestyles that place us at risk for premature death and avoidable disability. Allied health professions, by virtue of their education and vast numbers, are in a key position to provide quality health-promotion services to clients in the roles of caregiver, teacher, and health advocate.

SPECIAL HEALTH-PROMOTION CONCERNS OF THE AGED

Areas of disease prevention, health maintenance, and rehabilitation that affect physical and psychological functioning as part of the aging process are addressed in depth in other chapters. We can now look into some of these same activities within the context of health promotion. We also address the specific health-promotion issues that concern the elderly:

1. Protection from quackery, which victimizes many elderly
2. Access to health care providers who are skilled in the care of elderly clients and sensitive to their needs
3. Enhancement of people's ability to overcome barriers that inhibit successful participation in health-promotion programs, such as fear of injury or failure, denial of symptoms, perceptions of difficulty in attaining goals, and the belief in luck as the major determinant of good health

Quackery

According to the U.S. House of Representatives Subcommittee on Health and Long-Term Care, 60 percent of the victims of health care fraud are elderly people, even though they make up less than 15 percent of the population. About $14 billion is spent annually by individuals on remedies that are not only useless but also may be harmful or delay proper treatment. The indirect expenses for injuries to patients resulting from harmful or delayed treatment for arthritis alone exceeds $25 million.

The treatment of arthritis, cancer, and the physiologic changes related to aging seem to be areas common to quack medicine. Some reasons to seek alternate remedies include fear of pain and mutilation and a sense of hope and support that the quick practitioner may offer.[11]

According to the Arthritis Foundation, quackery succeeds with victims of this disease because there is no known cure and very little understanding about the condition. The person may also suffer extreme pain. Because arthritic pain usually follows intermittent patterns—appearing and then disappearing—bogus cures may appear to be effective, albeit temporary. Unfortunately, the penalty for selling unproven remedies is still relatively mild despite efforts by state and Federal governments to rectify this. Some of the unproven cures promoted in the past include copper and magnetic bracelets, megavitamin treatment, plant and herbal tonics, macrobiotic diet, blood washing, and changes in sexual techniques.

Cancer accounts for about one fifth of all deaths in this country. Its incidence rises with age and occurs most frequently in the age group over 65. Advances in technology and molecular biology have made earlier detection possible and have lengthened survival chances, but no cures seem to be on the horizon. Moreover, earlier detection and treatment advances have made cancer a chronic disease, not a terminal illness. Many more elderly people are now living with cancer or postcancer treatment than ever before. Age is not a criterion for treatment eligibility; patient choice and quality of life potential are the prime considerations. In some situations, the best solution treatment offers is symptomatic relief, especially in advanced stages of the disease. But older people can be diagnosed with early-stage disease. Other medical conditions may complicate disease symptoms or limit treatment options. It is not unusual for people with cancer and their families to go from doctor to doctor, treatment to treatment, looking for a cure. Such seeking may be part of the denial phase of normal grief, but ultimately there should be an acceptance of the inevitability of the prognosis. Popular unproven cures for cancer include Laetrile, a drug made from apricot pits, megadoses of vitamins A and C, macrobiotic diets, and coffee enemas.

When considering the physical and psychological effects of aging, think of all the bottles of tonic that have been sold in this country over the years purporting to cure everything from baldness to fatigue to impotence. Many such remedies are still part of a booming business and are legitimized today, even though we think of ourselves as a scientifically sophisticated society. The cosmetic industry is one of the most lucrative in the United States. Cosmetic products and advertising are federally regulated, but people who want to believe that there is a way to retain their youth through appearance still purchase a variety of creams. Manufacturers present them as antiwrinkle creams for the face, add an attractive package, and charge a high price for what is essentially a low-cost moisturizer. Although it is illegal to discriminate in hiring practices based on age, it is naive to pretend that the practice does not occur. Also, our society emphasizes a preference for young, attractive, slender people, making antiaging cures highly valued for social reasons. Other examples of antiaging remedies include mechanical facial exercisers, bust-firming creams, and tonics to stop hot flashes.

Senility is often jokingly called "old-timer's disease," but it is a frightening prospect to many of the aging. While it is not the only form of dementia, Alzheimer's disease is surely the most devastating; it is progressive, debilitating, and ultimately fatal. Everyday forgetfulness occurs regularly with aging. Perhaps the true liberation of aging would allow us to be ourselves and forget what is unimportant. We also forget more when we are stressed. If a person forgets where he or she left the house keys, this is not Alzheimer's disease. But when the person cannot remember what the house keys are for, it may be. Early diagnosis of Alzheimer's is extremely important. Some behavioral changes, such as loss of appetite, loss of interest in the environment, decreased emotional expression, and slowness of movement are seen in depression as well as some Alzheimer's cases. Older people who take psychotropic medications, particularly tranquilizers, can display similar behavioral changes. True differential diagnosis of Alzheimer's disease can be accomplished only by examination of brain tissue after death. However, when other possible causes for behavioral changes, such as multi-infarct dementia, have been excluded, the diagnosis of Alzheimer's can be made.

The person diagnosed as having Alzheimer's will, over the years, become more dependent on a caregiver for physical and emotional care. As a group, people with Alzheimer's disease are physically healthier than the aging population in general. The physical aspect of the loved one can remain the same for years after social and interpersonal characteristics have been lost. A health-promotion measure of providing a rich and varied, yet predictable and safe, environment for the person with Alzheimer's can be a difficult and draining endeavor. Encourage use of short-term stay, respite care, and day-care programs. Suggest that caregivers attend Alzheimer's support groups to help them maintain a positive outlook while doing the difficult job of assisting the loved one at home. Because our society places such an emphasis on intelligence, having a relative with Alzheimer's disease may be an embarrassment or perceived as a stigma by some family members. Thus, individuals and families risk delaying diagnosis and treatment from a lack of knowledge about the disease, and incur excessive financial loss because of useless quack treatments to "restore and improve memory."

Perhaps the best way to protect a person from falling prey to such quackery is to encourage him or her to seek another opinion from health or government sources before investing money or time in a questionable remedy. When the cure is for a specific disease, refer the person to any national organization concerned with that condition, such as the American Cancer Society. Certain health professions have specialist organizations such as the Oncology Nurses Society, which may be able to provide accurate, timely advice to patients. If the person is prone to buying products or memberships in special programs that appear questionable, advise him or her to make a habit of contracting government and consumer organizations that monitor business and advertising, such as those listed below.

Council of Better Business Bureaus
Attention: Standards and Practices
1515 Wilson Boulevard
Arlington, VA 22209

Federal Trade Commission
6th Street and Pennsylvania Avenue NW
Washington, DC 20580

Food and Drug Administration
HFE-88
5600 Fishers Lane
Rockville, MD 20857

Office of Consumer Affairs
(Check local telephone directory for location)

The National Institute on Aging[12] lists the following common ploys of dishonest health product promoters:

- Promising a quick cure
- Promising a painless cure
- Offering a secret formula that is available from only one company
- Presenting testimonials or case stories from satisfied customers
- Advertising that a product has many medical uses
- Claiming that they have made a medical breakthrough about which other scientists do not yet know

Finding the Right Health Care Professionals

As our knowledge of the special health needs of the elderly has grown, a separate and distinct health care field has evolved. Geriatric specialists in all health disciplines should understand the complex interaction between a person's health and his or her culture, beliefs, education, emotional state, and socioeconomic status. They should also be familiar with often subtle differences in disease manifestations between older and younger age groups (for example, in the elderly heart attacks may occur without the crushing chest pain usually experienced by younger people). Elderly patients may have multiple physical problems and require several different medications, so practitioners must be astute diagnosticians and skilled at monitoring the cumulative affects of multiple drug combinations. Increasing numbers of health graduates are choosing to specialize in geriatrics. But the field is new, and many people may have difficulty finding caregivers who are knowledgeable about the aging process and sensitive to the multiple concerns of the elderly. Unfortunately, too many practitioners still equate advancing years with mental and physical deterioration.

Most elderly people have lost their personal or family physician to death or retirement. Thus it is unlikely that they have someone who has known them for many years and who can assess health changes over time. Often they may see physicians and other health professionals in many different specialties because of problems affecting multiple systems.

Encourage patients to be cooperative and to report details accurately in relating to health care providers. Also, assure them of the right to be treated with earnest interest. Teach them ways to assess care and encourage assertiveness when they are not satisfied. The National Institute on Aging[13] suggests that patients and families consider the following points when selecting or evaluating health care providers:

- Are you comfortable discussing personal concerns, such as sexual and emotional problems, when they are relevant to care?
- Does the health care provider tend to attribute your symptoms or problems to "old age"?
- Does your health care provider take a thorough history, asking you about the health of relatives, an inventory of medicines you use, and other social factors that can affect your health?
- Does your physician seem to prescribe drugs automatically when you think there might be other ways to solve your problems?
- Do you sense that your physician has a long-term commitment to your care and that he or she will continue to treat you even if things become very difficult?

Enhancing Participation in Health-Promotion Activities

There are a number of barriers to health-promotion activities by older patients. The first barrier has to do with the patient's perception of how difficult participation might be, regardless of the possible benefits. Studies have shown that when people think an exercise regimen will be too difficult, they do not try to participate even when they know it could greatly improve their health. On the other hand, people will follow programs that have little benefit if they do not perceive them to be difficult. Although they know that cigarettes are the major cause of premature death and preventable illness in this country, many smokers do not try to stop unless the process is made to seem easy. This implies that, instead of emphasizing the benefits of health promotion programs, we would be more effective if we assessed the patient's perception of its *difficulty* and helped minimize the effect.[14]

Many people are afraid to engage in the mildest physical activity because they fear an accident could cause them catastrophic injury.[15] This fear can also limit opportunities for social activities outside the home. You can help by encouraging them to consider past accidents and those to which they now feel prone. Devise an accident-prevention plan consistent with their physical limitations and fears. For example, if someone has fallen in the past, would special shoes be helpful, or should carpeting be changed? The important thing is to help each person feel safe while he or she is following a health promotion plan.

Another barrier for some elderly people is their hesitation to try new activities, such as organized fitness programs. In some cases, fear of failure is linked to the notion that any display of weakness to care providers may indicate the need for institutionalization. Assure each person that his or her programs will be individualized according to strengths, not weaknesses.

Fear of illness can actually be a barrier to participation in health programs. Fear affects everyone in different and complex ways, and this is particularly true of the elderly with respect to health concerns. Sometimes scare tactics, such as showing pictures of black lung disease to smokers, has an unintended negative effect. People are so frightened of the consequences of their health problem that they deny disease symptoms or the possibility of disease. Research shows that low-intensity teaching programs and gentle, but consistent, encouragement to avoid risks and to practice health-promoting behaviors get the best results.[16]

A fourth barrier is external locus of control. Locus of control describes how much people think they can influence their own lives. People with an internal locus of control tend to believe that their behaviors, such as smoking or eating well-balanced meals, play a large part in determining their health. They are more likely to accept greater personal responsibility for their health and are more apt to engage in health-promoting activities. On the other hand, people with an external locus of control believe that they do not control most situations affecting their health and that illnesses are due primarily to luck or chance. For some people, the locus of control may be impossible to change, and the most positive approach to encouraging healthy behavior is to provide a consistent, low-key message as often as possible.[15]

The optimistic side is that most elderly people want instruction on how to maintain and improve their health, and with encouragement they will participate and enjoy both group and individual health promotion activities.

A PLAN FOR PROMOTING HEALTHY BEHAVIORS

The objective of health promotion is for each person to reach and maintain his or her optimal functioning. This may mean continuing and improving healthy behaviors. It usually entails changing some behaviors—either stopping activities, such as overeating or smoking, or starting others, such as exercising or being more assertive. For most people in the United States, these changes involve replacing one activity with another; for example, instead of watching television each morning, take a short walk. It sounds simple enough, but many habitual patterns have psychosocial aspects that must be considered. It is not unusual for people who give up a risky behavior, such as drinking too much alcohol, to find that they are isolated from friends and social situations that were part of that past behavior. Old drinking buddies may not want to socialize in new ways; they may not even like the new nondrinker. You can help your client avoid isolation by role-playing how a person might anticipate and deal with the reaction of friends to his or her new health practices. Also, direct the person to community support groups if they exist; you might even suggest forming a new support group or club.

To encourage behavior changes, plan your interventions in an organized step-by-step way. The following five steps can be used for diverse health-promotion activities, such as nutrition, exercise, stress management, and cancer self-detection screening.

1. Identify the problem to the patient and explain why it is a problem. Describe its implications, including all the short-term and long-term effects. Identify all behaviors that you think might influence the problem positively and negatively, giving a strong health message to the patient.
2. Determine the patient's readiness to participate in a program of change. Assess his or her past history of compliance with health plans, identifying strengths and weaknesses. Assess available support systems.
3. Develop an intervention plan with the patient that has specific goals and realistic time frames. Provide as much information about the risk and replacement behaviors as you think will be useful.
4. Begin the intervention, giving support to the patient and attention to his or her questions and concerns.
5. Evaluate the patient's success at maintaining health behaviors and eliminating risk behaviors. If successful, evaluate his or her potential sustaining the change over a long period of time. If unsuccessful, reevaluate the plan and start over again or refer the patient for more intensive interventions.

To illustrate, we can use the above steps to plan a smoking-cessation program:

1. Upon learning that a person is a smoker, tell him or her that you feel it is important to quit and that you can help. This may be the most important thing you can do for the patient because most people have never been taught how to quit by a health-care professional. Use a positive approach; tell the person that smoking is the leading cause of preventable hospitalizations and illness. Answer all questions honestly, but be positive. You may need to acknowledge that quitting smoking alone will not extend life, but it can improve the quality of the person's remaining years.

2. Ask the person about previous attempts to quit smoking. Was he or she successful? If so, for how long? What cessation techniques were useful? Why did the person return to smoking? Do significant others smoke? Will significant others assist or thwart cessation efforts?

3. Set a quitting date. Be clear that on the designated date the patient will discard all cigarettes and not smoke. Give the person all the information he or she will need to prepare for possible nicotine withdrawal symptoms: mild exercise might relieve nervousness; drinking extra water helps flush nicotine from the body; substituting low-calorie foods for rich snacks helps prevent weight gain, which might result from a temporary change in body metabolism. The physical withdrawal from nicotine lasts for just 3 to 4 days, although the psychological need to smoke may take months to conquer.

4. Contact the person on the quitting date and make arrangements to be available for support and follow-up as needed. Review progress and response to the withdrawal symptoms. Determine what behaviors are being used to replace smoking and encourage the positive ones, such as breathing exercises or taking short walks. Discourage negative behaviors such as overeating. Assure the person that one slip in the program—such as taking a few puffs from a cigarette—does not constitute total failure, so he or she should immediately restart cessation efforts.

5. If a person does not remain smoke-free, determine what the barriers are. If you feel that the person might be successful at another cessation attempt, suggest another quitting date to restart the program. Otherwise, refer him or her for more intensive treatment, such as group counseling, hypnosis, or medication.

THE ETHICS OF HEALTH PROMOTION

It is likely that research results will continue to support the efficacy of health promotion programs for the elderly aimed at the target behaviors discussed briefly in this chapter. Efforts are already under way to develop and enhance motivation for participation in public and private programs. The field of health promotion is currently receiving scholarly attention, as well as funding. For these reasons, the concept of health promotion raises ethical questions on many levels. Some broad questions should be asked of both researchers and practitioners involved in the care of aged clients. They are questions that each reader should consider, and, as such, they are presented here without answers. The list is by no means complete.

1. It is a fact that many recreation and health-promotion programs started in senior centers are unused and discontinued for various rea-

sons. Is it right to stimulate the interest and initial participation of people in programs that will not be sustained? Or is it just a form of dabbling?

2. Belief systems, locus of control, and religious preference are frequently linked to each other in ways that may support a person's self-esteem. Do we cause psychological injury when we try to promote health behaviors? If so, how? Can we justify such interventions?

3. Some health-risk behaviors may also be important coping behaviors. How do you weigh a person's need to continue risky behavior?

4. Certain cultural norms (such as those of the Gypsy society with regard to overeating) may conflict with desired behavioral outcomes. Are behaviors associated with cultural patterns to be regarded as sacred?

5. Statistics show that it is much cheaper to provide people with health-promotion programs than to pay for future curative care for diseases caused by the American lifestyle. Will there come a time when Americans are mandated by law to practice better health behaviors? Has this process already begun with the proliferation of antismoking laws? Have we begun to place blame on victims of ingrained lifestyle practices? How are values about health practices changing?

6. The passage (1920) and repeal (1933) of the Prohibition Amendment to the Constitution had economic and moral undertones. Can ethical lessons be learned from that experience that would provide perspective for making policy and planning and evaluating health-promotion programs?

REFERENCES

1. DuBois, R: Mirage of Health. Rutgers University Press, New Brunswick, NJ, 1959.
2. McKnight, K: Health in the Medical Era. Perspectives. London, 1982, p. 13.
3. Mechanic, D: From Advocacy to Allocation: The Evolving American Health Care System. Free Press, New York, 1986.
4. Hayflick, L: How and Why We Age. Ballantine Books, New York, 1994.
5. World Health Organization, Geneva, 1974.
6. Ryan, RS and Travis, JW: Wellness Workbook. Ten Speed Press, Berkeley, CA, 1981.
7. Orem, DE: Nursing Concepts of Practice, ed. 3. Mosby, St. Louis, MO, 1990.
8. Roos, NP and Havens, B: Predictors of successful aging: A twelve-year study of Manitoba elderly. Am J Pub Health 81(1):63–68, 1991.
9. Promoting Health/Prevention Disease: Objectives for the Nation. Healthy People: The Surgeon General's Report on Health Promotion and Disease Prevention. U.S. Public Health Service: U.S. Government Printing Office, Washington, DC, 1979.
10. 1990 Health Objectives for the Nation. U.S. Department of Health and Human Services, U.S. Public Health Service: U.S. Government Printing Office, Washington, DC, 1980.
11. Eisenberg, DM, et al.: Unconventional Medicine in the United States. New England J Med 328(4):246–252, 1993.
12. National Institute on Aging: Age Pages. U.S. Government Printing Office, Washington, DC, 1985.

13. Lubkin, IM: Chronic Illness Impact and Intervention, ed. 2. Jones and Bartlett, Boston/London, 1990.
14. Sennott-Miller, L and Miller, J: Difficulty: A neglected factor in health promotion, Nurs Res 36:268–272, 1987.
15. Speake, D: Health promotion activity in the well elderly. Health Values 2(6):29, 1987.
16. Job, RFS: Effective and ineffective use of fear in health promotion campaigns. Am J Pub Health 78:163, 1988.

SECTION THREE

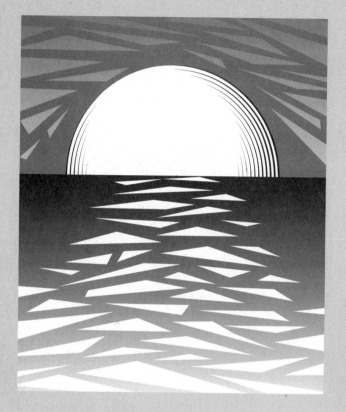

External Aspects
of Aging: The
Current Status

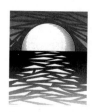

CHAPTER 12

Stress and Aging

Z. Annette Iglarsh, PT, PhD

BEHAVIORAL OBJECTIVES

Upon completion of this chapter, the reader will be able to:

1 Define stress and stressors.
2 Discuss current stress theories.
3 Classify and define types of stressors specific to older persons.
4 Identify coping mechanisms of older persons.
5 Design a treatment protocol for the elderly patient.
6 Select appropriate relaxation techniques for elderly patients.

This chapter serves to redefine many of the concepts presented in this text as stressors in the scheme of the mind-body connection. Stressors are the physiologic, psychologic, and social changes that occur as a person ages and force the individual to modify his or her behavior. These internal or external changes trigger a stress response in the body. Stressors do not commence abruptly with graying hair or menopause but are part of the gradual progression of aging. These changes are complex and may not be as overt as the classic symptoms of disease. Many individuals fear aging and its diseases, but few see it as a phase of great stress.

STRESS AND THE STRESS RESPONSE

Stress is not a new concept. Over 50 years ago, Dr. Hans Selye[1] first identified stress in hospitalized patients and described a mind-body connection. These patients manifested common physiologic and psychologic characteristics regardless of their diagnoses. These characteristics included decreasing appetite, dulling of psychologic affect, and increasing blood pressure. In a series of studies of laboratory rats, Selye[2] found similar physiologic changes in the rats when they were stressed. As a result, Selye[3] defined stress as "the non-specific response of the body to any demand placed upon it" (p. 8). Although researchers[4] disagree with Selye as to the nonspecific quality of the response, there is little dispute as to the physiologic changes caused by stressors. Selye labeled the body's response to these demands the general adaptation syndrome (GAS) (Fig. 12–1). This syndrome consists of three stages: alarm, resistance, and exhaustion. The initial response, the alarm reaction, is a response to sudden exposure to a stressor. The first part of this initial stage, the shock phase, consists of the following physiologic changes: an increase in heart rate and decreases in muscle tone, temperature, and blood pressure.

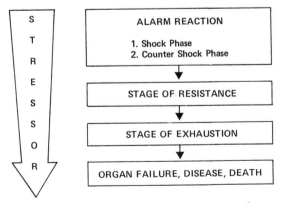

FIGURE 12–1. A schematic illustration of the general adaptation syndrome.

This is followed by the countershock phase, in which the body readies itself to meet the stressor by increasing corticoid hormone secretion. These hormones stimulate organs to increase blood pressure and to make stored energy more readily available. The stage of alarm is analogous to Cannon's fight-or-flight response.[5] In both the alarm stage and the fight-or-flight response, the body prepares either to meet physical harm or to run from the threat. Early researchers thought that the response stopped as soon as the physical threat disappeared. This is not true in modern society, where most of the stressors are psychological. These stressors, which are described later in this chapter, remain in the individual's mind, and therefore the stress response does not abruptly terminate. This sustained response leads to the remaining two stages of Selye's stress-response theory. The second stage, the stage of resistance, involves adaptation. Here the body adjusts organ function to counteract the physiologic changes in response to stress. These adjustments create a new homeostatic level of organ function in the body. In this new state, visible symptoms of stress may actually disappear. However, if the stressor persists, the final stage—the stage of exhaustion—occurs. Here symptoms of physiologic adaptation to stress reappear and the body's responses eventually fail with fatigue and disease. Organ failure and death may result.

The body's physiologic response to stress is summarized and simplified in the diagram of the neuroendocrine pathways (Fig. 12–2).[6] In this neu-

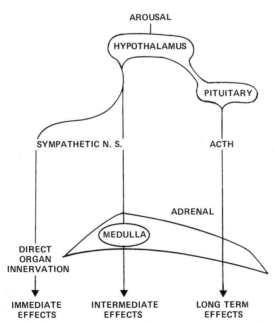

FIGURE 12–2. Neuroendocrine stress response pathways. (From Allen and Hyde,[6] with permission).

roendocrine response, the hypothalamus, a regulator of autonomic nervous system activity, prepares the body to meet stressors via hormone release. These hormones affect organ function and cause retrieval of needed materials from energy stores. These hormones also alter cardiovascular function to redirect blood to organs essential to the stress response and to survive blood loss from possibly injury. Other major physiologic effects of stress are increased secretion of growth hormone, adrenocorticotrophic hormone (ACTH), prolactin, adrenalin, and cortisol; lowered sensitivity to insulin; lowered tolerance to carbohydrates; stimulation of lipolysis and neutralization of fatty acids; hypercholesteremia; and stimulation of thrombus formation.[7] It is ironic that these physiologic reactions, which are lifesaving at the time of the potential threat, can lead to disease if prolonged. The same lifesaving physiologic changes in the body that enable a pedestrian to dart out of the path of a speeding car can be sustained and consequently cause disease. The individual may sustain these physiologic changes each time he or she mentally relives the near-accident when crossing the street or reflecting upon the traumatic event.

Researchers have also studied the physiologic stress response in the elderly. They analyzed the impact of major life stressors such as loss of a significant other or financial crises. Chronic stressors were not studied. The older individuals experienced decreased caloric intake, body weight, and lymphocyte count. Psychological distress and serum cortisol levels increased. These responses to major life stress returned to more normal baseline levels after a recovery period.[7]

Physiologic responses are often thought to occur only with negative stressors. Surprisingly, this is not true. The body responds in equal magnitude to negative and positive stressors.[3] That is, a similar physiologic reaction occurs in the person threatened by a mugger and the fortunate person winning the state lottery. In addition, some level of stress is necessary for effective daily function, that is, simply to maintain a level of attention or cognitive focus.[6] Each person has his or her own point at which this functional stress level becomes destructive. This point varies from moment to moment as environmental conditions and the individual's physical status vary. Many people say that they work better under pressure, but they also speak of the straw that breaks the camel's back. Disease, acute and chronic, can result from this prolonged or excessive stress state.

These diseases can actually be labeled diseases of adaptation[9] and are results of faulty responses to stress. These faulty responses are both excessive or diminished physiologic changes in the stress response. The aging process presents a dual problem to these responses. As a person ages, he or she is exposed to more incidents of stress as a mere function of time and experience, and each exposure leaves its mark and alters the degree of response system failure. The cardiovascular changes of aging vary with each individual. The variable factors include nutrition, smoking or alcohol abuse, and general physical status. Despite these variables, most individuals experience increasing vascular stiffness; increased systolic pulse and mean arterial pressure; and some degree of left ventricular hypertrophy.[10] Selye viewed these two aspects of aging (exposure to more stressors, and the scars of these exposures altering the stress response) as causing a gradual inability to remove the chemical scars of life and the stress response. In addition to the inability to remove these scars (for example, calcium deposits from blood vessels), the loss of irreplaceable tissue (for example, brain and heart tissue damage from microinfarcts or vascular failure) further limits adaptability with aging. A failure to effectively apply coping mechanisms increases the aging person's difficulty in dealing with life stressors.

STRESSORS: THE SOURCE OF STRESS

Researchers have attempted to identify individuals who are more prone to stress responses as they age. Poorly educated women who live alone are in greater jeopardy of physical strain when exposed to stress than individuals who do not manifest these characteristics. These more stress-prone individuals receive social support from very small networks of support. Therefore, they are exposed to limited social contact. Social *support* rather than social *contact* is positively related to stress. In addition, the strongest predictors of distress in these individuals are their state of health and level of independence in activities of daily living.[11] Women are more vulnerable to the effects of *chronic life strain* than to *stressful life events*.[12] The experiences of loss,[13–15] stress of later life, hopelessness, and depression can all lead to increased alcoholism and even suicide. Complications from alcoholism, fatal drug reactions from inappropriate doses of medications, and suicide are all being more frequently identified in the older population.[16]

Because aging is only one part of the entire life cycle, many stressors are not unique to the elderly. Furthermore, experiences may occur as stressors only when they appear in conjunction with normal aging events or physiologic changes. Events that may have heralded independence or maturity in one's youth may become life-threatening stressors in later years. Striking out on one's own, moving, meeting new people, or changes in day-to-day routines are examples of this dichotomy. Stressors are simply life demands that are environmental, physical, achievement-based, and socially oriented.

Environmental stressors are those demands that originate outside the individual's body.[17] These stressors can be as simple as a change in environment; for example, moving into a new home. In one's youth, this can be an exciting event; however, it can be a trauma for the older individual, especially if the move is determined by need or circumstance, not by choice. A loss of personal and familiar surroundings, separation from supportive friends, and change in daily routine may result from a change in location.

Increases in disease vulnerability or occurrence and mental disorientation may also result.[18] Health professionals are very familiar with the independently functional patient who cannot perform simple activities of daily life when hospitalized or admitted to a nursing home. The family who moves the aging parent into their home to care for the parent or the family that moves in with the older parent because neither can exist independently in difficult economic times may be creating more stressful or stress-potential situations than they realize. Crowding is another form of environmental stress that can lead to alienation and increased paranoia. This stressor is often encountered by people in urban areas and dwellers in high-rise apartment buildings.[19] A change in environment and overcrowding expose the aging individual to a large number of new stimuli. Unfortunately, the elderly person must cope with this barrage of stressors with an aging and decreasingly effective stress-control response. This is further exemplified by the older individual's response to physical stressors.

Stressors that originate within the body are classified as physical stressors. Fatigue, chronic illness, and failure of organ systems are common examples of these physical stressors.[20–24] Because dulling or decreased sensory integration capabilities, as well as diminished reception ability of the five senses, alter perception of stressors, the older person is prone to this category of stressors. The elderly individual may have distorted and often incorrect information, resulting in inaccurate assessment of the environment. Once again, the normal consequences of aging compound the physiologic effects of stressors; in this case, they alter the stress response at its earliest phase, perception. The entire neuroendocrine response system actually functions less effectively with aging.[25] An example of this deficit is the disruption of the neuroendocrine feedback system, the hypothalamic-pituitary response to hormonal feedback, which creates an additional burden to the stress-response system. Researchers[26,27] also show that repeated exposure to physical stressors can actually hasten aging. Conversely, the lack or limited exposure to physical stressors[28] can contribute to greater longevity or a slowing of the aging process.[29]

In an industrialized society, achievement-based stressors are numerous and the most subtle types of stressors. These stressors tend to be characterized by the individual's personality. The type A individual common to this society has been described by Rosenman and Friedman[30] as one who is:

1. Time urgent (time-conscious, deadline-oriented, impatient)
2. Quantitative (describes things in terms of numbers)
3. Polyphasic (does more than one activity at a time)
4. Competitive
5. Tense

As physical and possibly cognitive abilities diminish, the goal-oriented type A individual will not be able to achieve the goals on which he or she bases his or her value and self-worth.[31] Type A individuals do not change their ways but find themselves more frustrated. It is necessary for the older individual to reevaluate personal expectations; youthful goals may go unaccomplished. Sacrifices chosen for personal advancement in earlier years may be questioned as to their long-term value. Family, marriages, and relationships neglected to allow time and energy for personal professional growth may have suffered. They may not be viable social units when the individual finally has the time to assume these social responsibilities. Reinforcement that formerly came from the work environment must now be redesigned to maintain a sense of identity.

Often overlapping the achievement-based stressors are social stressors. As the husband finds time to direct attention to the family, he often finds his children moving away and his wife focusing more time on career development. Our transient society has weakened social bonds, such as the ones between growing children and aging parents. These weakened relationships become social stressors as adult children may be forced to move in with parents when they become unemployed or divorced, or when they live beyond their earnings. These social stressors also occur in reverse when aging parents move in with their adult children. This occurs when health impairs ability to function independently or when retirement financial plans are not sufficient to succeed in times of inflation. An opposite experience, the absence of social interaction, can be as stressful as excessive social relationships. Loneliness, a common social stressor, has also been correlated to a greater incidence of disease and high death rates.[32-34] Significant loss, especially of a loved one, has even caused sudden death, a severe stress response, as described in the giving-up syndrome.[35,36]

Retirement, often a long-awaited event, can be a harmful social stressor to many individuals.[9] Physical illness and premature organic brain syndrome can occur when an individual adjusts poorly to retirement. This occurs with such frequency that it has been labeled as "retirement disease." Retirement forces changes in an individual's relationship to his or her environment and the perception of his or her role in society. Consequently, the individual may face a change in personal income, potential for altered health as physical activity levels usually decrease, and lack of a daily schedule with a greater amount of free time.[37] Each of these major changes in the life of a retired person is a stressor. It is easy to see that the additive and interactive effects of these stressors can be overpowering and thus life-threatening for the aging individual.

All of the aforementioned stressors can also be categorized as life events. Holmes, Rahe, and Masuda[38-40] compiled a list of life events (Fig. 12–3) that stress an individual both positively and negatively. The numeric score attributed to the accumulation of the individual's life events over the preceding 24 months (some researchers and therapists use a 12-month period) will aid the therapist in identifying the person as prone to illness, acute or chronic (Figs. 12–4 and 12–5). Many of these identified sources of stress are com-

LIFE EVENT SCALE

Sex: ___F___   Age: ___68___

Score		Event
(100)		Death of spouse
(77)		Divorce
(65)		Marital separation
(63)		Jail term
(63)		Death of close family member
(53)	x	Personal injury or illness
(50)		Marriage
(47)		Fired from work
(45)		Marital reconciliation
(45)		Retirement
(44)		Change in family member's health
(40)		Pregnancy
(39)		Sex difficulties
(39)		Addition to family
(39)		Business readjustment
(38)		Change in financial status
(37)		Death of close friend
(36)		Change to different line of work
(35)		Change in number of marital arguments
(31)		Mortgage or loan over $10,000
(30)		Foreclosure of mortgage or loan
(29)		Change in work responsibilities
(29)		Son or daughter leaving home
(29)		Trouble with in-laws
(28)		Outstanding personal achievement
(26)	x	Spouse begins or stops work
(26)		Starting or finishing school
(25)		Change in living conditions
(24)		Revision of personal habits
(23)		Trouble with boss
(20)		Change in work hours, conditions
(20)		Change in residence
(20)		Change in schools
(19)		Change in recreational habits
(19)		Change in church activities
(18)		Change in social activities
(17)		Mortgage or loan under $10,000
(16)		Change in sleeping habits
(15)		Change in number of family gatherings
(15)		Change in eating habits
(13)	x	Vacation
(12)		Christmas season
(11)		Minor violation of the law

Score: ___92___   Stress Level: ___Mild___

FIGURE 12–3. Holmes and Rahe Life Event Scale showing score of individual experiencing mild life-event stressors.

LIFE EVENT SCALE

Sex: ___M___   Age: ___60___

(100)	x	Death of spouse
(77)		Divorce
(65)		Marital separation
(63)		Jail term
(63)		Death of close family member
(53)	x	Personal injury or illness
(50)		Marriage
(47)		Fired from work
(45)		Marital reconciliation
(45)		Retirement
(44)		Change in family member's health
(40)		Pregnancy
(39)		Sex difficulties
(39)		Addition to family
(39)		Business readjustment
(38)		Change in financial status
(37)		Death of close friend
(36)		Change to different line of work
(35)		Change in number of marital arguments
(31)	x	Mortgage or loan over $10,000
(30)		Foreclosure of mortgage or loan
(29)		Change in work responsibilities
(29)	x	Son or daughter leaving home
(29)		Trouble with in-laws
(28)		Outstanding personal achievement
(26)		Spouse begins or stops work
(26)		Starting or finishing school
(25)		Change in living conditions
(24)	x	Revision of personal habits
(23)		Trouble with boss
(20)		Change in work hours, conditions
(20)		Change in residence
(20)		Change in schools
(19)		Change in recreational habits
(19)		Change in church activities
(18)	x	Change in social activities
(17)		Mortgage or loan under $10,000
(16)		Change in sleeping habits
(15)		Change in number of family gatherings
(15)		Change in eating habits
(13)		Vacation
(12)	x	Christmas season
(11)		Minor violation of the law

Score: ___267___   Stress Level: ___Moderate___

FIGURE 12–4. Holmes and Rahe Life Event Scale showing score of individual experiencing moderate life-event stressors.

LIFE EVENT SCALE

Sex: ___F___   Age: ___70___

(100)		Death of spouse
(77)		Divorce
(65)	x	Marital separation
(63)		Jail term
(63)		Death of close family member
(53)	x	Personal injury or illness
(50)		Marriage
(47)		Fired from work
(45)		Marital reconciliation
(45)		Retirement
(44)		Change in family member's health
(40)		Pregnancy
(39)	x	Sex difficulties
(39)		Addition to family
(39)		Business readjustment
(38)	x	Change in financial status
(37)	x	Death of close friend
(36)		Change to different line of work
(35)	x	Change in number of marital arguments
(31)		Mortgage or loan over $10,000
(30)		Foreclosure of mortgage or loan
(29)		Change in work responsibilities
(29)		Son or daughter leaving home
(29)		Trouble with in-laws
(28)		Outstanding personal achievement
(26)		Spouse begins or stops work
(26)		Starting or finishing school
(25)	x	Change in living conditions
(24)	x	Revision of personal habits
(23)		Trouble with boss
(20)		Change in work hours, conditions
(20)	x	Change in residence
(20)		Change in schools
(19)	x	Change in recreational habits
(19)	x	Change in church activities
(18)	x	Change in social activities
(17)	x	Mortgage or loan under $10,000
(16)		Change in sleeping habits
(15)	x	Change in number of family gatherings
(15)	x	Change in eating habits
(13)		Vacation
(12)	x	Christmas season
(11)		Minor violation of the law

Score: ___451___   Stress Level: ___Excessive___

FIGURE 12–5. Holmes and Rahe Life Event Scale showing score of individual experiencing excessive life-event stressors.

mon events of the life cycle: mortgage, marriage, death or loss of spouse, change in residence, and so forth. As a function of time, the older individual will accumulate a large number of stressful events. Consequently, the older individual will compile a higher score on the Holmes and Rahe Life Event Scale and thus be more likely to suffer from stress-related illness (Fig. 12–6).

More recently, researchers have further categorized stressors as major life stressors, chronic stressors or chronic life strain, and hassles. Major life stressors for elderly individuals may be loss of friends or family members or loss of their identity (retirement); chronic stressors may include financial limitations or failing physical ability. Chronic stressors are highly correlated with depression.[41] The final stressor category, heated, protracted, arguments or hassles, involves minor stressors that are actually the most effective predictors of health status and physiologic response to stress.[42] In fact, individuals who consider their own health to be poor report that they experience more hassles. Appropriately, most of these reported conflicts were related to physical status.[43]

COPING MECHANISMS AND ADJUSTMENT TO THE STRESSORS OF AGING

People respond to stressful life events with different coping mechanisms. They often retreat to former or more immature coping mechanisms in the face of overpowering forces.[44] Common coping mechanisms are regression, conversion, denial, projection, and repression. Sigmund Freud listed examples of forces that may trigger these coping mechanisms as death of a loved one, separation, ill health, threatened body integrity (real or imagined), decreased cerebral and physiologic functioning, and environmental deprivation (owing to retirement or loss of money). Lowered sense of personal worth and loss of identity can lead to altered reality-testing ability, regression in behavior, and revival of infantile concerns. Health professionals are intimately aware of these changes in some elderly patients, especially those seen in nursing homes or retirement settings. As you read this paragraph, many of you have nodded as you remembered your patient who clung to her deceased husband's pipe (transitional object) as she wheeled around your clinic or another patient who became noncompliant in a treatment session because you were unable to begin the treatment session at the precise time it was scheduled.

There is great variability in the way people adapt to aging. Therefore, generalization or identification of an ideal lifestyle is not possible. However, by using common sense, you can formulate some basic, positive suggestions for an optimal lifestyle for the aging individual. Activity is obviously important, although the level may be limited to some degree by the physical re-

LIFE EVENT SCALE

Sex: ___M___   Age: ___80___

(100)		Death of spouse
(77)	x	Divorce
(65)		Marital separation
(63)		Jail term
(63)	x	Death of close family member
(53)	x	Personal injury or illness
(50)	x	Marriage
(47)		Fired from work
(45)		Marital reconciliation
(45)		Retirement
(44)		Change in family member's health
(40)		Pregnancy
(39)	x	Sex difficulties
(39)	x	Addition to family
(39)		Business readjustment
(38)	x	Change in financial status
(37)	x	Death of close friend
(36)		Change to different line of work
(35)	x	Change in number of marital arguments
(31)		Mortgage or loan over $10,000
(30)	x	Foreclosure of mortgage or loan
(29)		Change in work responsibilities
(29)	x	Son or daughter leaving home
(29)	x	Trouble with in-laws
(28)		Outstanding personal achievement
(26)	x	Spouse begins or stops work
(26)		Starting or finishing school
(25)	x	Change in living conditions
(24)	x	Revision of personal habits
(23)		Trouble with boss
(20)		Change in work hours, conditions
(20)	x	Change in residence
(20)		Change in schools
(19)	x	Change in recreational habits
(19)	x	Change in church activities
(18)	x	Change in social activities
(17)		Mortgage or loan under $10,000
(16)	x	Change in sleeping habits
(15)	x	Change in number of family gatherings
(15)	x	Change in eating habits
(13)	x	Vacation
(12)	x	Christmas season
(11)		Minor violation of the law

Score: ___741___   Stress Level: ___Excessive___

FIGURE 12–6. Holmes and Rahe Life Event Scale showing score of individual experiencing excessive life-event stressors. This individual is likely to suffer from stress-related illness.

strictions of aging. A positive, supportive social setting is also important. The individual should appropriately modify personal expectations and reflections of self. A comfortable but structured schedule is needed. The schedule should be subject to change but instituted to promote continued activity. As at any stage in life, planning or creation of a secure financial status[45] will reduce life's stressors to some extent.

Researchers[46] recommend the adoption of a pet. Pets can serve as transitional objects.[47] Researchers have also found that a pet dog can cause a subject to respond with less anxiety in a stressful environment[48,49] and that touching a pet can act as an antianxiety agent.[46] Pets also further reduce stress by directing the individual's attention away from stressful thoughts and forcing the individual to maintain a daily routine, often lacking in the retired individual.

To analyze appropriately methods to modify the lifestyle of the aging individual positively, strategies to adapt to retirement must also be considered. The individual should attempt to minimize the number and magnitude of changes that occur with retirement. Cultivating nonwork, leisure activities and early transition to the retirement income level are examples of this suggestion. The retirement process should be gradual, beginning with a reduction in the work week rather than a handshake and being "shown the door" on the last day. The retiring individual should attempt to participate in the retirement decisions rather than be the "victim of the deed." It would help if the individual decided the date of retirement and the retirement process. Individuals should plan their income and know their health (and how to maximize their physical abilities by such strategies as pacing physical activity and eating balanced diets). Involvement with other individuals who are retired and facing similar situations will help minimize loneliness, maintain identity, and solve some of the problems of experiences in this new lifestyle. Planning, positive attitudes toward retirement, successful experiences dealing with change, and flexibility will also contribute to a successful, healthy, and low-stress retirement.[37]

A single, close support figure can give an aging individual a sense of well-being.[50] Consequently, when an elderly person experiences high stress, he or she will be less likely to visit a physician if he or she has strong social support.[51] Strong social support increases the person's internal locus of control (the belief that control of one's state of life lies within the individual) and feelings of control. Social support improves the person's sense of personal control to a threshold level. Beyond this level, the individual may actually sense a loss of personal control.[52] People manifesting extremes of internal and external loci of control (the belief that external forces control one's life) are more vulnerable to the negative effects of life stress. Although internal locus of control is more effective when responding to stressful events, people who exhibit the extreme of this behavior often use avoidance to deal with certain stressors.[53] Avoidance is also a coping mechanism common to depressed individuals.[54]

STRESS MANAGEMENT IN THE CLINICAL SETTING

Establishing a Treatment Regimen

These suggestions for a maximal lifestyle and effective retirement will benefit the active, independent, aging individual. But how can you help the ill, dependent, aging individual being wheeled into your clinic for treatment? The aging patient experiencing stress will benefit from the following treatment sequence:

1. Identify major stressors; evaluate the stressors and determine whether the problems are within your capabilities or if it is more appropriate to refer the patient to another practitioner.
2. Identify and analyze the person's coping or adaptive mechanisms.
3. Instruct the patient in stress and stress-management theories.
4. Select and instruct the patient in the appropriate stress-management theory.

Identification of Stressors

Evaluation of stressors begins with a comprehensive intake interview with the patient and the patient's family members, if appropriate. Identify environmental (description of home setting and daily environment), physical (medical history and a review of current symptoms and health status), achievement-based (personal expectations and accomplishments), and social (marital status and interfamily relationships) stressors. If they feel comfortable with their interviewer, patients will often clearly outline their stressors, Listen with an open mind. This will enable the therapist to hear the patient self-diagnose his or her stress problems. The use of standardized tests, such as the Holmes and Rahe Life Event Scale,[38] Minnesota Multiphasic Personality Inventory,[55] and the Cornell Medical Index,[56] can assist the health professional in identifying a patient's stressors if the patient is not communicating effectively. After analyzing the patient's intake and test data, the therapist can decide whether he or she can treat the patient effectively for stress management in conjunction with the therapy regimen or if a referral to a psychologist, psychiatrist, or social worker is more appropriate. For example, a person with severe personality disorders would be treated most successfully by a psychiatrist, and a person requiring a new residence modified for nonambulatory people would best be served by a social worker. Multiprofessional treatment approaches to stress management can be most effective, giving the patient the strength of each discipline. Communication among the professionals and the patient becomes more complex but also more integral to treatment success.

Identification of Coping Mechanisms

Once the stressors are identified, the next step is to identify the individual's current coping mechanism for each stressor or group of stressors.

Has the individual chosen an effective or destructive coping mechanism? Is the patient aware of the stressor and the effects of the coping mechanism being used? Not all mechanisms selected are negative. Sometimes an infantile mechanism can shield an individual from a stressor until a time at which that person is better able to deal with it. Your patient may primp each day for a visit from her husband who died a few weeks ago; another patient may "bargain" to live until a grandson's wedding day and apparently maintain his health status until that day but die soon after; and yet another patient refuses instruction in the use of assistive devices because he claims he is not going to need them when he recovers from his flaccid paralysis after a massive cerebral vascular accident. Each stressor, despite the coping mechanism utilized, must be dealt with at some time because it may cause a subliminal stress response.

Instruction in Stress and Stress-Management Theory

Identification of the stressor has limited value to the health professional unless the patient is aware of its existence. The patient will respond more effectively if he or she shares in the responsibility of recognizing and evaluating the coping mechanism being utilized and subsequently designing the treatment strategy. If the therapist identifies the patient's fear of financial uncertainty as a stressor but the patient repeatedly smiles and proudly states that her husband left her secure and free from want or concern, the therapist's treatment is rendered ineffective. It is obvious from this example that the patient is not aware of her stressor because of her denial. It is important to teach the patient responsibility for self, the existence of the mind-body connection, and the potential for modification of this mind-body connection in a positive manner to learn to relax at will or need. The practitioner can implement this goal by definition of stress terminology, graphic representations of the mind-body connection, and simplified relaxation experiences (for example, a slowed breathing pattern will allow the person to feel less tense and more in control of a physiologic parameter, respiration). If the patient is interested in additional information, refer the patient to selections from this chapter's bibliography or to less academic articles, which often appear in popular magazines. This patient involvement will extend beyond the clinical settings, beyond the length of the treatment program, and into the patient's day-to-day life experiences.

Relaxation Techniques

Once the coping mechanism is identified, the health professional and the patient can select the appropriate relaxation technique. A common-sense approach should be used when selecting the appropriate relaxation techniques. The therapist's comfort with the techniques, the patient's personality, the patient's specific stress problem, and the environment in which the technique will occur should all be considered. There is an endless list of techniques and combinations of techniques from which to choose. Some of these are:

- Meditation
- Progressive relaxation
- Selected awareness: hypnosis, autogenic training, and guided imagery
- Biofeedback
- Breath control
- Systematic desensitization
- Exercise or physical activity

Meditation

Meditation is described as the focusing and maintaining of awareness on a repetitive or unchanging stimulus.[6] It is a combination of a physiologic state, a psychologic feeling, a philosophy, a religious technique, and a state of mind. Meditation is not successful for all people, but it does help all people to varying degrees. It originated in Eastern culture, and in this country had been associated with cults and movements popular during the 1960s and 1970s. Consequently, this technique is often rejected by the older population. However, if the therapist selects a comfortable or familiar object of meditation, such as the internal object of the patient's own breathing or an external object such as a picture of a grandchild or the sound of a number, the patient may be more accepting of this technique. Taking a moment to discuss which object of focus would allow the aging patient to feel most comfortable may help the patient accept this technique. The aging patient may prefer a sitting or reclining posture in a quiet, secluded environment. Meditation is an effective relaxation technique because it induces a relaxation response,[57] which produces a physiologic state opposite to the physiologic changes of the stress response, and reduces somatic organ arousal.[58]

Progressive Relaxation

Progressive relaxation is a technique classically taught in most physical and occupational therapy programs. It was developed by E. Jacobson[59] and is intended to induce deep muscle relaxation. It is helpful for some people because it allows the subject to feel muscle tension. It is a good technique for type A people because they can compete with themselves in their ability to maintain relaxation while tensing another part of their body. It is also an effective technique for subjects with good body awareness, such as athletes and dancers, because they can easily recognize tension and fatigue in muscles. The technique is a combination of 5 seconds of tension and 45 seconds of gradual relaxation in a series of muscle groups. The therapist instructs the patients (individually or in small groups) to begin contracting the agonist muscles, followed by contracting the antagonist muscle groups (for example, contraction and relaxation of the biceps is followed by contraction and relaxation of the triceps). The entire sequence begins at the head and progresses downward or begins at the toes and progresses to the head and neck area. Once the technique is learned, the patient can recognize parts of the body that are tense, and then can progress to relaxation of these areas without tensing all the muscle groups of the body in sequence. This technique is often well accepted by the geriatric population because it clearly consists of a descriptive task followed by a physical action.

Selected Awareness

Selected awareness utilizes the biologic limitations of people to respond to a limited number of stimuli at one time.[6] Normally, the individual perceives and appraises the most threatening or interesting stimuli in the environment, which contains an endless number of stimuli. The therapist can direct the patient to perceive selected stimuli to induce a state of relaxation. Hypnosis, autogenic training, and guided imagery are all types of selected awareness techniques.

During hypnosis, the therapist creates a relaxed atmosphere by giving the subject a mental task or a repetitive stimulus. Both activities will alter perception. The hypnotist restricts the subject's awareness and then focuses the awareness on a mental image. In addition, the hypnotist tells the subject what he or she will be feeling—overt physiologic changes in the relaxation response—to build credibility and trusting rapport. Once the patient has successfully experienced a hypnotic state, he or she can be instructed to reproduce the state without the presence of the hypnotist.[60]

Autogenic training is similar to hypnosis in its utilization of a therapist who directs attention. However, unlike hypnosis, the focus is on the patient's physiologic function. The patient concentrates on the sensations of the relaxation response. The patient is taught how the body is altered in the relaxation response and then tries to create those changes by imagining sensations such as warmth or heaviness.[61] This technique increases the effectiveness of progressive neuromuscular relaxation and biofeedback.

In another selected-awareness technique, guided imagery, the focus is on the subject's imagination. The therapist asks the patient to concentrate and to visualize a place, real or imagined, that helps the patient feel relaxed. The place can be exotic and foreign or a quiet, private room at home. The feeling of relaxation attained and the image can be reproduced by the patient as needed. This technique is often very difficult for the type A patient and may be rejected as a time waster. To overcome this problem, the therapist can establish a contract with the patient. Two possible strategies are (1) asking the patient to perform the technique for a very short period of time— 5 minutes—which can be extended as patient comfort increases with successful relaxation experiences, and (2) by acknowledging to the patient that the therapist is aware of the patient's potential difficulty in relaxing and asking for the patient's cooperation in spite of this difficulty.

Biofeedback

Biofeedback is a much more overt form of relaxation therapy than those discussed as examples of selected awareness. In biofeedback, the individual receives information on the dynamic state of several possible physiologic functions to help gain control over that function.[62] These functions range from muscle tension to heart rate and blood pressure. Allied health professionals use electromyography (EMG) (muscle tension) biofeedback to reeducate muscle function impaired by disease or trauma. Electromyogram biofeedback can also be used to induce general muscle tension, reducing the muscle tension secondary to the stress response. In all types of biofeedback, a device is used as a transducer, converting a physical state into a monitorable mode via oscilloscope, audio signal, or digital readout. Once the physical state is perceived by the patient, the patient can then alter it into the desired physiologic response. In many settings, mechanical devices are not available, but biofeedback need not be ignored. By holding a patient's hand, you can monitor changes in hand temperature. By palpating a patient's upper trapezius or other areas of muscle spasm, you can perceive the changing levels of muscle tension that can be verbally relayed to the patient.

The preceding techniques can be conducted by the therapist or by using a recorded tape. Researchers[63] have found that the therapist's live voice is a more effective tool, but a tape is appropriate for homework sessions and for use in sessions once the patient is familiar with the technique. The elderly patient may be intimidated by the operation of the tape recorder, and detailed instruction may be necessary. The patient should be able to choose from a variety of voices (both male and female) because some may be more conducive to relaxation for the individual than others. The therapist should try to listen to the content, as well as to experience each tape. Some tapes will contain phrases and approaches to relaxation that will be more appealing than others. Asking an elderly patient to let the abdominal muscle "sag and feel flabby" or to try "to be mellow" may be inappropriate.

Breath Control

A simple, non-device-oriented technique is breath control. This is an essential feature of yoga instruction and can be simple or complex. An individual can be trained to breathe in different levels of the lungs, to modify the timing or rhythm of the breath, or to alternate the nostril utilized.[64] A simple modification of the breathing pattern—elongation of the expiration phase of the breath—will promote relaxation. Prolongation of the momentary pause between the inhalation and exhalation will allow the patient to feel in control of the breath and thus more in control of the self. Often the patient can be taught to think of something positive, relaxing, or encouraging during the pause. This simple technique allows the patient quickly to gain control of a physiologic parameter—respiratory rate—which will induce a greater feeling of relaxation. Modification of breathing patterns can also be used with other relaxation techniques, such as progressive neuromuscular relaxation or biofeedback.

Systematic Desensitization

Systemic desensitization is actually a problem-solving strategy.[65] In this technique, the patient is asked to write down a list of personal problems, fears, or stressors (Fig. 12–7). The list is then rewritten in order of subjective magnitude of difficulty, beginning with the least stressful item. Once the list is formulated, the patient is asked to solve those stressors with feasible solutions. The stressors remaining are dealt with by utilizing any of the previously described relaxation techniques, beginning with the least-threatening unsolved item. Once this item can be thought of without producing a stress response, the individual can move on to the next, more difficult item. By utilizing this technique, the patient has productively dealt with some of his or her problems and can think about the unsolvable problems without inducing a stress response. The patient usually feels a sense of accomplishment and control over the self. These are rare achievements in elderly individuals, who often feel a loss of independence and self-determination.

Exercise or Other Physical Activity

The final relaxation technique is an activity that researchers only recently have identified as a stress-reducing event.[66,67] Exercise has always been recommended as an activity to improve and to maintain general body function, with special emphasis on the cardiopulmonary system.[68] Physical exercise removes the metabolic by-products of stress, minimizes response to new stressors, and gives the individual a sense of well-being.[66] However, these positive effects will occur only if the physical activity is noncompetitive, because competitive activity itself can be a stressor. This relaxation technique should not be ignored when treating elderly patients. Many individuals who have been active throughout their lives continue this lifestyle as they age. This is exemplified by the number of retirees who complete the Boston Marathon each year. Obviously, the majority of the patients are not silver-haired marathon runners, but what about walkers, bikers, and dancers? A clinician[68] has found that rhythmic movements performed by wheelchair patients stimulate cardiovascular function and induce a pleasant relaxation state. Physical activity performed in small groups can accomplish

A. *Problem List*
money
loneliness
sad, depressed
general aches and pains
scared to go out alone
fear of falling
fear of dying
can't handle my bank statement
don't like to eat alone
can't sleep well

B. *Organized Problem List*
1. don't like to eat alone
2. can't handle my bank statement
3. can't sleep well
4. scared to go out alone
5. fear of falling
6. fear of dying
7. general aches and pains
8. sad, depressed
9. money
10. loneliness

C. *Possible Solutions*
1. don't like to eat alone: Join an organized eat-together program or simply arrange to eat with friends on a frequent basis.
2. can't handle bank statement: Ask a friend or your bank's manager for assistance.
*3. can't sleep well: Maintain some activity level during the day, limit daytime naps, and practice relaxation just before going to sleep.
*4. scared to go out alone: Arrange walks and shopping trips with friends, join organized community activities, and follow police suggestions to maximize safety.
*5. fear of falling: Use adaptive devices (glasses or care) as needed; limit travel in inclement weather; when walking, concentrate on foot placement and potential obstacles.
*6. fear of dying: Join discussions with friends, community groups, and religious counseling sessions.
*7. general aches and pains: Schedule a complete physical with a physician and maintain an activity level but do not overdo it.
*8. sad, depressed: Participate in counseling sessions, keep busy.
*9. money limitations: Watch for sales, participate in community and government support programs as needed, and get investment counseling.
*10. loneliness: Participate in community activities and get a pet.

*The starred items have solutions to some degree, but the individual must use relaxation strategies to minimize the residual stressor effects to safer (non-disease-prone) physiologic levels.

FIGURE 12–7. Outline of the systematic desensitization process.

relaxation as well as socialization. As with any event of therapist-patient interaction, the therapist's enthusiasm for the activity is essential and will encourage greater patient involvement.

The following outline may assist the therapist and the patient in choosing one of these relaxation techniques:

1. Meditation
   a. General relaxation technique.
   b. Easier to learn in quiet environments.
   c. When teaching older patients, consider minimizing the training techniques so that patients do not feel out of place doing extroverted or faddish-seeming things.
   d. Example of effective application: The patient is anxious about living with his or her children but is unable to live alone and must learn to relax in his or her stressful environment.
2. Progressive relaxation
   a. Can be general or specific technique.
   b. Good to replace maladaptive behavior (such as overeating).
   c. Good for patients with good body awareness.
   d. Good for type A person—relaxation becomes goal.
   e. Example of effective application: The patient is recently retired and finds himself or herself feeling tense in non-goal-oriented routine.
3. Selected awareness
   a. Can be general or specific technique.
   b. Select approach based on therapist's or patient's comfort.
   c. May need to convince the patient of the value of such a cognitive technique.
   d. Example of effective application: The patient has rheumatoid arthritis and would benefit from directing thoughts away from his or her painful joint condition.
4. Biofeedback
   a. Type selected depends on patient problem and equipment available.
   b. Can be general or specific.
   c. Train patient to the equipment and then wean the patient so that he or she can relax without the monitoring device.
   d. Often the devices and gadgets motivate the patient.
   e. Patient must be capable of monitoring the physiologic event and capable of altering the physiologic state (neurologic cognitive abilities).
   f. Example of effective application: The patient suffers from muscle tension headaches and has intact cognitive ability.
5. Breath control
   a. Can be used with other techniques.

    b. Can be used as an immediate stress-intervention technique without anyone else being aware of its being used.

    c. Allows the patient to regain control over a physiologic function when the patient may feel he or she is losing control of self.

    d. Example of effective application: The patient is overwhelmed by the concept of learning how to relax and needs to feel quick reduction of tension and control of self.

6. Systematic desensitization

    a. Should be used formally or informally with all patients.

    b. Promotes use of more productive coping mechanisms.

    c. Example of effective application: See Figure 12–7.

7. Exercise

    a. Extent of utilization will depend on patient status, but creative thought will allow the therapist to apply it to all patients in varying degrees.

    b. Group teaching and musical accompaniment promote more effective patient involvement.

    c. Group activities may reduce social stressors.

    d. One example of effective application: A group of physically capable but physically uninvolved women would benefit from an early-morning brisk walking activity.

The therapist will be able to select an appropriate relaxation treatment for any patient from the previous list of stress-management techniques. However, the therapist should not apply these techniques without the same prudent judgment that would be used when applying a more traditional clinical modality. The therapist should analyze the effect of relaxation therapy on the patient's physiologic status, which is altered by normal aging and disease states. What will be the effect of altered blood pressure, heart rate, respiratory rate and depth, oxygen consumption, and blood content (glucose and hormone levels)[6] on the patient's physical condition? Patients with diagnoses such as hypertension, hypotension, diabetes,[69] hypoglycemia, and epilepsy should be evaluated by their physician before relaxation therapy begins and then monitored periodically by their physician as relaxation therapy continues. In addition, the therapist should have the patient describe any changes in physiologic status during, after, and between treatment sessions. Including these descriptions with the objective data from EMG biofeedback, thermometer, or blood pressure devices in the patient's records is essential for treatment documentation.

Instruction in relaxation techniques for outpatients follows a simple progression. Each series should begin with the patient's being instructed in stress, the mind-body connection, and the relaxation technique. The therapist should familiarize the patient with the technique, the environment, and any devices that will be used. The sessions begin with close patient-therapist interaction. Homework or patient assignments should be given after each session and reviewed at the beginning of each new session. These assignments range from keeping a stress diary to practicing the techniques using tapes supplied by the therapist. Accordingly, these assignments will reinforce the training sessions and encourage the patient to use the techniques in daily activities. Training sessions continue until the patient approaches a level of relaxation below which he or she can no longer reduce tension: the relaxation potential. At that time, the therapist begins to spend less time with the patient during the session and allows the patient to perform the techniques independently. As the series comes to a close after 5 to 7 weeks, the patient and therapist should discuss training termination and future patient responsibilities. Patients appear to be more compliant with the relaxation program if periodic return visits are conducted to evaluate patients' ongoing competence at controlling stress. This training sequence can be carried out in conjunction with standard therapy treatment and can be integrated into treatment regimens.

You may be even more effective using relaxation therapy with your inpatients. Fortunately, unnecessary stressors in the inpatient setting can be reduced, and the inpatient may have greater opportunity for relaxation therapy practice in this structured setting. All the patient's caregivers should be involved in stress identification and reduction of stressors with the patient. Inasmuch as health professionals may be stressors or "stress inducers" as well as "stress reducers," helping the patient recognize his or her stressors may inadvertently reveal to the caregiver that person's role as stressor. The caregivers can encourage the patient to practice the relaxation techniques and positively reinforce the patient's control of stress throughout the day if they are knowledgeable about stress theory. Small-group in-service presentations on relaxation principles will help the health professional assist the patient to manage stress and give the caretaker insight into his or her stress status.

An additional benefit of relaxation exists for the therapist. In order to teach relaxation to others, the therapist also must relax prior to the instructional session and will feel more relaxed as the relaxation session progresses. This positive aspect of relaxation therapy can make these sessions the highlight of the working day and can also reduce professional burnout.[70]

SUMMARY

This chapter has given the therapist an added responsibility in the course of clinical practice. Stress and stress-management theories are appropriate concerns of therapists treating the older patient for physical dysfunction and the associated psychophysiologic problems or complications. It challenges the therapist to look beyond the patient's loss of motion or disruption of cognitive function to identify the patient's stressors. Once the stressors are identified, the therapist can refer to other appropriate members of the health care team for solutions to or treatment of these stressors. Concurrently, the therapist educates the patient about his or her stress status and teaches the patient stress-control techniques. These new treatment modalities should not be thought of as added techniques but as complementary techniques that treat the whole patient. This will dramatically add to the therapist's treatment effectiveness and thus improve the elderly patient's prognosis. In addition, the therapist may discover a new dimension to the aging patient: a patient experiencing the stressors of a lifetime.

To cope with these stressors of a lifetime, Selye[9] formulated a "code of behavior . . . to minimize distress and maximize eustress" (functional stress):

1. Find your natural stress level.
2. "Altruistic egoism . . . love of our neighbor is the most efficient way to give vent to our pent-up energy and create enjoyable, beautiful or useful things."
3. "Earn they neighbor's love."
4. "Fight for your highest attainable aim, but do not put up resistance in vain." (p. 93)

These final concepts should cultivate further your thoughts regarding stress and your aging patients. They are concepts related to patient care but can also be generalized to enhance the quality of your life and your patient's life.

REFERENCES

1. Selye, H: A syndrome produced by diverse nocuous agents. Nature 138:32, 1936.
2. Selye, H: Stress and aging. Geriatr Soc 18:9, 1970.
3. Selye, H: The Stress of Life. McGraw-Hill, New York, 1959.
4. Lazaras, RS: Psychological Stress and the Coping Process. McGraw-Hill, New York, 1966.
5. Cannon, W: Traumatic Shock: Surgical Monographs. D. Appleton, New York, 1923.
6. Allen, R and Hyde, D: Investigation in Stress Control. Burgess Publishing, Minnesota, 1982.
7. Dilman, VM: Transformation of development: Program in the mechanism of aging pathology. Practitioner 4:465, 1979.
8. Willis, L, Thomas, P, Garny, PJ, and Goodwin, JS: A prospective study of response to stressful life events in initially healthy elders. J Gerontol 42(6):627–630, 1987.
9. Selye, H: Stress, aging and retirement. Journal of Mind and Behavior 1(1):93, 1980.
10. Lakatta, EG: Hemodynamic adaptations to stress with advancing age. ACTA Med Scand (Suppl)711:39–52, 1986.
11. Arling, G: Strain, social support, and distress in old age. J Gerontol 42(1):107–113, 1987.
12. Kraus, N: Stress and sex differences in depressive symptoms among older adults. J Gerontol 41(6):727–731, 1986.
13. Hays, JC, Kasl, S, and Jacobs, S: Past personal history of dysphoria, social support, and psychological distress following conjugal bereavement. J Am Geriatr Soc 42(7):712–718, 1994.
14. Tudiver, F, Hilditch, J, and Permaul, JA: A comparison of psychosocial characteristics of new widowers and married men. Family Medicine 23(7):501–505, 1991.
15. Koller, PA: Family needs and coping strategies during illness crisis. AACN Clinical Issues in Critical Care Nursing 2(2):338–345, 1991.
16. Osgood, NJ: The alcohol-suicide connection in late life. Postgrad Med 81(4):379–384, 1987.
17. Pahkala, K, Kivela, SL, and Laippala, P: Social and environmental factors and dysthymic disorder in old age. J Clin Epidemiol 45(7):775–783, 1992.

18. Riegle, GD and Hess, GD: Chronic and acute suppression of stress in young and old rats. Neuroendocrinology 9:175, 1972.

19. Milgram, S: The experience of living in cities. Science 167:1461, 1970.

20. Hunskaar, S and Sandvik, H: One hundred and fifty men with urinary incontinence. Vol. 3: Psychosocial consequences. Scandinavian Journal of Primary Health Care 11(3):193–196, 1993.

21. Halstead, MT and Fernsler, JI: Coping strategies of long-term cancer survivors. Cancer Nursing 17(2):94–100, 1994.

22. Angeleri, F, Angeleri, VA, Foschi, N, Giaquinto, S, and Nolfe, G: The influence of depression, social activity, and family stress on functional outcomes after stroke. Stroke 24(10):1478–1483, 1993.

23. Yates, BC and Booton-Hiser, DA: Comparison of psychologic stress response in patients and spouses ten weeks after a cardiac illness event. Progress in Cardiovascular Nursing 7(4):25–33, 1992.

24. Downe-Wamboldt, B: Stress, emotions, and coping: A study of elderly women with osteoarthritis. Health Care for Women International 12(1):85–98, 1991.

25. Rangell, L: Discussion of Buffalo Creek disaster: Course of psychic trauma. Am J Psychiatry 133:313, 1976.

26. Curtis, HJ: Biological mechanisms underlying the aging process. Science 141:686, 1963.

27. Timeras, P: Aging. In Cox, H (ed): The Physiology of Aging. Dushkin, Guilford, CN, 1980.

28. Davis, R: Stress homeostatic mechanisms. In Eliot, RS (ed): Stress and the Heart: Contemporary Problems in Cardiology. Futura, Mount Kisco, NY 1974.

29. Trujillo, TT: A study of radiation induced aging. Radiat Res 16:144, 1962.

30. Rosenman, R and Friedman, M: Overt behavior pattern in coronary disease: Detection of overt behavior pattern A in patients with coronary disease by new psychophysiological procedure. JAMA 173:1320, 1960.

31. Howard, J, et al: Adapting to retirement. J Am Geriat Soc 30:488, 1982.

32. Maddison, D and Viola, A: The health of widows in the year following bereavement. J Psychosom Res 12:239, 1968.

33. Clayton, PJ: Mortality and morbidity in the first year of widowhood. Arch Gen Psychiatry 30:747, 1974.

34. Lynch, J and Convey, W: Loneliness, disease, and death: Alternative approaches. Psychosomatics 20:702, 1979.

35. Engel, G: A life setting conducive to illness: The giving up—given up complex. Ann Inter Med 69:293, 1968.

36. Kennedy, GJ and Fischer, JD: Aging, stress and sudden cardiac death. Mt Sinai J Med (NY) 54(1):56–62, 1987.

37. Howard, J, Marshall, J, and Rechnitzer, P: Adapting to retirement. J Am Geriatr Soc 30:488, 1982.

38. Holmes, T and Rahe, R: The social readjustment rating scale. J Psychosom Res 11:213, 1967.

39. Rahe, R: Life events and mental illness: An overview. J Human Stress 5:2, 1979.

40. Holmes, T and Masuda, M: Life changes and illness susceptibility. In Dohrenwend, BS and Dohrenwend, BF (eds): Stressful Life Events: The Nature and Effects. W Ley, New York, 1974.

41. Kraus, N: Life stress as a correlate of depression among older adults. Psychiatry Res 18(3):227–237, 1986.

42. Weinberger, M, Hiner, SL, and Tierney, WM: In support of hassles as a measure of stress in predicting health outcomes. J Behav Med 10(1):19–31, 1987.

43. Ewedemi, F and Linn, MW: Health and hassles in older and younger men. J Clin Psychol 43(4):347–353, 1987.

44. McGrae, R: Age differences in the use of coping mechanisms. J Gerontol 37:454, 1982.

45. Barfield, R and Morgan J: Trends in satisfaction with retirement. Gerontologist 18:19, 1978.

46. Katcher, A and Friedmann, E: Potential health value of pet ownership. Compendium on Continuing Education 11:2, 1980.

47. Winnicot, DW: Transitional objectives and transitional phenomena. Int J Psychoanal 34:89, 1953.

48. Sebkova, J: Anxiety levels as affected by the presence of a dog. Unpublished thesis, Lancaster, PA, 1977.

49. Friedmann, E: Pet ownership and coronary heart disease. Circulation 168(Suppl 2):57, 1978.

50. Levitt, J, Clark, MC, Rotton, J, and Finley, GE: Social support perceived control, and well-being: A study of an environmentally stressed population. Int J Aging Hum Dev 25(4):247–258, 1987.

51. Kraus, N: Stressful life events and physician utilization. J Gerontol 43(2):553–561, 1988.

52. Kraus, N: Understanding the stress process: Linking social support with locus of control beliefs. J Gerontol 42(6):589–593, 1987.

53. Kraus, N: Stress and coping: Reconceptualizing the role of locus of control beliefs. J Gerontol 41(5):617–622, 1986.

54. Foster, JM and Gallagher, D: An exploratory study comparing depressed and nondepressed elders' coping strategies. J Gerontol 41(1):91–93, 1986.

55. Dahlstrom, W, Welseh, G, and Dahlstrom, L: An MMPI Handbook, Vol I, Clinical Interpretation (rev ed), vol 2, Research Applications. University of Minnesota Press, Minneapolis, 1974.

56. Brodman, K, Erdmann, A, and Wolff, H: Cornell Medical Index Health Questionnaire. Cornell University Medical College, New York, 1949.

57. Benson, H, Beary, J, Carol, M: The relaxation response. Psychiatry 37:37, 1974.

58. Girdano, D and Everly, G: Controlling Stress and Tension: A Holistic Approach. Prentice-Hall, Englewood Cliffs, NJ, 1979.

59. Jacobson, E: Progressive Relaxation. University of Chicago Press, Chicago, 1938.

60. Barber, T: Physiological Effects of Hypnosis. Psychol Bull 58:360, 1961.

61. Luthe, W (ed): Autogenic Therapy: Vol 5. Grune & Stratton, New York, 1969.

62. Gaardner, I and Montgomery, P: Clinical Biofeedback: A Procedural Manual Behavioral Medicine. Williams & Wilkins, Baltimore, 1981.

63. Paul, G and Trimble, R: Recorded vs. live relaxation training and hypnotic suggestion: Comparative effectiveness for reducing physiological arousal and inhibiting stress response. Behavioral Thearpy 1:285, 1970.

64. Rama, S, Ballentine, R, Hymes, A: The Science of Breath. Himalayan International Institute, Honesdale, PA, 1979.

65. Goldfriend, M: Systematic desensitization as training in self-control. J Consult Clin Psychol 37:228, 1971.

66. Dusek-Girdano, D: Stress reduction through physical activity. In Girdano, D and Everly, G (eds): Controlling Stress and Tension: A Holistic Approach. Prentice-Hall, Englewood Cliffs, NJ, 1979.

67. Krause, N, Goldenhar, L, Liang, J, Jay, G, and Meada, D: Stress and exercise among the Japanese elderly. Social Science and Medicine 26(11):1429–1441, 1993.

68. Switkes, B: Senior-Cize: Exercises and Dances in a Chair. Betty Switkes, Washington, DC, 1982.

69. Fowler, J, Budzynski, T, and Vandenbergh, R: Effects of an EMG biofeedback relaxation program on the control of diabetics. Biofeedback Self Regul 1:105, 1976.

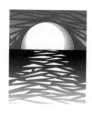

CHAPTER 13

Nutritional Rehabilitation and the Elderly

Ronni Chernoff, PhD, RD

BEHAVIORAL OBJECTIVES

Upon completion of this chapter, the reader will be able to:

1 Identify at least three physiologic changes of normal aging that affect nutritional requirements in the elderly.
2 Discuss the problems of assessing the nutritional status of the elderly.
3 Recognize the effect on nutritional status of sensory changes associated with advancing age.
4 Describe the symptoms of protein energy malnutrition in the elderly.
5 Identify nutrition support interventions that can be used in elderly patients.
6 Discuss nutritional needs in older people.

Nutrition is a vital factor in all phases of the life cycle. Growth, development, maturity, and acute and chronic illnesses all have inherent nutritional requirements that must be filled to best meet dynamic metabolic states. Nutritional needs vary according to changing physiologic conditions. Nutrient intake necessary to maintain health and prevent disease may be different from that required by the treatment of chronic medical conditions or for the recovery of health following an acute medical episode. Nutritional needs of an elderly individual who requires rehabilitation will be unique, and may change with alterations in physical condition over time. Additionally, the nutritional requirements of older people are affected by the normal aging process, regardless of disease or rehabilitation demands.[1]

Normal aging is associated with physiologic changes that contribute to modifications in nutrient requirements. The major changes are a reduction in total body protein, a decrease in total body water, an increase in total body fat with a redistribution of fat stores, and a loss in bone density. Although these changes occur in all people as they age, they occur at different rates among individuals and may be affected by chronic disease processes. Aging is a uniquely individual process that may be impacted by nutritional intake throughout earlier life stages.[1]

Some of the changes in the nutritional requirements of individuals can be accommodated if the clinician is alert to their presentations and etiologies. Distinguishing between physiologic age-induced changes and nutritional deficiencies may be difficult. Observing nutritional intake, physical strength, functional status, and physiologic alterations that occur with time will yield important clues to potential nutritional problems in elderly people. The demands of chronic disease, the extraordinary needs of acute illness, and the basal requirements to maintain homeostasis make the provision of nutritional care to elderly, chronically ill patients a challenge for their caregivers.

ASSESSMENT OF NUTRITIONAL STATUS

One of the more difficult determinations in elderly people is the accurate assessment of their nutritional status; due to the physiologic changes that occur with normal aging, many of the commonly used assessment standards are not reliable in this population.[2]

Anthropometric Measures

Anthropometric measures, including height, weight, and skinfold measures, are usually important components of a nutritional assessment. These parameters are the ones most affected by the aging process.[3] The most apparent age-related change occurs in height. Height decreases as people get older due to changes in skeletal integrity, most noticeably affecting the spinal column. Loss of height may be the result of thinning of the vertebrae, compression of the vertebral discs, development of kyphosis, and the effects of osteomalacia and osteoporosis.[4] Loss of height occurs in both men and women, although it may happen more rapidly to elderly women with osteoporosis. Therefore, stature changes and body appearance may be altered as older people lose their ability to stand erect; the organs in the thoracic cavity will become displaced, and breathing and gastrointestinal problems may ensue.[5]

Loss of height may range from 1 to 2.5 cm per decade after maturity. Also, height is difficult to measure in individuals who are unable to stand erect. Height measurements cannot be obtained from people who cannot stand unaided; who cannot stand at all because of neuromuscular disorders, paralysis, or loss of lower limbs; or who are bedbound because of muscle contractures or other problems. The best estimate of stature in these individuals is obtained by measuring their recumbent height or choosing selected anthropometric sites (that is, bony prominences) and measuring the distance between a number of selected points.[6] Such measurements will provide an estimate of height to use in determining appropriate body weight.

Weight is another important anthropometric measure that is altered with advancing age. Weight tends to increase into middle age (40 to 50 years), stabilize for 15 to 20 years, and then decrease progressively thereafter.[3] It is important to note that these changes occur at different rates among elderly people. Use of most standard height and weight tables is not valid in older people because most reference tables do not include elderly people in their subject pool, and most are not age-adjusted. The most appropriate tables can be compiled from the Health and Nutrition Examination Surveys (Table 13–1).[7] They provide average weight-for-height data and rank individuals on percentiles relative to others in their age group.

A more commonly used measure is the body mass index (BMI), which evaluates relative weight for height using a mathematical ratio of weight (in kilograms) divided by height (in square meters).

$$Wt \ (Kg)/Ht \ (M)^2$$

This formula yields a whole number that should be greater than 21 and less than approximately 35.[8] However, nomograms and tables are available that minimize the need for calculation. There is some controversy among experts regarding the range of acceptable BMI measures in elderly people.[9]

Skinfold measurements (triceps, biceps, subscapular, suprailiac, thigh) are often included in a thorough nutritional assessment. Loss of muscle mass, shifts in body fat compartments, changes in skin compressibility and elasticity, and lack of age-adjusted references serve to decrease the reliability of skinfold measures in the assessment of nutritional status in elderly

Table 13–1. **Percentiles of Weight for Height for Men and Women, 55–74 Yrs Old**

Ht (cm)	Percentile Wt (kg)						
	5	**10**	**15**	**50**	**85**	**90**	**95**
				MEN			
157	45–54*	49–59	56–63	61–77	68–91	73–95	77–100
160	47–55	49–60	51–64	62–80	71–92	71–96	79–101
163	47–57	50–62	54–65	63–77	72–94	74–97	80–102
165	48–58	54–63	59–73	70–79	80–89	90–98	90–103
168	51–59	55–67	59–73	68–80	77–101	80–102	84–105
170	55–65	60–71	61–73	69–85	79–103	81–108	88–112
173	54–67	54–71	58–73	70–83	79–95	81–98	86–111
175	56–65	59–70	63–74	75–84	81–96	84–98	88–105
178	57–68	61–73	63–77	76–87	83–102	86–104	89–117
180	59–65	62–70	65–70	69–84	85–102	87–109	99–111
183	60–67	64–76	66–81	76–90	86–108	89–112	92–112
185	62–68	65–73	68–76	78–88	88–105	90–108	94–113
188	63–69	67–74	69–78	77–89	89–106	92–109	95–114
				WOMEN			
147	39–53	46–59	48–63	54–92	63–95	65–99	71–104
150	41–54	45–59	48–63	55–78	66–95	68–99	74–105
152	43–54	45–65	47–69	54–78	67–87	70–88	73–105
155	43–64	43–68	45–69	56–79	65–94	70–95	71–106
157	47–59	49–61	52–63	58–82	67–93	69–101	73–111
160	42–61	45–65	49–67	58–80	67–100	68–102	74–118
163	43–60	47–65	49–67	60–77	68–97	70–102	75–119
165	43–60	47–66	49–69	60–80	69–98	72–102	75–111
168	44–57	48–60	50–63	68–82	70–98	72–105	76–109
170	45–58	48–64	51–68	61–80	71–105	73–104	77–109
173	45–58	49–64	51–68	61–79	71–100	74–104	77–110
175	46–59	49–65	52–69	62–85	72–101	74–105	78–110
178	47–60	50–65	52–69	63–85	73–101	75–105	79–111

*Lower limit for small frames; higher limit for large frames.
Source: Adapted from Frisancho.[7]

people. The reference populations used in the derivation of skinfold standards do not include older people and do not adjust for age-related changes. Skinfold measures provide only gross estimates of body composition under the best conditions; with elderly subjects, these measures can provide baseline information against which changes can be assessed over time.[10]

Biochemical Measures

Biochemical assessment parameters are also affected by advancing age, although not as dramatically as anthropometric indexes.[2] Laboratory measures may be affected by an age-related decline in renal function, fluid imbalances or hydration status, long-term chronic illnesses, and drug-drug or drug-nutrient interactions. Among the commonly used biochemical markers, serum transferrin is one that is markedly affected by advancing age. Since tissue iron stores increase with age, circulating serum transferrin levels are reduced. Iron stores and transferrin are related in an inverse relationship. Therefore, a below-normal serum transferrin should be evaluated in relation to other biochemical measures and serum iron levels, if obtainable.[11,12]

The most reliable predictor of nutritional status in elderly people is serum albumin. It is uncommon to find a serum albumin below 4 g/dL unless the subject is overhydrated; has cancer, renal, or hepatic disease; or is taking medications that may interfere with hepatic function. Recent evidence suggests that serum albumin is a prognostic indicator of potential infectious complications and other nosocomial problems in hospitalized, frail, or dependent elderly individuals.[13,14] It is a primary prognostic indicator of rehospitalization, extended lengths of stay, and other complications associated with protein energy malnutrition in elderly people.[15] Unless there is drug interference or an existing chronic disease process, most biochemical measures should remain within normal limits.

Immunologic Assessment

Tests for immunocompetence are often included as part of a nutritional assessment because malnutrition results in compromised host-defense mechanisms. However, the incidence of anergy is reported to increase with advanced age, and the response to skin test antigens appears to peak after longer intervals in older people.[16] It is difficult to distinguish between alterations related to protein energy malnutrition and those related to a depressed immune response from other causes.[17] The value of these tests is therefore limited in elderly people.

Evaluation of Socioeconomic Status

Accurate nutrition assessment of an elderly person who is suspected of being malnourished requires a comprehensive evaluation. Social history, economic status, drug history, oral health condition, family and living situations, and alcohol use should be evaluated along with the physical and physiologic measures usually assessed.[2] Although the parameters commonly used to assess nutritional status are unreliable because of the lack of age-adjusted standards, they do contribute information to develop a comprehensive picture of an individual's health and nutrition status and can be used to effectively track changes that occur in people over time.

It is also useful to assess elderly individuals' ability to perform the activities of daily living (ADL) and instrumental activities of daily living (IADL).[18,19] Table 13–2 lists ADL and IADL.

Table 13–2. Activities of Daily Living and Instrumental Activities of Daily Living

Activities of Daily Living	Instrumental Activities of Daily Living
Bathing	Use of telephone
Dressing	Shopping
Going to toilet	Food preparation
Transferring	Housekeeping
Continence	Laundry
Feeding	Transportation
	Medications management
	Financial management

NUTRITIONAL NEEDS OF THE ELDERLY

Energy Needs

The most well-documented change that occurs over time, and which has been alluded to several times already, is the decrease in energy metabolism.[20] This reduction in energy needs is related to a decrease in the protein mass rather than to a reduction in the metabolic activity of aging tissue. Basal energy requirements reflect the energy needed for all the metabolic processes that are involved in maintaining cell function; the reduction of active metabolic mass will result in lowered energy needs.

Energy requirements are markedly affected by physical activity. Results of experiments conducted as part of the Baltimore Longitudinal Study on Aging indicate that there is an age-related decline in physical activity in both men and women.[21,22] Decreases in physical activity may be related to the onset of bone and joint diseases, the progression of chronic diseases of the heart and lungs, neurologic disorders, failing vision, or fractures related to poor balance or osteoporosis. It is noteworthy that the lowered energy requirements are more closely associated with this decrease in activity energy expenditure than with a decrease in basal energy rate.[21]

There is increasing evidence that frail, older adults can benefit from strength-training exercises. Muscle strength can be rehabilitated by regular training, and greater independence fostered by increased confidence in functional ability.[23] Regular exercise stimulates protein turnover, maintains muscle mass, and burns more calories.[24,25]

Protein

Protein requirements in elderly individuals might be expected to decrease to accommodate a lower total lean body mass. However, recent studies indicate that protein requirements may be slightly higher in older subjects.[26] One explanation is that lower calorie intake contributes to reduced retention of dietary nitrogen, therefore requiring more dietary protein to achieve nitrogen balance.

Protein needs are also affected by immobility,[27] which contributes to negative nitrogen balance. Elderly people who are bedbound, wheelchair-bound, or otherwise immobilized require higher levels of dietary protein to achieve nitrogen equilibrium.

For healthy, free-living elderly people, protein requirements have not been shown to increase or decrease significantly. However, protein requirements are affected by the presence of chronic or acute illnesses. Surgery, sepsis, long-bone fractures, and unusual losses such as those that occur with burns or gastrointestinal disease increase the need for dietary protein. Some clinicians have been wary of providing high levels of protein for fear of precipitating renal disease in elderly individuals. Research has shown no evidence that dietary protein induces deterioration of renal function in individuals who have no evidence of renal disease.[28,29] For elderly patients who have a measurable decline in renal function, therapeutic regimens should be followed.

Dietary Fat

Fat in the diet contributes energy and essential fatty acids and is necessary to absorb fat-soluble vitamins. Since only small amounts of fat are needed to provide essential fatty acids, and since fat-soluble vitamins are available from other dietary sources, the primary contribution from dietary fat is calories. For older people, restricting dietary fat, thereby reducing calorie intake, is a reasonable strategy to maintain calorie balance without restricting intake of other nutrients; however, in some individuals too-rigid restrictions on dietary fat may contribute to energy deficits.

There are major differences of opinion regarding the type and amount of dietary fat that adults over age 65 should ingest.[30-32] Cardiologists are firm believers in the benefits of diets restricted in fat, regardless of the age of the individual. Geriatricians are somewhat more focused on health maintenance and quality-of-life issues and tend to be more conservative in prescribing low-fat diets. Evidence indicates that risk factors for heart disease change with advancing age and that management of systolic hypertension may be more important than lowering serum cholesterol unless cholesterol levels are well over 250 mg/dL.

Carbohydrates

Carbohydrate intake in the diets of elderly people should be approximately 55 to 60 percent of the total caloric intake, with an emphasis on complex carbohydrates. The ability to metabolize carbohydrates appears to decline with advancing age.[10] Fasting blood glucose levels tend to increase slowly over time, with 140 mg/dL the mean for individuals over age 65; therefore, it has been suggested that glucose tolerance tests be compared to age-cohorts using age-adjusted glucose tolerance tables.[33]

Complex carbohydrate intake is important in elderly people because it provides fiber, a constituent of the diet that enhances bowel motility, which tends to decrease over time. Fresh fruits and vegetables are difficult to chew if oral health status is not optimal or dentures do not fit properly, and these foods are expensive when they are out of season. Cereal fibers should be encouraged as an alternative, but it is difficult to obtain adequate fiber from cereal foods alone.

Vitamins

Vitamin requirements for people over 65 are mostly speculative at present, although there is much ongoing research. The recommended dietary allowances (RDA) suggest intake levels for individuals over 51, but this allows a lot of variability in requirements for people in middle through old age.[34]

Vitamin deficiencies may exist subclinically in elderly persons, particularly for some of the water-soluble vitamins. When the stress of an illness or an injury occurs, depleted reserve capacity may not be able to compensate for rapid depletion of tissue stores and the individual may become overtly deficient. Subclinical deficiencies may exist in people who have adequate but not excess dietary intake, because the absorption and utilization of these vitamins may be compromised by the use of multiple medications or single nutrient supplements. A drug profile, including both prescription and over-the-counter medications, should be part of every history taken of an elderly person.[10]

The water-soluble vitamins that are often discussed include vitamin C (ascorbic acid) and vitamin B_{12}. Although there appears to be no age-related alteration in vitamin C absorption, this vitamin is often linked with wound-healing problems or easy bruisability. Vitamin C is an essential factor needed to make collagen, the protein matrix that holds cells together and is therefore necessary when new tissue is being formed. The RDA for vitamin C is 60 mg/day, a level far exceeded in most American diets. With large doses of supplemental vitamin C, tissue saturation is reached rapidly and the excess vitamin is excreted in urine. Very large doses (greater than 1g/day) may contribute to some serious side effects such as the formation of kidney stones or chronic diarrhea in sensitive individuals. There is little evidence that massive doses of vitamin C aid in wound healing, ward off the common cold, or cure cancer.[35]

Many older adults may be at risk for deficiency in vitamin B_{12}. The major dietary sources for vitamin B_{12} are red meat and organ meats, which many elderly people have eliminated from their diets because of the fat and cholesterol content. In addition to dietary inadequacy, some older adults have a condition called atrophic gastritis, in which gastric acid production is decreased. Gastric acid is necessary for vitamin B_{12} to be released from a series of protein carriers and absorbed. Symptoms of vitamin B_{12} deficiency are generally nonspecific but include irritability, lethargy, and mild dementia.

It is less likely that elderly people will be deficient in fat-soluble vitamins (A, D, E, K) because these can be stored in liver tissue. Limited exposure to sunlight, the use of sunscreens, and an inadequate intake of dairy products can contribute to deficiency in vitamin D, particularly in the homebound or institutionalized elderly. It is also known that the amount of vitamin D precursor in skin, which is stimulated by sunlight, particularly ultraviolet rays, decreases with age. Dietary vitamin D goes through several conversions in liver and kidney to become the active form of the vitamin; the kidney becomes less efficient at the final step of conversion with advanced age. Since vitamin D is an important nutrient in bone mineralization and in immune function, it is wise to encourage the inclusion of foods rich in vitamin D in the diets of elderly individuals who may be at risk of deficiency.

Vitamin K deficiencies may occur, usually in association with the use of sulfa drugs, antibiotics, or vitamin K antagonists in anticoagulation therapy.

The risk of vitamin A toxicity is greater than the risk of vitamin A deficiency.[37] This is especially true in older people who are taking over-the-counter vitamin supplements, many of which have very high levels of vitamin A. Beta carotene, a vitamin A precursor, has received a great deal of attention in recent years because of its apparent protective effect against various types of neoplasms. The long-term effects of high doses of beta carotene have not been adequately explored, and since most cancers take 20 years or more to develop, the long-range benefits for older people are difficult to assess.

Minerals

Requirements for most minerals do not change with age. The need for iron decreases because of a tendency to increase tissue iron stores with advancing age and a cessation of menstrual blood loss in women. Calcium requirements have attracted much attention in recent years. Investigators have suggested that dietary calcium intake recommendations increase from 800 mg/day to 1200 or 1500 mg/day to reduce the risk of osteoporosis. The controversy surrounding calcium requirements in older people has not yet been settled.[38] Many investigators do not think that requirements should be changed; others believe that they should be increased.

For most other major minerals, such as sodium and potassium, requirements are not changed by the aging process but are affected by the presence of acute or chronic diseases and their treatments. Serum levels of minerals or electrolytes should be maintained within normal limits or controlled as part of disease management. In elderly people, drastic shifts in electrolyte levels and hydration status can be very debilitating because they take longer to adapt or compensate than younger people. There does not appear to be any significant change in requirements for other minerals, such as zinc, chromium, copper, manganese, or selenium in normal, healthy elderly people. However, various disease states, along with inadequate diet, such as occurs with alcoholism, drug-nutrient interactions, severe chronic malabsorption, or chronic malnutrition, may lead to deficiencies in all micronutrients.

Fluids

Water is an important nutrient for older people. Inadequate fluid intake may lead to rapid dehydration and precipitate the associated problems: hypotension, elevated body temperature, constipation, nausea, vomiting, mucosal dryness, decreased urine output, and mental confusion. What is particularly noteworthy is that these problems are rarely attributed to fluid imbalances, which are easily corrected. Fluid intake should be adequate to compensate for normal losses (through kidneys, bowel, lungs, and skin) and for unusual losses associated with increased body temperature, vomiting, diarrhea, or hemorrhage. A reasonable estimate of fluid needs is approximately 1 mL/kcal ingested or 30 mL/kg actual body weight. The minimum intake for all older adults regardless of their size or caloric intake should be approximately 1500 mL/day. Fluid needs can be met with water, juices, beverages such as tea or coffee, gelatin desserts, and other foods that would be liquid at room temperature. Tube-feeding formulas contain approximately 750 mL of water per liter of solution; it is wise to compensate for the solids displacement by adding 25 percent of the volume of the tube feeding as additional free water.

There are many reasons why an elderly person may become dehydrated besides not drinking adequate volumes of fluid. Osmoreceptors decrease with advancing age, thereby making the elderly individual less sensitive to fluid needs; fever, infection, and excess climatic heat contribute to increased fluid needs, which may not be met with voluntary dietary fluids; institutionalized, immobile, demented, arthritic, or comatose individuals do not have free access to dietary fluid; incontinent persons may voluntarily restrict their fluid intake; and nutrition-support-dependent patients may be underhydrated simply because they are receiving inadequate volumes of nutrient solutions and adequate free water is not provided as part of their nutrition regimen.[39]

WEIGHT LOSS AND CACHEXIA

One of the most difficult nutritional problems to correctly identify and treat in elderly individuals is the chronic weight loss and cachexia often associated with chronic disease and institutionalization. Cachexia is a syndrome characterized by anorexia, muscle wasting, early satiety, and possible changes in energy metabolism. Cachexia is associated with systemic illness and may occur with infectious syndromes; cardiac, renal, hepatic, and pulmonary dysfunction; autoimmune disease; and cancer. Weight loss can be dangerous, and even life-threatening if aggressive nutritional intervention is not instituted. It has been well documented that weight tends to increase until middle age, stabilizes for 10 to 15 years, and then decreases progressively.[3,7,40] Although the cause of this weight loss has not been adequately explained, it has been observed by many investigators. Loss of lean body mass occurs as part of normal aging; therefore, unchecked weight loss can become a serious problem. It is important to note that all protein compartments shrink with advancing age. This includes muscle tissue (which is most noticeable), organ tissue, blood components, blood vessels, immune bodies, hormones, enzymes, and collagen. These losses occur as part of normal aging, but may be affected by chronic disease; immobilization in a bed or chair; altered metabolic responses associated with acute illness; and increased nutritional demands due to stress, surgery, bone fractures, and sepsis.

One consequence of lean body mass reduction is its impact on energy metabolism. Because protein tissue is the most metabolically active body compartment, it demands the greatest energy resources to maintain its mass, make new tissue to replace old, and repair surgical wounds, pressure ulcers, fractures, or injured tissue. When the total mass of body protein is reduced, energy demands decrease accordingly.[41] Therefore, as people grow older, less energy is required to maintain metabolically active body mass. However, requirements for macronutrients other than energy sources (protein, carbohydrate, fat) do not decrease significantly if at all. This contributes to a situation in which less food is needed to meet requirements, but the needs for protein, vitamins, and minerals remain fairly constant or may increase, leading to a potentially deficient intake of these nutrients or a weight gain. Weight gain may stress the cardiopulmonary system, make mobility difficult for individuals who have bone or joint disease, make control of chronic conditions such as diabetes or hypertension more difficult, and contribute to the development of other chronic conditions. It is often difficult for elderly, chronically ill, average-weight individuals (BMI 21–29) to avoid weight gain and still get adequate essential nutrients.

However, the problem most often encountered in the chronically ill, elderly population is that of chronic weight loss of unknown etiology. Although the explanation may appear simple—less energy is ingested than is needed to maintain body weight—the reasons why this occurs may be more obscure. They may be related to the fact that the changes that are associated with advancing age and chronic disease are complex and often interrelated.[42,43]

The most profound change that occurs is the loss of lean body mass previously described; other physiologic changes take place that also affect nutritional intake of elderly individuals. For example, sensory changes occur over time.[41,44] Loss of visual acuity and peripheral vision may contribute to impaired mobility. Going to the grocery store or restaurant may be difficult because of problems with driving, limitations in night vision, and a decrease in response time to changes in light. Presbyopia makes reading menus, price tags, recipes, or directions more difficult. Visual discrimination may decrease, thus contributing to difficulty in distinguishing specific food items or fluid levels in containers. Hand-eye coordination is affected, potentially contributing to difficulty in pouring liquids or handling hot food containers. Fear of burning oneself, being embarrassed by having an accident, or not having the coordination or strength to open food containers may lead to the avoidance of certain foods or food preparation methods. All of these scenarios contribute to decreased dietary intake.

Taste and smell sensitivity may decrease with age.[41,44,45] Many studies have attempted to examine changes in taste sensation in older people, but these studies are difficult to interpret. Taste studies are usually conducted using various-strength solutions representing each of the basic four taste sensations: sweet, salt, sour, and bitter. Food has many flavor components that offer varying taste sensations, thereby making extrapolation of data from usual taste studies to taste perceptions of food difficult. However, if food is perceived as tasteless by the individual, it will not be eaten. External factors contribute to alterations in taste perception and affect the quantity of food ingested. Omission of flavoring agents such as salt, use of multiple medications, and the effects of chronic illnesses all contribute to the decreased palatability of food.

Psychological changes occur in elderly people due to changing social circumstances, loss of emotional support systems, stresses of chronic illnesses, isolation from family and friends, and institutionalization; these changes may lead to a precarious nutritional state.[46] Depression is the most common psychological disorder in elderly women[47] and is known to affect appetite and eating habits. Depression may also cause alcoholism and drug dependency in elderly women. These circumstances definitely have an effect on eating patterns and subsequent nutritional status.

Alcoholism and drug dependency may also be major factors contributing to the incidence of falls, injuries, and accidents in older people.[48] These kinds of injuries increase the need for certain essential nutrients and lead to hospitalization or placement in long-term care facilities, increasing the risk of malnutrition. Chronic subclinical malnutrition leads to a diminished reserve capacity, making a rapid, adequate response to physical injury unlikely and possibly worsening the medical condition by allowing opportunistic infection;[49] malnutrition makes recuperation and rehabilitation slower and more prolonged, consumes more resources, requires more health care, and perhaps hampers the achievement of complete recovery.

PROTEIN ENERGY MALNUTRITION

Protein energy malnutrition in the hospitalized elderly individual is usually associated with a primary disease, either chronic or acute, including cancer, chronic cardiac failure, chronic pulmonary disease, renal failure, hepatic failure, and gastrointestinal problems.[50] One of the most serious consequences of undetected protein energy malnutrition in elderly people is impairment of the immune system. Already affected by advanced age, immune responses may be even more compromised by protein energy malnutrition.[17] Complications associated with this problem are increased risk of infection and decreased ability to mobilize host defenses, leading to increased morbidity and mortality.

The most frequent symptom of protein energy malnutrition is confusion or a recent history of alterations in mental status. This symptom, which may be present on admission or develop during hospitalization, can usually be linked to a history of chronic weight loss. The probable mechanism for confusion is dehydration, which is often present and usually related to inadequate fluid intake.[51]

Once protein energy malnutrition has been identified, clinical judgment is important in setting therapeutic priorities and appropriate initiation of nutritional intervention. Once the acute phase has subsided and recuperation is under way, daily calorie counts should be instituted and the patient encouraged to consume an adequate diet.

Unfortunately, because of cuts in hospital reimbursement in recent years, elderly convalescent patients are being sent to nursing homes rather than recovering in the hospital. Today, nursing home patients are often quite sick and require skilled care. Nursing home diets need adjustment to provide higher-density nutritional foods to accommodate patients who are still in the recovery phase of their illness. When their nutritional requirements are not met, patients are at greater risk of becoming malnourished. One effect of this problem is that nursing home patients are frequently being readmitted to hospitals with urinary tract, upper-respiratory, and other infections and pressure ulcers.[52,53]

Primary Protein Energy Malnutrition

There is evidence that as many as 40 percent of institutionalized and hospitalized elderly are below the 15th percentile of their weight for height. In addition to the obvious depletion of protein stores that has been previously described, elderly people suffering from primary protein energy malnutrition also sustain a reduction in fat stores. In the absence of intercurrent illnesses, visceral protein stores and immunologic function are maintained. However, a marked depletion of reserve capacity will occur; when a stress such as an acute illness occurs, hypoalbuminemic protein energy malnutrition develops rapidly.[54]

Primary protein energy malnutrition can be correctly diagnosed by means of a good history indicating a recent and significant weight loss, in association with a serum albumin of less than 3 g/dL that is not related to hepatic or renal disease or overhydration causing serum dilution. The presence of anemia, lymphocytopenia, and anergy provides confirmation of the diagnosis of protein energy malnutrition.

The patient should be encouraged to eat as much as possible, as previously stated. Smaller, more frequent meals may be accepted more readily by elderly patients with smaller appetites and early satiety. Oral liquid supplements can be added to solid food consumption if fluid overload is not contraindicated. The goal of refeeding should be to provide 35 kcal/kg of the patient's actual weight and at least 1 gram of protein per kilogram. Our experience has demonstrated that only 10 percent of elderly people who have protein energy malnutrition can consume adequate calories to correct their nutritional deficiencies; most subjects therefore require more aggressive nutritional intervention.[55] Others have shown that protein energy malnutrition that is not corrected will contribute to medical complications and an increased rate of morbidity and mortality in this group of individuals.[56,57]

If the malnourished patient cannot consume adequate calories orally, enteral or parenteral feeding should be considered. Except for patients who have nonfunctioning gastrointestinal tracts, enteral feeding by tube is the intervention of choice. Feeding can be accomplished using pliable, small-bore (8–12 Fr) feeding tubes placed nasogastrically or nasoenterically (into the duodenum or proximal jejunum), through a gastrostomy or jejunostomy. For long-term feeding, indwelling tubes should be considered for use because they reduce the possibility of aspiration and are less likely to be pulled out by a confused or combative patient.

Enteral nutrition support provides a reasonably safe, cost-effective method of providing adequate protein, calories, vitamins, and minerals and meeting fluid requirements for a patient who is not able to meet his or her own needs by eating. Ensuring appropriate nutrient intake will contribute to the individual's recovery from acute illnesses, improve the prognosis for chronic conditions that may hamper rehabilitation, and correct subclinical or overt nutrient deficiencies.[58,59] It is important to note that most standard tube-feeding formulas require 1500 to 2000 mL to provide 100 percent of the RDA for most nutrients. Table 13–3 lists guidelines for safe use of enteral nutrition support.

For severely debilitated, malnourished individuals who have dysfunctional gastrointestinal tracts, parenteral feeding may be the only option. Intravenous feeding in elderly, sick patients requires very careful monitoring, particularly to maintain fluid and electrolyte equilibrium. Blood glucose levels must be checked regularly to avoid hyperglycemia. If fat emulsions are included as part of the regimen, serum lipid levels must also be carefully monitored.[60] Parenteral nutrition should be provided only if there is an ex-

Table 13–3. **Guidelines for Enteral Nutrition Support**

Select Appropriate Tube

- Short term: use nasogastric or nasoenteric tube; long term: use indwelling tube (gastrostomy, jejunostomy)
- Soft, pliable, nonirritating material
- Lumen diameter (8–12Fr)

Select Formulas That Meet Nutritional Needs

- Protein requirements: maintenance 0.8 g/kg body weight; Repletion 1.0–1.5 g/kg body weight
- Energy requirements: maintenance 30–35 kcal/kg body weight; repletion 35–40 kcal/kg body weight
- Vitamin requirements: meet at least 100% RDA
- Fluid requirements: at least 1 mL/kcal (Enteral formulas are 75% water; therefore, 25% total volume should be added as free water)

Select Administration Regimen

- Continuous infusion: if there is limited absorptive surface or gastric dysfunction, place a tube in the small bowel
- Intermittent feeding: if the stomach and bowel function are normal, place tube in stomach
- Rate of administration: to achieve adequate volume to meet requirements, start slowly (50 mL/h) and increase as tolerated

perienced health care professional available; the safest place for provision of parenteral feeding is the acute-care hospital. Extended-care facilities often lack professional staff with knowledge or experience in parenteral feeding.

CANCER: A CHRONIC DISEASE

Individuals who have cancer have many medical problems relating to their illness and its treatments. There are many debilitating side effects; however, the dangers of infections are particularly serious in cancer patients who may be receiving chemotherapy. Many chemotherapeutic agents render immune systems weak or unresponsive. Malnutrition also depresses immune responses and contributes to the potentially life-threatening nature of infections in cancer patients. Malnutrition has other consequences for cancer patients in addition to its impact on immune function.[61]

Weight loss and cachexia are the most common manifestations of malnutrition in elderly cancer patients.[62] Chronic weight loss in elderly patients is a difficult process to reverse, often requiring extraordinary amounts of calories and other nutrients to reverse the weight loss and to restore lost body mass. Regained weight should be carefully evaluated to avoid an excess of fat tissue and to encourage the synthesis of protein tissue. This requires a careful balance of adequate protein to meet needs and form new tissue, sufficient calories to avoid the use of protein substrate for energy, and exercise to stimulate new protein tissue synthesis. Careful monitoring is also needed to manage potential shifts in fluid balance; over- or underhydration can cause rapid shifts of weight as fluid accumulates or is lost.

Maintenance of fluid and electrolyte balance is critical in elderly cancer patients.[63] Inadequate intake of fluid is common in elderly people; they have diminished thirst sensations associated with aging and changes in osmoregulatory mechanisms, often related to chronic disease processes.[64] Dehydration related to nausea and vomiting, diarrhea, and unusual losses (fistula, burns, radiation enteritis) can occur, leading to electrolyte imbalances that may be life-threatening (hyperkalemia, hypercalcemia, hypernatremia). It is important not to hydrate patients too quickly because overhydration may occur with equal rapidity. Overhydration can lead to congestive heart failure, hypertension, edema, or ascites. One common cause of overhydration in elderly cancer patients is uncoordinated intravenous therapy, which may occur if medical care is being provided by several different teams of clinicians.

Chronic weight loss, fluid and electrolyte problems, and chronic undernutrition will also contribute to vitamin deficiencies, most likely water-soluble vitamins that are needed to maintain healthy tissue.[63] Cancer therapies are designed to kill cells in rapidly dividing neoplasms, but they will also damage healthy tissue and are potentially more toxic to the patient if normal function of other tissue is not maintained. A delicate balance can be achieved between antimetabolite drug therapy and adequate nutritional substrate for normal functioning if the primary clinician is attuned to the nutritional status and needs of the patient.

Managing elderly cancer patients and protecting their nutritional status is difficult under the best circumstances but requires an awareness of the importance of nutrition in the treatment and recovery phases of cancer therapies.

OTHER CHRONIC CONDITIONS

There are other chronic conditions in which nutrition plays an important role in rehabilitation. These include problems such as chronic anemias, alcoholism, and pressure ulcers. These, among others, are linked to nutritional intake and status and require nutritional intervention to facilitate recovery and rehabilitation.

There is an unexplained anemia that occurs in some elderly people that is not precipitated by the most common etiologic factors, such as chronic diseases and their processes and treatments. Epidemiologic evidence indicates that nutrition may be an important etiologic factor; anemias are more prevalent in poor elderly people, who have a greater risk of malnutrition.[65]

A remarkable similarity between the hematopoietic and immunologic changes that occur with aging and those that occur with protein deprivation has been demonstrated. Nutritional deficiencies respond to nutritional rehabilitation (refeeding with a diet rich in nutrients); the anemia of senescence is not noticeably affected by refeeding the individual. Correcting other serum parameters affected by malnutrition may not correct immune or hematopoietic function, but reserve capacity improves and the patient may develop a sense of well-being, feel stronger, and respond more positively to therapy.[66]

Alcoholism is a serious problem that severely compromises nutritional intake. Alcoholism affects dietary intake because alcohol, a rich source of calories, replaces nutrient-dense foods. However, alcohol contributes no other nutrients and precludes the alcoholic from eating other foods. Alcoholics are often deficient in water-soluble vitamins and are protein-malnourished. The chronic problems they develop are often related to chronic nutritional deficiencies.[66] Certainly, replacing alcohol with nutritious food will correct simple deficiencies, but some changes, such as an enlarged liver, are irreversible. Nutritional rehabilitation contributes to better health in elderly alcoholics.

Pressure (decubitus) ulcers are potentially serious in frail, elderly, chronically ill people. They are easier to prevent than to cure, but the patients most susceptible are those who are among the most debilitated, those confined to a bed or wheelchair.[67] Pressure ulcers develop due to prolonged direct pressure over bony prominences. Chronic weight loss leads to a decrease in subcutaneous fat, fragile epidermis, decreased blood flow in both large and superficial dermal vessels, and depressed immune function. Once breaks in the skin occur, irritation due to incontinence, exposure to bacterial contaminants, and compromised blood flow contribute to further skin, subcutaneous fat, and muscle breakdown. There are many common treatments: turning patients frequently, air- or fluid-filled mattresses, surgical debridement, antibiotics, dressing changes, hormones, and other agents reported in the literature.[68] However, restoration of nutritional status is essential to healing decubitus ulcers. Achieving nitrogen balance by providing sufficient protein to form new tissue, with adequate levels of calories to protect the protein from being used for energy, are primary goals. Also, vitamin C and zinc are essential for forming new tissue and closing wounds. There is no doubt that healing pressure ulcers is among the greatest challenges for a chronic-care patient, avoidance of ulceration involves maintaining nutritional status and preventing weight loss with reduction of subcutaneous fat compartments. Nutrition is a crucial component in the prevention and treatment of decubitus ulcers.

SUMMARY

Nutrition plays a very important role in the maintenance of health, prevention of disease, and rehabilitation potential of sick people, especially the elderly. Protein, vitamins, minerals, and fluid intakes should be adequate to meet basic needs and to restore depleted reserves. Increased levels of some nutrients may be needed to correct deficiencies, heal injured tissue and broken bones, fight infection, and promote a feeling of well-being and strength.

REFERENCES

1. Chernoff, R and Lipschitz, DA: Nutrition and aging. In Shils, ME and Young, VR (eds): Modern Nutrition in Health and Disease, ed 7. Lea & Febiger, Philadelphia, 1988.
2. Mitchell, CO and Chernoff, R: Nutritional assessment of the elderly. In Chernoff, R (ed): Geriatric Nutrition: The Health Professional's Handbook. Aspen, Gaithersburg, MD, 1991.
3. Mitchell, CO and Lipschitz, DA: Detection of protein-calorie malnutrition in the elderly. Am J Clin Nutr 35:398–406, 1982.
4. Chumlea, WC, Garry, PJ, Hunt, WC, and Rhyne, RL: Serial changes in stature and weight in a healthy elderly population. Hum Biol 60:918–925, 1988.
5. Silverberg, SJ and Lindsay, R: Postmenopausal osteoporosis. Med Clin N Amer 71(1):41–57, 1987.
6. Martin, AD, Carter, JEL, Hendy, KC, and Malina, RM: Segment lengths. In Lohman, TG, Roche, AF, and Martorell, R (eds): Anthropometric Standardization Reference Manual. Human Kinetics, Champaign, IL, 1988.
7. Frisancho, AR: New standards of weight and body composition by frame size and height for assessment of nutritional status of adults and the elderly. Am J Clin Nutr 40:808–819, 1984.
8. Dwyer, JT: Screening Older American's Nutritional Health: Current Practices and Future Possibilities. Nutrition Screening Initiative, Washington, DC, 1991.
9. Potter, JF, Schafer, DF, and Bohi, RL: In-hospital mortality as a function of body mass index: An age-dependent variable. J Gerontol:Med Sci 43(4):M59–M3, 1988.
10. Chernoff, R, Mitchell, CO, and Lipschitz, DA: Assessment of the nutritional status of the geriatric patient. Ger Med Today 3(5):129–141, 1984.
11. Lipschitz, DA, Cook, JD, and Finch, CA: The clinical evaluation of serum ferritin as an index of iron stores. N Engl J Med 290:1213–1216, 1974.
12. Bothwell, TH, Charlton, R, Cook, JD, and Finch, CA: Iron Metabolism in Man. Blackwell Scientific Publishers, Oxford, England, 1979.
13. Morrow, FD: Assessment of nutritional status in the elderly: Application and interpretation of nutritional biochemistries. Clin Nutr 5:112–120, 1986.
14. Finucane, P, Rudra, T, Hsu, R, Tomlinson, K, Hutton, RD, and Pathy, MS: Markers of the nutritional status in acutely ill elderly patients. Gerontology 34:304–309, 1988.
15. Sullivan, DH, Walls, RC, and Lipschitz, DA: Protein-energy undernutrition and the risk of mortality within 1 yr of hospital discharge in a select population of geriatric rehabilitation patients. Am J Clin Nutr 53:599–605, 1991.
16. Cohn, JR, Buckley, CE, Hohl, CA, Tyson, GB, and Neish, DD: Persistent cutaneous cellular immune responsiveness in a nursing home population. J Am Ger Soc 31(5):261–264, 1983.
17. Goodwin, JS and Burns, EL: Aging, nutrition and immune function. Clin Appl Nutr 1(1):85–94, 1991.
18. Katz, S: Assessing self-maintenance: Activities of daily living, mobility, and instrumental activities of daily living. J Am Geriatr Soc 31:721–727, 1983.
19. Spector, WD: Functional disability scales. In Spilker, B (ed): Quality Life Assessments in Clinical Trials, Raven, New York, 1990.
20. Shock, NW, Gruelich, RC, Andres, R, Arenberg, D, Costa, PT, Jr., Lakaata, EG, and Tokin, JD: Normal Human Aging: The Longitudinal Study of Aging, NIH Publ No: 84–2450. National Institutes of Health, Washington, DC, 1984.
21. McGandy, RB, Barrows, CH, Jr, Spanias, A, Meredith, A, Stone, JL, and Norris, AH: Nutrient intakes and energy expenditures in men of different ages. J Gerontol 21:581, 1966.

22. La Porte, RE, Black-Sandler, R, Cauley, JA, Link, M, Bayles, C, and Marks, B: The assessment of physical activity in older women: Analysis of the interrelationships and reliability of activity monitoring, activity surveys, and caloric intake. J Gerontol 38:394–397, 1983.

23. Fiatarone, MA, Marks, EC, Ryan, ND, Meredith, CN, Lipsitz, LA, and Evans, WJ: High-intensity strength training in nonagenarians: Effects on skeletal muscle. JAMA 263(22):3029–3034, 1990.

24. Butterworth, DE, Neiman, DC, Perkins, R, Warren, BJ, and Dotson, RG: Exercise training and nutrient intake in elderly women. J Amer Dietet Assoc 93:653–657, 1993.

25. Fiatarone, MA, O'Neill, EF, Doyle, ND, Clements, KM, Roberts, SB, Kehayias, JJ, Lipsitz, LA, and Evans, WJ: The Boston FICSIT Study: The effects of resistance training and nutritional supplementation on physical frailty in the oldest old. J Am Geriatr Soc 41:333–337, 1993.

26. Gersovitz, M, Motil, K, Munro, H, Scrimshaw, NS, and Young, VR: Human protein requirements: Assessment of the adequacy of the current recommended dietary allowance for dietary protein in elderly men and women. Am J Clin Nutr 35:6–14, 1982.

27. Fiatarone, MA, O'Neill, EF, Ryan, ND, Clements, KM, Solares, GR, Nelson, ME, Roberts, SB, Kehayias, JJ, Lipsitz, LA, and Evans, WJ: Exercise training and nutritional supplementation for physical frailty in very elderly people. N Engl J Med 330(25):1769–1775, 1994.

28. Tobin, J and Spector, D: Dietary protein has no effect on future creatinine clearance. Gerontologist 26:59A, 1986.

29. Lindeman, RD: The aging renal system. In Chernoff, R (ed): Geriatric Nutrition: The Health Professional's Handbook. Aspen, Gaithersburg, MD, 1991.

30. Berg, RL and Cassells, JS (eds): The Second Fifty Years: Promoting Health and Preventing Disability. National Academy Press, Washington, DC, 1990.

31. Kaiser, FE: Cholesterol, heart disease, and the older adult. Clin Appl Nutr 2(1):35–43, 1992.

32. Schaefer, EJ, Moussa, PB, Wilson, WF, McGee, D, Dallal, G, and Castelli, WP: Plasma lipoproteins in healthy octogenarians: Lack of reduced high density lipoprotein cholesterol levels. Results from the Framingham Heart Study. Metabolism 38:293–296, 1989.

33. Andres, R: Aging and diabetes. Med Clin N Amer 55:835–846, 1971.

34. Blumberg, JB: Changing nutrient requirements in older adults. Nutr Today Sept/Oct: 15–20, 1992.

35. Jacob, RA: Vitamin C. In Shils, ME, Olson, JA, and Shike, M (eds): Modern Nutrition in Health and Disease, ed 8, pt 1. Lea & Febiger, Philadelphia, 1994.

36. Pedrosa, MC and Russell, RM: Folate and vitamin B_{12} absorption in atrophic gastritis. In Holt, PR and Russell, RM (eds): Chronic Gastritis and Hypochlorhydria in the Elderly. CRC Press, Boca Raton, 1993.

37. Krasinski, SD, Russell, RM, Otradovec, CL, Sadowski, JA, Hartz, SC, Jacob, RA, and McGandy, RB: Relationship of vitamin A and vitamin E to fasting plasma retinol, retinol-binding protein, retinyl esters, carotene, α-tocopherol, and cholesterol among elderly people and young adults: Increased plasma retinyl esters among the vitamin A supplement users. Am J Clin Nutr 49:112–120, 1989.

38. Heaney, RP: Calcium intake and bone health in the adult: A critical review of recent investigations. Clin Appl Nutr 2(4):10–29, 1992.

39. Chernoff, R: Thirst and fluid requirements in the elderly. Nutr Rev 52:83–85, 1994.

40. Master, AM, Lasser, RP, and Beckman, G: Tables of average weight and height of Americans aged 65 to 94 years. J Am Med Assoc 172:658–662, 1960.

41. Shock, NW, Gruelich, RC, Andres, R, Arenberg, D, Costa, PT, Jr., Lakaata, EG, and Tokin, JD: Normal Human Aging. Op cit.

42. Martin, KI, Sox, HC, and Krupp, JR: Involuntary weight loss: Diagnostic and prognostic significance. Ann Intern Med 95:568, 1981.

43. Rabinovitz, M, Pitlik, SD, Leifer, M, Garty, M, and Resenfeld, JB: Unintentional weight loss: A retrospective analysis of 154 cases. Arch Intern Med 146:186, 1986.

44. Schiffman, SS: Perception of taste and smell in elderly persons. Crit Rev Food Sci Nutr 33(1):17–26, 1993.

45. Young, EA and Urban, E: Aging, the aged, and the gastrointestinal tract. In Young, EA (ed): Nutrition, Aging, and Health. Alan R Liss, New York, 1986.

46. Dwyer, JT, Gallo, JJ, and Reichel, W: Assessing nutritional status in elderly patients. Am Fam Phys 47(3):613–620, 1993.

47. Women's Health: Report of the Public Health Service Task Force on Women's Health Issues, vol 1. Public Health Reports 100(1):73–106, 1985.

48. Rowe, JW: Falls. In Rowe, JW and Besdine, RW (eds): Health and Disease in Old Age. Little, Brown, Boston, 1982.

49. Bower, RH: Malnutrition and immune function. Clin Appl Nutr 1(1):15–24, 1991.

50. Lipschitz, DA: Protein calorie malnutrition in the hospitalized elderly. Primary Care 9(3): 531–543, 1982.

51. Hoffman, NB: Dehydration in the elderly: Insidious and manageable. Geriatrics 46(4):35–38, 1991.

52. Sullivan, D, Chernoff, R, and Lipschitz, DA: Nutritional support in long-term care facilities. Nutr Clin Prac 2(1):6–13, 1987.

53. Breslow, RA, Hallfrisch, J, Guy, DG, Crawley, B, and Goldberg, AP: The importance of dietary protein in healing pressure ulcers. J Am Geriatr Soc 41:357–362, 1993.

54. Lipschitz, DA: Protein calorie malnutrition in the hospitalized elderly. Primary Care 9:531–543, 1982.

55. Lipschitz, DA and Mitchell, CO: The correctability of the nutritional, immune, and hematopoietic manifestations of protein calorie malnutrition in the elderly. J Am Coll Nutr 1:17–25, 1982.

56. Morley, JE: Nutritional status of the elderly. Am J Med 81:679–695, 1986.

57. Shaver, JH, Loper, JA, and Lutes, R: Nutritional status of nursing home patients. JPEN 4: 367–370, 1980.

58. Chernoff, R and Lipschitz, DA: Enteral feeding and the geriatric patient. In Rombeau, JL and Caldwell, MD (eds): Clinical Nutrition. vol 1: Enteral and Tube Feeding, ed 2. WB Saunders, Philadelphia, 1990.

59. Ouslander, JG, Tymchuk, AJ, and Krynski, MD: Decisions about enteral tube feeding among the elderly. J Am Geriatr Soc 41:70–77, 1993.

60. Chernoff, R and Lipschitz, DA: Total parenteral nutrition: Considerations in the elderly. In Rombeau, JL and Caldwell, MD (eds): Clinical Nutrition. vol 2: Parenteral Nutrition. WB Saunders, Philadelphia, 1986.

61. Chernoff, R and Ropka, M: The unique nutritional needs of the elderly patients with cancer. Sem Oncol Nurs 4(3):189–197, 1988.

62. Hardy, C, Wallace, C, Khansur, T, Vance, RB, Thigpen, JT, and Balducci, L: Nutrition, cancer and aging: An annotated review. II: Cancer cachexia and aging. J Am Ger Soc 32: 219–228, 1986.

63. Chernoff, R: Nutrition and chemotherapy in the elderly. In Dunkle, RE, Petot, GJ, and Ford, AB (eds): Food, Drugs, and Aging. Springer, New York, 1986.

64. Reiff, TR: Water and aging. Clin Ger Med 3(2):403–411, 1987.

65. Lipschitz, DA, Mitchell, CO, and Thompson, C: The anemia of senescence. Am J Hematol 11:47–54, 1981.

66. Barboriak, JJ and Rooney, CB: Alcohol and its effects on the nutrition of the elderly. In Watson, RR (ed): Handbook of Nutrition in the Aged. CRC Press, Boca Raton, 1985.

67. Pinchofsky-Devin, GD and Kaminski, MV: Correlation of pressure sores and nutritional status. J Am Ger Soc 34:435–440, 1986.

68. Gilchrest, BA: Skin. In Rowe, JW and Besdine, RW (eds): Health and Disease in Old Age, Little, Brown, Boston, 1982.

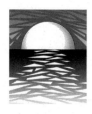

CHAPTER 14

Medication Management and Appropriate Substance Use for the Elderly

Barbara W.K. Yee, PhD
Betty J. Williams, PhD

BEHAVIORAL OBJECTIVES

Upon completion of this chapter, the reader will be able to:

1   Explain why the elderly are a high-risk population with regard to drug use.
2   Describe the normal physiologic changes that occur with aging and how these changes affect drug action.
3   Recognize how drugs function (for example, drug interactions).
4   List complications seen with drugs commonly taken by older patients.
5   Describe some of the consequences of alcohol abuse, and identify early warning signs.
6   Identify key factors that contribute to noncompliance, and discuss effective strategies to increase compliance.
7   Outline how elderly consumers and caregivers can help minimize the potential for adverse drug reactions.

Common Drug Therapies
Cardiovascular Disease
  Hypertension
  Congestive Heart Failure
  Angina Pectoris
  Cardiac Arrhythmias
  Atherosclerosis
Conditions of the Nervous System
  Insomnia and Anxiety
  Depression
  Psychiatric Diseases
  Alzheimer's Disease
Respiratory Disease
Joint Disease
Diabetes
Compliance Issues
Types of Compliance
Factors Linked to Noncompliance
  Number of Medications Taken

  Inadequate Information and
    Instructions
  Cultural Background
  Social Isolation
  Cost of Drugs
  Duration of Drug Therapy
  Limitations Due to Chronic Illness
    and Physical and Mental
    Impairments
Strategies for Reducing Noncompliance
What a Rehabilitation Specialist Can Do
Alcohol Use among the Elderly
Chronic Alcohol Use
Obstacles to Rehabilitation
References
Bibliography
Appendix 14–1: Checklist for Elderly
  Consumers and Their Caregivers
Appendix 14–2: Resources

Appropriately using both prescribed and over-the-counter medications, as well as enjoying an occasional drink, may significantly enhance the quality of life for older individuals. Rational medication practices are essential for optimal bodily function, physical and mental activity, recovery from illness and injury, control of chronic conditions, and maintenance of health throughout life, especially during the later years.

In this chapter, we will discuss the following: (1) why the elderly are at greater risk for medication and substance misuse or abuse than younger people; (2) common drug therapies for chronic diseases and ailments of older adults; (3) compliance issues that influence medication management and substance use; (4) issues related to alcohol use and abuse; and (5) obstacles to rehabilitation. A list of resources is provided for further information and assistance.

Certain factors place the elderly at greater risk for medication and substance misuse or abuse than other age groups.[1] These can be divided into two major categories: internal factors, related to the elderly person, and external factors, related to the elderly person's drugs or to health professionals who care for elderly persons. Compliance issues, because of their special importance, are discussed in a separate section of the chapter.

INTERNAL FACTORS

Chronic and Multiple Diseases

Elderly persons have more chronic diseases, and are more likely to have multiple diseases and experience more symptoms from these diseases, than younger people, thereby increasing the number of prescribed and over-the-counter medications taken simultaneously.[2,3]

Although older Americans comprise only 12 percent of the U.S. population, they fill about 25 percent of the prescriptions written annually. The average older person fills more than twice as many prescriptions as a person under the age of 65.[4] An average of 10.7 prescription medications are obtained by noninstitutionalized elderly each year. Fifty-four percent of all prescription drug costs are paid out-of-pocket by the elderly.[5,6]

In a year-long sample survey of the nation's office-based physicians, Nelson[7] found that patients aged 65 and older (22 percent of sample) used over 28 percent of the drugs studied. More importantly, patients aged 75 or older were provided with or had prescribed for them three or more medications than their younger counterparts. Black patients had more medications prescribed for them than their white counterparts. These drug consumption patterns suggest that appropriate drug management is critical during the later years.

Patients with chronic diseases receive a broader range of medications than those with acute illnesses. In addition, physicians treating chronic conditions are more likely than those treating acute conditions to consult colleagues about methods of treatment. The implications are that physicians treating chronic conditions are likely to be influenced by their consulting colleagues and often bring in specialists when treating their elderly patients. This situation increases the number of prescribers, the number of drugs prescribed, and the amount of coordination required to manage effective and safe drug therapy for elderly individuals suffering from multiple chronic conditions.[8] Potent medications are prescribed for older patients more frequently than for younger patients, potentially leading to harmful effects, such as adverse drug reactions or dangerous drug interactions.[7,9] For example, some common prescription drugs taken by the elderly, such as digoxin and warfarin, have been associated with a high incidence of drug-induced hospital admissions.

Physiologic Changes

There is a commonly held belief that the elderly are more sensitive to the effects of drugs than are younger adults. In fact, the aged are more sensitive to the effects of some drugs, but less sensitive to the effects of others. Additionally, the elderly may react more or less vigorously than younger individuals to the same drug due to the influence of factors associated with the aging process. The reaction of any elderly person to a drug may be difficult to predict because of age-related changes in the body. These changes are of two types: pharmacokinetic and homeostatic.

Pharmacokinetic Parameters

The factors that influence how the body handles drugs are called *pharmacokinetic parameters*.[10–13] These factors include absorption, distribution, metabolism, and excretion of the drug. The rates at which these steps occur determine not only how fast a drug works and how long the drug effect lasts but also the blood concentration that will be reached and, therefore, the magnitude of the therapeutic or toxic effect.

The pharmacokinetics of a drug vary from individual to individual, but do not vary in a single patient unless affected by other factors, such as disease or the presence of other chemicals in the body. Individual variations in pharmacokinetics can explain the observation that one person may be strongly affected by a dose of a drug that causes negligible effects in another. The process of aging produces changes in the body that will alter pharmacokinetic parameters and therefore cause changes in the apparent sensitivity to various drugs. The types of changes to be expected are considered below.

Absorption. There is little evidence that aging alters the rate at which drugs are absorbed from the gastrointestinal tract. Absorption may, however, be altered by some conditions associated with aging. Poor nutrition may increase drug absorption, whereas excessive laxative or antacid use may retard absorption.

Distribution. The distribution of a drug depends on its chemical composition. Some drugs are water-soluble and distribute themselves primarily in the water compartments of the body: blood, extracellular fluid, etc. Other drugs are fat-soluble and may concentrate in adipose tissue. Still others have a particular affinity for protein and may bind to protein in muscle or serum.

Several physiologic changes that occur in aging may alter drug distribution. The elderly have less lean body mass, less body water, and more fat as a percentage of total body mass. Because of the relative alterations in the size of body compartments, a drug dosage calculated on the basis of a patient's body weight may produce an unexpectedly high blood concentration and excessive effect. Allowing a patient to become dehydrated can further complicate the situation. Drugs that accumulate in body fat may require above-normal doses when therapy is initiated to fill the adipose tissue reservoir, and may linger in the body longer than expected when therapy is terminated. One can imagine a situation in which additional drugs must be given because of increased body fat; a small miscalculation brings the drug level to the toxic concentration, but because a large amount of the drug is stored in fat, it takes a long time to rid the body of the drug and eliminate the toxicity.

Metabolism. Metabolism or biotransformation of drugs takes place to some small extent in virtually every tissue of the body, but by far the greatest amount of drug metabolism occurs in the liver. Although aging may impair the liver's ability to metabolize some drugs, other factors consistent with aging are probably of more importance. Among these are a decreased liver blood flow and a decline in the ability of the liver to recover from disease or injury, such as that caused by alcohol or hepatitis. Reduction in liver blood flow decreases the rate of extraction of drug from the blood by the liver; injury reduces all liver function. Additionally, congestive heart failure or severe nutritional deficiencies reduce liver function and the rate of drug metabolism.

Excretion. Although some drugs are excreted in the feces—and to a very minor extent, in sweat, in tears, and via the lungs—the kidney is the major organ of drug excretion. Renal function declines with age, reducing the rate of excretion of drugs and their metabolites. Reduced excretion has the effect of allowing drugs and their metabolites to accumulate in the body, possibly causing toxicity but undoubtedly increasing the duration of action. Of equal importance are diseases common to the elderly that impair renal function. In congestive heart failure, cardiac output is reduced and the kidney is less effective in clearing the blood of foreign material. The elevated renal pressure seen in hypertension can, it left untreated, produce irreversible damage to the kidney and therefore reduce the ability of the kidney to deal with drugs and their metabolites.

Homeostatic Mechanisms

Many drugs, especially those affecting the cardiovascular system, are administered with the full expectation that compensatory reflexes will come into play and participate in the overall effect. The compensatory reflexes, like all homeostatic mechanisms, become blunted with age. Drugs that normally evoke compensatory changes, therefore, appear overly effective in the elderly. For example, if a vasodilator drug is given in an emergency situation in which rapid reduction of blood pressure is needed (for example, hypertensive crisis), a young adult will respond with compensatory reflexes that will modulate the fall in blood pressure. In an elderly person, however, these reflexes do not operate as briskly, and the blood pressure may drop to a lower level with the same drug dose.

Similarly, elderly diabetics may experience a hypoglycemic attack if they do not eat within a short time after taking their medication, because their bodies do not respond with sufficient speed to the lowering of blood sugar. Exercise also will tend to reduce blood sugar and can be dangerous in elderly diabetics unless care is taken to ensure that medication and food are taken on schedule.

Inherited Traits

Inherited traits that influence the absorption, metabolism, distribution, and excretion of a drug may be more devastating in old age because the elderly often lack sufficient reserve capacity to bounce back from health problems or drug-induced complications. Inherited factors may also alter tissue sensitivity. Inherited traits, coupled with the changes that occur with age, such as drug use, may be significantly different from young adult norms.

Age

Age is another major factor, even within the elderly population. The young old, those younger than 70, are very different in a number of characteristics in comparison to the old old, those over the age of 75. For example, the old old are more likely to be frail, suffer from many health conditions, and be treated with drugs; they are therefore at greater risk for drug-induced problems.

Sullivan and Korman[14] warn that both prescribed and over-the-counter drugs may produce iatrogenic effects (negative health conditions produced by therapeutic interventions), such as confusional states, in older persons. The danger in attributing these confusional states to the normative processes of aging, or to irreversible rather than remedial processes, is that nothing is done to remedy the situation. Effective therapies are difficult to implement when the elderly patient is confused and cognitively impaired. Unfortunately, in large number of these cases, careful drug review and monitoring could have averted or lessened the negative impact of these tragedies.

Gender

The gender of the patient also influences drug usage. It appears that elderly women use 19.6 prescriptions a year in comparison to 15.3 for elderly men.[7,15] This gender difference can be attributed to a number of factors. The two main reasons are that women live longer than men, thereby increasing the number of chronic conditions to be treated, and women visit their physicians more frequently than men and are therefore given more prescriptions.

Nutrition

Science has increasingly focused on how nutrition influences one's health over the life course, particularly during the second half of life. The nutritional status of older people is influenced adversely by poverty, social isolation, lack of adequate exercise, ignorance of what constitutes good nutrition, and biologic changes associated with aging and disease. For example, loss of teeth or poorly fitted dentures may encourage the older person to rely on soft processed foods. Loss of appetite due to reduced sensitivity of taste buds or lack of company during mealtime may encourage these elderly people to skip meals or eat quickly prepared foods. These conditions may lead to malnutrition.

Malnutrition plays a critical role in the morbidity and mortality of the very old. It significantly decreases the human immunological competence, making these malnourished elders more susceptible to infections. Malnutrition also increases the susceptibility of the patient to nonhealing decubitus ulcers. It reduces the effectiveness of drugs as well.[16] Drug and alcohol consumption can also influence the nutritional status of the elderly.

Drugs are capable of altering nutrient intake or utilization in four ways. First, drugs may impair absorption of nutrients when used for prolonged periods of time. For example, some drugs that lower blood cholesterol, such as neomycin, have been associated with diminished vitamin B_{12} and iron absorption.[17] Regular use of mineral oil as a laxative may decrease absorption of vitamins A, D, E, and K.[18]

Second, drugs may also impair the body's utilization of nutrients. For example, treatment of epilepsy with phenytoin or phenobarbital has been found to impair folic acid utilization.[19] Pyridoxine utilization is affected by isoniazid used in the treatment of tuberculosis. Neurologic symptoms may develop with long-term pyridoxine depletion.

Lastly, drugs may act to reduce food intake by producing gastric irritation or nausea and create a significant loss of appetite. Drugs also may affect the senses of smell and taste, leading to a decrease in food intake as well. Examples of such drugs are penicillin tablets and sympathomimetic nasal sprays.[20]

High alcohol consumption also influences the nutritional status of elderly people by filling them with too many empty calories. More will be said about the relationship between alcoholism, drug misuse, and the elderly in a later section.

Certain medications can also interfere with mineral metabolism, for example, decreasing calcium absorption, increasing bone loss, and making the elderly person more prone to osteoporosis.[21]

Symptomatology

Because the elderly have more health conditions that require professional intervention, they seek medical care more frequently than younger people and, as a result, more medications are prescribed for these problems. The number of medications prescribed seems to be related to the frequency of office visits to a physician by older persons.[22]

A study of ambulatory elderly found a stronger relationship between symptoms and diseases than between age and symptoms.[23] This study suggests that symptomatology is more likely than the age of the patient in predicting higher drug usage. Sharpe and Smith[24] also supported this notion, observing that the strongest direct effect on prescription drug use was perceived morbidity or anxiety about the morbidity. Higher consumption of prescription drugs has been demonstrated to be related to lower life and health satisfaction.[25]

Age Cohort Influences

Alcohol and drug abuse remain in the closet among the elderly cohort because these vices are very stigmatizing for those over 65. Drug abuse is not a problem that one usually associates with the elderly population. Indeed, the drug abuse problem in this age group is quite different from that featured typically in the national news. However, there is a problem of excessive and compulsive drug use by the elderly, a problem that centers primarily around the use of laxatives. Not only can the abuse of laxatives lead to the diminished effect of particular drugs; it can change the effects of other drugs that are being taken by altering gastrointestinal function.

Over-the-Counter Drug Use

The elderly consume more *over-the-counter (OTC) drugs* than younger people. Of persons over 60, 40 percent use OTC preparations every day. On average, two of every five drugs taken by the elderly are OTC drugs—a rate seven times greater than that of younger adults. Approximately one third of all expenditures for medications by the elderly are for nonprescription drugs.[26] The amount spent on nonprescription drugs by the elderly in 1981 was estimated to be about $7 billion.

The OTC drugs commonly used by the elderly include analgesics (aspirin, Tylenol), laxatives, antihistamines and anticholinergics, sympathomimetics (cold or allergy medication), alcohol-based OTC medication (cough syrup), and caffeine. Use of analgesics is greatest among people over 60 because of arthritis or frequent headaches.[27] Thirty percent of the elderly over 60 are regular users of laxatives, while 3 percent seriously overuse these OTC drugs.[28] Four of five older men drink a caffeinated beverage daily, with one of five consuming four or more cups of coffee every day. Although the frequency of overuse is unclear, caffeine can produce physical dependence. OTC drugs are often used by the elderly without consultation from their physicians and, perhaps of more concern, without the knowledge of their physicians.

A more dangerous situation for the elderly consumer is the fact that nearly 80 percent of daily OTC drug users take them in combination with alcohol, prescribed drugs, or both.[29] Unfortunately, many elderly consumers and their physicians do not view over-the-counter medications as potentially dangerous drugs that should be used judiciously according to specific label directions.[16] More will be said about the interactions between drugs later.

For a variety of reasons, the elderly often choose to self-medicate for some health conditions, such as arthritis, insomnia, or constipation. Some elderly choose to self-medicate with OTC drugs rather than visit a physician because of limited mobility or fixed incomes, unavailability of a familiar physician due to retirement or death, the increase in the number of OTC drugs on the market, the rise in health consumerism and greater exposure to drug use to treat health conditions in the elderly population, or the attitude that these health conditions are not serious enough to visit a doctor.[30] (See review in Fincham.[31]) OTC drugs can be used safely and effectively in accordance with specific label directions and in consultation with a primary-care physician. The elderly have more health reasons than younger people to use OTC drugs but are at much greater risk of developing special problems associated with chronic OTC drug use, such as increased sensitivity to adverse side effects or metabolic derangement.

While drug abuse and alcoholism in older patients tend to present non-specifically as medical or metabolic problems, or with decreased levels of functioning,[32] diagnosis of OTC misuse or abuse can be made only if clinicians are aware of the extent of potential drug abuse and alcoholism by their elderly patients. Patients with the following characteristics should be screened for potential OTC misuse: those with no previous relationship with a physician; poor patients; and patients with chronic symptoms, somatization disorders, or a history of drug or alcohol abuse.[29]

EXTERNAL FACTORS

Drug Interactions

Because of the likelihood of multiple diseases, there is a significant possibility that elderly people may be taking several different drugs simultaneously. Many times, the drugs have been prescribed by different physicians with little regard for other drug use. Drug interactions can pose a significant problem in all patients. The problem becomes more acute in the elderly because of the number of different drugs they usually take. It is important to recognize that drug interactions can occur not only among prescription medications but also among prescription and nonprescription drugs.

Whenever two or more drugs are being taken simultaneously, there is a risk of drug interaction. Drug interactions take one of two forms, the *pharmacokinetic interaction*, where one drug causes changes in the way the body handles the other drug, and the *pharmacodynamic interactions*, in which the action of one drug enhances or interferes with the action of the other. Of the two, the pharmacokinetic interactions are the most prevalent, and in some cases, the more difficult to predict.

No attempt is made here comprehensively to list drug interactions. Several books, some of which are listed in the bibliography (Shinn and Shrewsbury, 1985; Hansten, 1985), compile documented instances of drug interaction and discuss the mechanisms of those interactions.

Pharmacokinetic Interactions

Pharmacokinetic interactions can occur between any two drugs, regardless of their chemical composition. Mechanisms by which pharmacokinetic interactions occur include interference with drug metabolism, enhancement of drug metabolism, competition for protein-binding sites, and enhancement of excretion.

Interference

Interference with drug metabolism is probably the most common way in which one drug may alter the action of another. A drug that inhibits the metabolism of a second drug can cause the second drug to have an abnormally great effect and a longer duration. For example, some of the drugs that are used in the treatment of depression, the monoamine oxidase inhibitors such as amitriptyline (Elavil), have as their mechanism of action inhibition of an enzyme that metabolizes normal body constituents. This enzyme also functions in the metabolism of some other drugs and chemicals, such as alcohol and tyramine, a component of many cheeses and other foods. When a patient is taking a monoamine oxidase inhibitor, it is likely that alcohol will produce a more profound effect than normally seen. It is also possible that eating cheese containing tyramine will provide a hypertensive crisis because of the abnormally large and prolonged effect of the tyramine, which is a vasoconstrictor. Consumption of large amounts of green, leafy vegetables may alter a person's response to coumarin anticoagulants because the vitamin K contained in those vegetables reduces the anticoagulant effect.

Enhancement

Enhancement of drug metabolism is usually accomplished by increasing the amount of enzyme in the specialized liver microsomal system. This enzyme induction may occur as a result of the action of a number of different types of chemicals. Probably the most well-studied of these chemicals are the barbiturates, a group of common sedative-hypnotic agents. These drugs are themselves metabolized by the liver microsomal system, and can cause an accelerated rate of metabolism in both themselves and other drugs. This is thought to be one reason why patients develop "tolerance" to the effects of barbiturates. Tolerance, in pharmacologic terms, refers to the phenomenon in which, with continued administration, larger doses are required to produce the same effect. It is a common factor in compulsive drug use and abuse. Additionally, the concomitant use of barbiturates may accelerate the metabolism of anticoagulants (such as Dicumarol), anticonvulsants (such as Dilantin), and many other drugs. In each case, the result is the reduction of the effect of the drug, indicating that the dose of the anticoagulant being used to prevent thrombus formation may no longer be adequate or that the anticonvulsant dosage can no longer control the epilepsy. Enzyme induction is a reversible effect, making it equally dangerous when therapy with barbiturates or some other enzyme inducer is terminated. At that time, the rate of drug metabolism will be reduced to normal levels, causing a relative increase in the amount of unmetabolized drug in the body.

Competition for Sites

Many drugs are carried in the plasma as protein-bound molecules. Different proteins seem to bind acidic drugs, basic drugs, and relatively uncharged drugs, but within those groups, there is no real specificity of the binding sites for one or another drug. Since the number of binding sites is finite, if two drugs that bind to the same protein sites are in the body simultaneously, the two drugs will compete for the available sites. The drug that binds with the greater affinity will occupy the greater number of binding sites, leaving more than the usual amount of the other drug unbound (or free). Free drug is the only form that is active, since it is the only form that can leave the blood. Therefore, the more of any drug that remains free in the blood, the greater its effect. In addition, free drug is the only form that can go to the liver or the kidney for metabolism and excretion.

When a drug is bound to a less than normal extent, its effect should be expected to be greater, but of shorter duration. Aspirin is an example of a drug that binds to plasma protein. By competing with uric acid for plasma protein binding sites, thereby promoting the excretion of uric acid, aspirin can be effective in the treatment of gout, which results from the accumulation of urate crystals in the joints. Unfortunately, some other drugs, for example, probenecid (Benemid) that are used to treat gout also bind to plasma protein, and this binding is competitive with aspirin. The result is that the combination is no more effective in the treatment of gout than either agent alone, and since each drug causes its own characteristic toxicities, more symptoms of toxicity may appear.

Excretion

Excretion of drugs occurs primarily via the kidneys, but to a lesser extent through the gastrointestinal tract. Any drug that alters the function of either organ can alter the rate at which drug is excreted. Diuretics, such as hydrochlorothiazide (Hydrodiuril), are used commonly to treat congestive heart failure, hypertension, and renal disease in the elderly. Because diuretics increase the rate of water loss via the kidney, any drug that is excreted dissolved in the urine will be lost from the body at a faster rate. Laxatives shorten transit time through the gastrointestinal tract and speed up the excretion of drugs by this route. Drugs that could be affected include the digitalis glycosides (digoxin and digitoxin), used in the treatment of congestive heart failure, cholestyramine (Questran) used to lower blood triglycerides and cholesterol, and steroids.

Pharmacodynamic Interactions

Pharmacodynamic interactions usually occur among drugs that are chemically similar or have similar therapeutic effects. There are three types of pharmacodynamic interactions.

Pharmacologic Antagonism

Propranolol is a drug that is used in the treatment of various cardiovascular diseases including hypertension and angina pectoris. This drug acts by preventing access of the normal body constituents, epinephrine and norepinephrine, to some of their sites of action (receptors), thereby preventing their effects. Propranolol is said to be a blocking drug, and can interfere with the action of any drug that acts at those same receptors. This type of pharmacodynamic interaction is called *pharmacologic antagonism.*

Physiologic Antagonism

A second type of pharmacodynamic interaction occurs when two drugs that are administered produce opposing physiologic effects. The effect produced will be that of neither drug, but will be somewhere in between the two. This type of interaction is usually called *physiologic antagonism.*

Synergism

A third type of pharmacodynamic interaction occurs when two drugs that each produce a similar action, when given together, produce an effect that is greater than the sum of their individual actions. This is the effect seen when sedatives such as diazepam (Valium) and alcohol are consumed together. Either agent produces sedation and general central nervous system depression; together, the combination is deadly. This enhanced effect, produced by coadministration of two drugs that cause the same effect, is called *synergism.*

Because elderly people commonly take many drugs simultaneously—and in many cases, drugs prescribed by different physicians—it is important that at least one individual be aware of all the drugs being used and the forms of those drugs in use. One possibility is the pharmacist. A pharmacist is trained to recognize the potential for drug interactions and should be able to inform the physician if a problem of this sort exists. For this reason, it is advisable to use a single pharmacy for all prescriptions so that a record may be maintained of all current medications. The pharmacist will also work with the physician(s) to make sure that medication instructions are as clear and simple as possible.

Prescribing Behavior of Physicians

The prescribing behavior of physicians is influenced by personal characteristics such as age, medical school attended, attitudes concerning the value of medication in the management of acute and chronic disease, and outside pressures, such as pharmaceutical representatives, journals, advertising, colleagues, and demands from patients.[33]

The pharmaceutical industry is estimated to spend more than $2 billion a year on advertising its products.[34] Advertising encourages physicians to prescribe more drugs and consumers to take more medications. Mass media advertising provides the strongest influence on the drug-use behavior of health professionals and consumers.

Physicians and their elderly patients may also be psychologically predisposed to use medications to provide relief for chronic disease symptoms and do so on a long-term basis.[24] Because both doctors and their older patients perceive medications to be the answer to the patients' health problems, older patients are more likely to receive medications than other therapeutic solutions, which may be equally or more effective at relieving the symptoms of many chronic conditions. Overprescribing often leads to problems among the elderly.

Simonson[35] states that physicians are caught in a dilemma. On one hand, elderly individuals may exert a significant amount of pressure on physicians to prescribe the medications that they, the patients, want. On the other hand, the rejection of unreasonable requests for medication could seriously damage the prescriber-patient relationship. Prescription writing may be a means of terminating the interview in a fashion that is accepted by both physician and patient, or the fulfillment of the unwritten contract.[36] The patients, especially older persons with numerous somatic complaints, may feel, when no prescription is written, that the doctor has failed to cure them or doesn't care to help cure their health problems. These patients may feel less satisfied with these types of physicians and may "doctor-shop" until they find a physician who is willing to prescribe medications to treat their ailments.

Lack of Geriatric Training in Physician Education

In 1982, only 600 physicians in the United States described themselves as having expertise in geriatrics. One study has indicated that 34,000 to 53,000 geriatricians will be needed in the United States by the year 2010.[37]

There is a serious lack of geriatric training in medical education, even now. Although many educators and governmental agencies recognize how serious this problem is, the large majority of medical education programs in the United States have not mainstreamed geriatrics in their curriculum. A small minority of programs have a geriatric elective, but most programs have been slow to systematically include geriatrics in their curriculum. The large majority of newly trained physicians get their geriatrics education on the job by trial or error, often at the expense of the older patient.

One major problem is the absence of a comprehensive body of knowledge on drug usage in the elderly. As a result, physicians have no prescription guidelines on which to rely.[38] Although some physicians recommend doses that are 30 to 50 percent of those used for younger adults,[39] a preferable method is to calculate the dose carefully on an individual basis and, when possible, to monitor drug concentrations in the blood.[40] When monitoring is not possible, a useful rule of thumb, when prescribing for a patient over 70 years of age, is to use one third of that used for a subject of the same weight who is half the patient's age.[41]

The implications of inadequately trained physicians for geriatric patients are serious and may lead to unrecognized and untreated health conditions or inappropriate drug therapy for misdiagnosed conditions. This creates a whole host of other problems, such as adverse drug interactions or exacerbation of the underlying condition. Another implication of the inadequate training of physicians in geriatrics is the issue of undermedicating, and of overlooking chronic conditions in the elderly, such as depression, arthritis, diabetes mellitus, and osteoporosis. For instance, physicians often fail to treat depression in elderly patients because it can exhibit atypical symptoms, such as mental confusion. Another instance of failure to treat depression by physicians may be created because the health professional may regard depression as an emotion that accompanies old age.

Societal Issues

Only recently have adverse reactions to drugs become well documented and routinely recognized. Many adverse reactions to drugs, such as confusion or dizziness in the elderly population, were attributed to other causes, associated with either aging or disease conditions such as dementias, normative depopulation of brain cells, or deterioration of the vestibular system.

Currently, the Food and Drug Administration requires that companies demonstrate safety and efficacy for the malady a drug is claimed to treat before it can be approved for marketing. Most studies demonstrating safety and efficacy are limited largely to people between the ages of 20 and 60. Many experts have called for an amendment to the Food, Drug and Cosmetic Act of 1962, which would require drug companies to determine drug safety and efficacy for children and for adults over 60.[42] Efficacy studies for elderly patients are currently under way.[43] This policy change could lessen one source of drug problems for elderly people.

COMMON DRUG THERAPIES

A discussion of the action of drugs used to treat all disease conditions of the elderly is far beyond the scope of this chapter. For detailed information on any specific drug, consult the bibliography at the end of the chapter (see Craig and Stitzel, 1994; Gilman, Rall, Nies, and Taylor, 1990; Katzung, 1992). For a more detailed discussion of rapidly changing antibiotic drugs, see the review in Craig and Stitzel (1994). Reviews of medication management issues for Parkinson's disease can be found in Korman and James (1993), for chronic pain in Rowland and Fallon (1993), and for the use of anti-inflammatory drugs in Chapron.[44]

It can generally be said that the same drugs are used to treat the same conditions, whether the patient is young or elderly. The differences in therapy usually consist of differences in dosages, with the usual dose being gradually reduced with age. In some instances, a different drug is preferred for the elderly than that used for younger adults because it is more effective or less likely to cause disturbing side effects.

From the standpoint of health care providers other than physicians, two questions regarding drug therapy should be of concern: Is drug therapy adequate? Is drug therapy excessive? Adequate drug therapy is signaled by the disappearance or control of the original symptoms. An indication of excessive drug therapy may be the appearance of new symptoms. These symptoms may seem totally unrelated to the original condition and may be so subtle that the patient is not even aware of their presence (for example, changes in behavior). In either case, the patient should be advised to see a physician and to clearly and completely describe the condition.

Drug toxicities come in many types. Some toxicities, such as gastrointestinal distress, nausea, or vomiting, are very general and nonspecific, in that they may be caused by many different types of drugs. Other toxicities are very specific, and are seen only with specific drugs, such as the blurred vision sometimes seen with ibuprofen (Motrin, Advil, Nuprin) and the "pseudo-Parkinsonism" seen with some agents used to treat emotional and mental disease, such as haloperidol (Haldol).

Cardiovascular Disease

Hypertension

Hypertension is a significant problem in the elderly, especially in Western cultures. Hypertension itself can be a virtually "silent," symptomless disease; its main danger is its possible sequelae—stroke, heart attack, and renal disease. A number of different types of drugs are available to treat hypertension: vasodilators such as hydralazine (Apresoline), calcium channel blockers such as nifedipine (Procardia), beta-adrenergic blocking agents such as propranolol (Inderal), centrally acting adrenergic agents such as clonidine (Catapres), renin system inhibitors such as enalapril (Vasotec), and diuretics.

Each type of agent acts through a different mechanism and has its own toxicities. Because of safety, many physicians will try nondrug therapy initially (weight reduction, salt restriction). Thiazide diuretics (for example, Diuril) are considered a reasonable first step in therapy, but these drugs have the liability that they are likely to produce some degree of hypokalemia, hyperglycemia, and hyperuricemia. These effects may be particularly problematic in the elderly, since hypokalemia may provoke cardiac rhythm disturbances, and the elderly have a higher-than-normal incidence of arrhythmias. There is a high incidence of late-onset diabetes in the elderly. The production of hyperglycemia can exacerbate the problem, but can also complicate treatment of the diabetes. Gout is another problem that is more prevalent in the elderly than in the general population, and production of hyperuricemia can trigger an attack.

Calcium channel blockers and beta-adrenergic blocking agents are both very effective agents in the general population; however, in older patients, calcium channel blockers are more effective than beta blockers. Either type of drug is effective in treating angina pectoris and would be a particularly good choice in patients who have both angina and hypertension. Both have the liability that they can slow and even stop the heart in overdose. Patients with congestive heart failure are particularly sensitive to this effect, and these drugs should be avoided in these situations, if possible. The beta blockers can also cause some problems in asthmatics (provoke attacks and reduce effectiveness of some drug treatments) and in diabetics (reduced compensatory response to low blood sugar).

The other drugs mentioned above also have specific toxicities, but none seems to be more prevalent in the elderly than in younger patients.

Congestive Heart Failure

Congestive heart failure is a significant health problem in the elderly, made even more frightening by the fact that some of the drugs used to treat this condition are extremely toxic. Congestive heart failure is a condition in which the heart does not pump with enough force to supply blood to all parts of the body. The major symptoms of this condition are shortness of breath, the feeling that you cannot breathe deeply enough to take in all the oxygen you need, a general feeling of tiredness, and an inability to exert oneself. Congestive heart failure is treated either with cardiac glycosides (for example, digoxin and digitoxin) or vasodilators. The cardiac glycosides are plant alkaloids that have a powerful stimulant effect on the heart. Under the influence of the glycosides, the weakened heart is able to pump more forcefully and increase the cardiac output. These agents are not curative, and thus must be given for life if they are used as the treatment modality.

The problem with using cardiac glycosides is that they are very toxic compounds and have a very narrow safety margin. The safety margin is a measure of the difference between the dose that will produce the therapeutic effect and the dose that will cause toxicity. The dose of these agents is, therefore, crucial, and it is not unusual for small, seemingly insignificant changes in body function to allow enough of the drug to accumulate in the body to cause toxicity. The removal of digoxin from the body seems to be slower in the geriatric population than in younger adults, particularly in the presence of renal disease. Early symptoms of toxicity—blurred vision, slowed heart rate—may not seem particularly severe but may progress to significant cardiac rhythm disturbances, nausea, and vomiting and can be life-threatening. Hypokalemia, hypomagnesemia, and hypoxemia all increase the incidence of digitalis-induced arrhythmias. In the elderly, unlike their younger counterparts, the earliest symptom of toxocity may manifest itself as confusion. Unfortunately, this symptom can easily be mistaken for age-related forgetfulness. Thus, it is important for health care providers and the family of the patient to be alert for changes in behavior that may signal drug toxicity.

In recent years, some physicians have chosen to treat congestive heart failure with vasodilators. These drugs are felt to be effective because they reduce the resistance of the vasculature and, thereby, the pressure against which the weakened heart must pump, allowing it to pump more blood with each stroke. These drugs are certainly less toxic than the digitalis glycosides, but they may not be effective in all cases. Symptoms of vasodilator overdose are somewhat similar to the symptoms of congestive heart failure—specifically, tiredness and lack of energy.

Angina Pectoris

Angina pectoris is a condition in which areas of the heart suffer temporarily from oxygen lack, producing severe substernal pain that radiates across the chest and down the arm. Patients often describes the pain as a crushing sensation. Although there is no single, well-defined cause of angina, it seems to be satisfactorily treated by the use of vasodilator drugs such as nitroglycerin and amyl nitrite. These drugs are usually used when a rapid drug effect is needed, and the route of their administration is somewhat unique. Nitroglycerin is administered by putting a tablet under the tongue. Blood vessels are very close to the surface in this area, and the drug can be absorbed quickly and travel to its site of action, the heart. Amyl nitrite is supplied in a crushable glass ampule. For administration, the ampule is crushed, and the drug is inhaled as a vapor. Other drugs, such as the calcium channel blockers and beta blockers, are useful when given prophylactically to prevent recurrences of anginal attacks.

Cardiac Arrhythmias

Cardiac arrhythmias are disturbances in the normal rhythm of the heart. These changes may take the form of abnormally slow, abnormally fast, or uncoordinated beats. Depending on the type of rhythm alteration, different drugs are used for therapy. Among these drugs are quinidine, procainamide, lidocaine, disopyramide, and beta blockers. The rates of removal from the body of procainamide, quinidine, and lidocaine seem to be reduced in the elderly, and disopyramide has effects on bladder function leading to voiding problems, particularly in elderly men.

Atherosclerosis

Atherosclerosis is a condition in which plaques of lipid material collect in the inner walls of blood vessels. When this condition becomes sufficiently advanced, blood flow to the affected area of the body can become seriously compromised. Vascular compliance is reduced and blood pressure increases. The heart may also be affected, either due to atherosclerotic lesions in the vessels of the heart or as a result of continued pumping against high resistance.

Most therapy for atherosclerosis is aimed at preventing the development of plaques by reducing the blood levels of certain lipids, notably cholesterol. Lovastatin (Mevacor) is a drug widely promoted for reduction of serum cholesterol by inhibiting one enzymatic step in the synthesis of cholesterol. Since this drug is relatively new, it is not yet clear what, if any, long-term toxicities may occur, but experience thus far has shown little toxic effect. Niacin, in amounts much higher than those used for its vitamin properties, is quite effective in reducing serum lipids. The agent produces some effects that are quite unpleasant for the patient, such as flushing, itching, and gastrointestinal distress, and may cause some liver toxicity if liver function is already compromised. The itching, flushing, and gastrointestinal distress are usually a problem only for the first few days when the medication is taken, but some more serious problems may persist. Exacerbation of the condition may occur in diabetics taking this drug, and patients with pre-existing gout may experience acute gouty attacks. Cholestyramine (Questran) is a resin that is given orally but is not absorbed into the body. It acts by binding cholesterol and promoting its excretion in the feces. Because of the frequency of laxative use in the elderly, the passage through the gastrointestinal tract of cholestyramine, and thus its effect, may be unpredictable. In addition, cholestyramine may bind and promote the excretion of some fat-soluble vitamins (A, E, and K), an effect that can be serious if nutritional status is already marginal.

Conditions of the Nervous System

Insomnia and Anxiety

Insomnia is a frequently reported complaint among the elderly. Sedatives and hypnotics, such as the barbiturates and benzodiazepines (for example, Valium), seem to have quite variable effects in elderly persons because decline in liver and kidney function cause their retention in the body for as much as three times longer than in younger patients. There also appears to be an age-related increase in pharmacodynamic sensitivity to these drugs. These drugs, particularly the benzodiazepines, are even more frequently prescribed for anxiety. All the sedative-hypnotics have potential for producing tolerance (as reduced effect in response to the same dose) and compulsive drug use. Furthermore, these agents cause markedly enhanced CNS depression when taken with alcohol.

Depression

Depression in the elderly is often misdiagnosed as senile dementia and thus may not be treated appropriately. The same drugs used for this condition in younger individuals, tricyclics, such as amitriptyline (Elavil), and monoamine oxidase inhibitors, such as phenelzine (Nardil), are effective in the elderly. Both these agents are metabolized by the liver and excreted with their metabolites via the kidneys; thus, they may have a longer duration and greater incidence of toxicity in the elderly.

Symptoms of toxicity to these drugs may be hard to identify because they consist primarily of disease symptoms commonly seen with depression, for example, sedation, confusion, lassitude, tremor, and blurred vision, but they may also include cardiac rhythm disturbances and difficulty in urinating. As mentioned earlier, the monoamine oxidase inhibitors may interfere with the metabolism of alcohol and other drugs and may cause the appearance of symptoms of toxicity from the other drugs.

A newer group of drugs, the serotonin uptake inhibitors, for example, fluoxetine (Prozac), has gained a great deal of popularity in the treatment of depression. From all indications, fluoxetine poses no greater problem in the elderly than in the population at large, except that the elderly are likely to take longer to metabolize and excrete the drug, prolonging the effect. It should be mentioned that in the case of fluoxetine, as well as most other drugs mentioned in this chapter, observations about effects and dangers in the elderly come primarily from experience. Very few clinical drug studies have included the elderly as a segment of the test population. Common adverse effects seen with fluoxetine include anxiety, nervousness, insomnia, and nausea. News accounts of bizarre and hostile behavior in patients taking fluoxetine cannot, at this time, be causally linked. However, it is worth noting that caregivers and relatives should be alert to changes in behavior seen with this as well as with other medications.

Psychiatric Diseases

A variety of psychiatric diseases in the elderly are treated by the use of two classes of antipsychotic drugs, the phenothiazines, for example, chlorpromazine (Thorazine) and the butyrophenones, for example, haloperidol (Haldol). These drugs are undoubtedly useful in the management of schizophrenia of old age as well as some of the symptoms associated with delirium or dementia, such as agitation or combativeness. Much of the effectiveness of the drugs in agitated patients is probably due to their sedative effects. Chlorpromazine is frequently used for the elderly but may not be completely satisfactory for the geriatric patient. Unfortunately, it is not advisable to try to increase the effectiveness of the phenothiazines simply by increasing the dose, since there is too great a possibility of producing toxic effects. Chlorpromazine may produce orthostatic hypotension, as well as the movement disorders pseudo-Parkinsonism and tardive dyskinesia. Haloperidol has fewer effects on blood pressure than the phenothiazines and produces less sedation, but it is even more likely to produce movement disorders.

Sherman[45] argues that psychoactive drugs are among the most frequently prescribed agents for the elderly. These include antipsychotic medications, antianxiety drugs, sedative-hypnotics, and antidepressants. The most troubling misprescribing can be found in long-term care facilities. For instance, although 46 to 75 percent of long-term care residents have behavioral, social, emotional, and mental disorders and receive psychoactive drugs to deal with these disorders, few have psychiatric diagnoses that justify these prescriptions.[46] The Omnibus Reconciliation Act of 1987 has addressed the problem of psychoactive drug misuse. Shorr and associates[47] found a 26.7 decrease over a 30-month period in antipsychotic drug use among long-term care residents. Depression[48] and anxiety disorders[49] may be the most prevalent but underaddressed problem of nursing home residents.

Alzheimer's Disease

Alzheimer's disease and other senile dementias seem to be associated with a profound and rather selective loss of cholinergic (acetylcholine-secreting) neurons in the central nervous system. Cholinergic neurons appear to play an important part in cognitive function, especially memory. Although the antipsychotic drugs (discussed above) may produce some symptomatic improvement in such things as disturbed behavior, emotional lability, and abnormal sleep-wake cycles, they do not improve the basic disorder. In addition, there is some indication that they may worsen memory impairment and intellectual functioning. Currently, there is active research in the area of drug therapy of Alzheimer's disease, but no drug that has yet emerged is of clear benefit to the patient.

Respiratory Disease

Asthma and other respiratory diseases are treated in much the same way in the elderly as in younger patients, but some of the drugs pose serious hazards to the elderly. The drugs used fall into three classes: those that prevent the immune response that results in the asthmatic attack, and thus must be given prophylactically; those that cause the relaxation of bronchiolar smooth muscle, allowing less restricted breathing; and the glucocorticoids, which act in an unknown way to provide relief.

Prophylactic treatment of asthmatics with cromolyn sodium (Intal) is effective in reducing the number and severity of asthmatic attacks in young patients, and in some older patients, although the elderly seem less responsive to this drug. The drug is poorly absorbed after oral administration and is usually given by inhalation of a microfine powder. Probably because it is so poorly absorbed, systemic toxicities are rare; most side effects involve the area of administration for example, sore throat, cough, dry mouth.

Relaxation of the bronchiolar smooth muscle can be accomplished by either of two drug classes, the methylxanthines, of which theophylline seems to be the most effective, and the β-adrenergic agonists, for example, albuterol (Proventil). Theophylline is a close chemical relative of caffeine, and like caffeine, is found in tea and coffee. Theophylline causes increased alertness, nervousness, and insomnia, but not to the degree seen with caffeine. Similarly, both caffeine and theophylline cause relaxation of airway smooth muscle, but in this instance, theophylline is the more effective. Theophylline is metabolized by the liver, and its metabolism can be more rapid when hepatic enzymes are induced. Cigarette smoking has a drastic effect on the rate of theophylline metabolism. In smokers, a significant increase in dose is needed to produce the same active blood concentration. In the presence of heart or liver disease, the normal dose of theophylline may have to be decreased to avoid toxicity. Theophylline is also used in chronic obstructive lung disease (for example, emphysema), not only because of the relaxation of smooth muscle but also because it seems to have an effect on skeletal muscle, which results in improved diaphragmatic performance. Toxicities that might be anticipated with theophylline can include seizures and cardiac arrhythmias, but more commonly consist of anxiety, nausea, abdominal discomfort, and headache.

Albuterol is one of a group of similar drugs used either by oral administration for prophylaxis of asthmatic attacks, or acutely, by inhalation. In either case, the drug acts on the smooth muscle of the bronchioles to open the airway and allow freer breathing. Because these drugs are closely related to the cardiac stimulant adrenoceptor agonists, they can cause palpitations and cardiac arrhythmias and are effective in lowering blood pressure. As might be anticipated, these systemic effects are much less prevalent when the drug is administered by inhalation than when it is given orally, but may be problematic in older patients with cardiovascular disease.

Because of severe adverse effects when administered chronically, the use of corticosteroids (glucocorticoids such as prednisone) in asthma or obstructive lung disease is usually reserved for patients who do not improve adequately when given bronchodilators alone, or whose condition continues to worsen despite other therapies. The problem of severe chronic toxicity can be alleviated if the steroid is given by inhalation. Corticosteroids given by this route are very effective in many cases of mild asthma. With more severe disease, inhaled corticosteroids may be administered along with a bronchodilator for enhanced effect. The major toxicity to be expected with inhaled glucocorticoids is a propensity for the development of oral yeast infections, which can usually be avoided if the patient gargles after using the inhaler. Systemic adverse effects of corticosteroids are discussed below.

Joint Disease

Virtually all members of the elderly community suffer from some form of inflammatory joint disease, such as rheumatoid arthritis or osteoarthritis. The drugs must commonly used in the treatment of arthritis are the nonsteroidal antiflammatory drugs (NSAIDs). The most commonly recommended of the NSAIDs, for mild to moderate arthritis, is aspirin. All of the beneficial effects provided by the newer NSAIDs such as ibuprofen (Motrin, Advil, Nuprin) are also provided by aspirin. There are, however, differences in adverse effects and in pharmacokinetic parameters (duration of action, major inactivation pathway, etc.) among the drugs, which may lead to the selection of one or the other for a particular patient. Acetaminophen (Tylenol), on the other hand, has no anti-inflammatory action and therefore is of little or no use in the treatment of arthritis. It may provide some small pain relief but no relief of the inflammation and swelling. One effect of aspirin that does not seem to be duplicated by other members of the NSAID group is its apparent value in the prophylaxis of coronary artery disease. The FDA currently recommends one aspirin per day to reduce the probability of heart attack, especially if the patient has had a previous heart attack, but also warns that such treatment is not without risk, particularly the exacerbation of peptic ulcer.

The major problem associated with the use of aspirin on a chronic basis is the gastric irritation that many people experience. Aspirin may cause gastric bleeding in some individuals or activate a preexisting ulcer. Ibuprofen and the newer NSAIDs may also cause gastric irritation, but the ratio of beneficial (anti-inflammatory) to detrimental (gastric irritation) effects is greater with ibuprofen than aspirin. Aspirin, in general, is quite a safe drug; in massive overdose, it can be quite dangerous, but it provides its own "warning signal." One early sign of aspirin toxicity is tinnitus, ringing in the ears, which is completely reversible, but occurs early enough in toxicity to be of diagnostic value. The major toxicity of aspirin is acid-base disturbance, which can be a severe problem in the elderly due to their diminished ability to compensate for insults to body chemistry.

The effect of glucocorticoids (such as prednisone) on rheumatoid arthritis is prompt and dramatic. These drugs, like the NSAIDs discussed above, do not alter the course of the disease, but merely decrease the inflammation caused by the bone and cartilage damage. While the relief of symptoms provided by glucocorticoids can allow significant increase in mobility and a subsequent elevation of mood, their chronic use can lead to serious and disabling effects. Chronic systemic administration (oral or by injection) can cause the production or the worsening of peptic ulcer, osteoporosis, or diabetes. Some patients may exhibit bizarre, psychotic behavior, and vision problems, such as glaucoma or cataracts, may be induced. These effects can be particularly devastating in the elderly, a population in which many of these conditions are already prevalent.

Diabetes

Diabetes mellitus can be classified as Type 1 (insulin-dependent diabetes mellitus) or Type 2 (non-insulin-dependent diabetes mellitus). Type 1 is usually thought of as juvenile diabetes, although it occurs infrequently in adults. Among adults, Type 1 occurs most frequently in the elderly. Type 2, or adult-onset diabetes, is more commonly seen in all adults, including the elderly.

The treatment for Type 1 diabetes is insulin, which, because it is degraded in the stomach, cannot be given orally but must be injected. The only differences among the available insulins are their durations of action and their sources. Duration of action of the particular insulin used is very important because it must fit into the lifestyle of the patient. For example, the time of a meal in relation to when the insulin injection is given is very important for good control of the blood sugar. This is particularly important in the elderly, in whom the normal homeostatic controls may be blunted or lost. It is necessary, therefore, that a schedule be developed by the patient or a caregiver that is relatively closely maintained. The source of the insulin (beef, pork, or synthetic human) is unimportant unless allergy or resistance to one insulin has developed. Generally, beef, pork, or beef-pork mixtures are less expensive than the synthetic form.

Other than allergic reactions, the primary toxicity associated with the use of insulin is hypoglycemia. Hypoglycemia, particularly in the elderly, can cause mental confusion, bizarre behavior, and ultimately, coma. Hypoglycemia in a Type 1 diabetic should be considered a medical emergency, and someone in the household should be trained by a physician to deal with it.

Type 2 diabetes is not treated with insulin, but is treated with one of the oral hypoglycemics, such as tolbutamide (Orinase). Of the oral agents, tolbutamide is probably the safest to use in the elderly because of its relatively short duration of action. Toxicity to tolbutamide is relatively rare, with a skin rash being the major manifestation. Prolonged action of tolbutamide (hypoglycemia) may occur when it is given concurrently with other drugs metabolized by the same enzymes; a physician or pharmacist should be able to help the patient avoid this potential problem.

COMPLIANCE ISSUES

There is some controversy in the literature as to whether the elderly are less compliant than younger cohorts in the population. Estimates of noncompliance by elderly persons have ranged from 2 to 95 percent.[35] In their recent review, Green and associates[50] found no conclusive evidence that the elderly are less compliant. Weintrab[51] also noted that the rate of compliance in the elderly is no different than that of other patients. Yet, in their review, Lipton and Lee[40] reported that noncompliance is widespread among elderly patients. Varying views about the extent of noncompliance in the elderly may be due to differing methodologies in reviewing the available literature. Although these authors disagree about the extent of noncompliance, they do agree that the elderly are potentially at greater risk for being noncompliant than any other segment of the population. And more importantly, the consequences of noncompliance in the elderly may be more severe and less easily resolved than in younger persons.[16] Noncompliance engenders some calculable and incalculable consequences. On the economic side, it has been reported that 15 percent of geriatric hospital admissions result from noncompliance.[52] The incalculable costs of noncompliance include impaired health, less than ideal quality of life, and needless death.[40]

Types of Compliance

Compliance has generally been viewed as more than a dichotomous (yes-no) event. Rather, the more accepted position is to view compliance in terms of a continuum of behaviors. Finchman and Wertheimer[53] have proposed four behavior (or anchor) points in the compliance continuum. Initial noncompliance refers to instances in which patients do not get their new prescriptions filled or do not pick up new prescriptions once they have been left to fill. Varying noncompliance refers to instances in which patients intermittently consume the prescribed medications as instructed. Appropriate compliance refers to instances in which patients consistently consume medications exactly as they are prescribed. Hypercompliance refers to instances in which patients consume more than the prescribed dosage. Most of the studies on compliance have focused on the initial and appropriate compliance points on the continuum.[54] Studies have shown that 20 percent of the elderly do not have their prescriptions filled initially. Kendrick and Bayne[56] found an average compliance rate of 57 percent in their study on varying compliance. It has been suggested that, in some cases, elderly patients have deliberately underused medications to avoid overmedicating themselves. (See review of medication compliance in Ascione.[56])

Factors Linked to Noncompliance

Many factors have been linked to noncompliance in the elderly, including

- Number of medications taken
- Inadequate information or instructions
- Cultural background
- Social isolation
- Cost of drugs
- Duration of drug treatment
- Limitations due to chronic illness and physical and mental impairments

Number of Medications Taken

As mentioned previously in this chapter, elderly persons take more drugs because they have more chronic diseases. Taking three or more drugs increases the likelihood that a person will be noncompliant.[40] The elderly are at risk for noncompliance because 25 percent of them take three or more drugs a day.[5]

The greater the complexity of drug regimens, such as number of drugs or dosing requirements, the more drug-drug interactions and medication errors will occur.[44,57]

Inadequate Information and Instructions

In addition to being unsure about basic information regarding the drugs they are taking (name, purpose, dosage schedule, side effects), elderly persons frequently hesitate to ask for information.[58] This, coupled with the failure of physicians to provide the necessary information about the drug regimen,[59] increases the likelihood of noncompliance by the elderly. In a study conducted by the American Association of Retired Persons,[5] it was reported that elderly people are less satisfied than younger people with the medication information they receive from health professionals.

Another serious problem is variation in interpretation of directions on prescription labels by elderly patients or undocumented changes in prescription instructions.[60] Resolution of these issues could assist the elderly patient, the pharmacist, or the caregiver to correctly monitor drug regimens.

Another related factor is the fact that elderly patients have long and somewhat complicated medical histories. These patients may not remember or volunteer all the relevant facts, which makes the physician's job much more difficult. Communication must be improved between the health care providers of each patient. More time must be devoted to collecting the critical information on each patient in order to improve the quality of health care for elderly patients.

Cultural Background

Cultural background can also influence therapeutic regimens or a patient's health behaviors significantly. For example, illness perceptions can create barriers to treatment regimens. Prescribed treatment regimens that do not account for a patient's beliefs about the causes of illnesses or diseases often may lead to noncompliance because the patient feels that the prescribed treatment is not going to be effective. These cultural health beliefs are strongly held by the elderly portion of ethnic communities, and some evidence indicates that these beliefs grow stronger with age.

Social Isolation

Twenty-five percent of the elderly population live alone. Social isolation is a common phenomenon among elderly persons. Compliance problems become more common when elderly persons are socially isolated.[61]

Cost of Drugs

The available literature on the relationship between noncompliance and drug costs indicates that drug costs are a factor in noncompliance.[62,63] Because many elderly are on fixed incomes, and drug costs are high, some patients may discontinue medication "when they feel better," instead of waiting for a physician's order. In some cases, there may be little effect, but in others it can be disastrous. For example, hypertension is normally without overt symptoms, but its danger is the possible sequelae of untreated hypertension, namely, stroke, heart attack, and kidney failure. A person who discontinues antihypertensive medication runs a very serious risk.

A second problem that arises from trying to cut financial corners is drug hoarding. Saving the last few unused tablets from an antibiotic prescription is not uncommon in the elderly. These "saved pills" may be used later when elderly people have what they consider to be the "same problem," or may be "shared" with a friend who has "the same thing." Several problems are associated with these practices: the condition may not be the same, in which case the drug may have no beneficial effect, but could be toxic; the drug may be outdated and ineffective, or toxic; and use of the drug may give the patient a false sense of security, and prevent him or her from seeking proper attention.

Duration of Drug Therapy

Studies have shown that the level of compliance decreases over time. This has been found to be particularly true for persons with chronic diseases, which are more prevalent among the elderly.[64]

Limitations Due to Chronic Illness and Physical and Mental Impairments

Limited mobility due to arthritis and heart disease, as well as sensory impairments, all contribute to noncompliance in elderly persons.

Chronic Illness. Limited mobility can inhibit a person's ability to have prescriptions filled, and arthritic hands make it difficult to open and close medication containers.[65]

Sensory Impairments. Another problem that interferes with the elderly person's ability to carry out drug regimens accurately are vision and hearing impairments. According to Rupp,[66] approximately two thirds of people 80 and older have impaired hearing, and fewer than 15 percent have 20/20 vision.[67]

In a study conducted for the Food and Drug Administration, 32 percent of the respondents aged 65 and over did not or were not able to read the labels on the OTC drug packages.[68] The ability to differentiate drug tablets by color becomes more difficult with sight impairment, especially blue-green or white-yellow.[69]

Hearing loss has been blamed for elderly persons' reluctance to ask questions for fear that they will not be able to hear the answers.[70, 71]

Cognitive Impairments. Approximately 11 percent of people over 65 have some cognitive impairment.[72] Many have the responsibility for managing their own medications during the early stages of dementia despite problems of forgetfulness and confusion. Cognitive impairments, such as decrements in the ability to process and retrieve drug information, can lead to serious medication misuse.

Changes in the brain, such as cellular brain mass and cerebral blood flow, or increased permeability of the blood-brain barrier, may result in decreased physical coordination, prolonged reaction time, and impairment of short-term memory, which are manifested by an increased number of falls and increased frequency of confusion. The brains of older people appear to be more sensitive to the side effects of drugs and alcohol.[73]

Strategies for Reducing Noncompliance

In their review of the literature on interventions designed to reduce noncompliance in the elderly, Green and associates[49] found that interpersonal communication methods, together with written or audiovisual materials and self-help memory aids, are effective in increasing knowledge and reducing noncompliance in the elderly. Lipton and Lee[40] review specific strategies that can be used to improve compliance. Simonson,[35] Higbee,[74] and Cooper[1] discuss ways in which health professionals, caregivers, and patients themselves can encourage better compliance and decrease medication errors:

1. Simplify the drug therapy.
2. Provide proper patient education.
3. Use special medication packaging and labeling techniques.
4. Use compliance aids such as memory aids.

Although these strategies are mainly targeted at physicians, pharmacists, and nurses, all health professionals will benefit from using them.

What a Rehabilitation Specialist Can Do

One of the roles a rehabilitation specialist can play is in identifying a person who may be noncompliant. Haynes and associates[61] have identified eight factors that tend to be present in noncompliant persons:

1. Illness fails to respond to therapy.
2. Patient is socially isolated.
3. Patient is forgetful or confused.
4. Sensory deficits are present.
5. Drug therapy is complex.
6. Patient fails to keep appointments.
7. Drug therapy is expensive.
8. Patient fails to obtain timely prescription refills.

Haynes and associates[61] recommend that these factors be used as a rough barometer to assist health professionals in identifying noncompliant patients. Simonson[35] observed that asking a patient whether he or she is complying is a good first step.

Although much of the responsibility for compliance lies with the elderly person or his or her family, physicians, pharmacists, and perhaps nurses, a rehabilitation specialist should be aware of the issues and not minimize his or her own importance as a source of influence with an elderly person.

ALCOHOL USE AMONG THE ELDERLY

Excessive or prolonged consumption of alcohol by older people can lead to serious health problems. Men who have three drinks a day and women who consume one and a half drinks a day are at higher risk of developing liver cirrhosis.[75] Moos and associates[76] found that problem drinkers in the 55-to-65-year-old age group were more likely to use cognitive and behavioral avoidance responses to cope with stress. These elderly problem drinkers drank to avoid thinking about the stress in their lives. Yee and Thu[78] also found that Vietnamese adults used smoking and drinking to cope with the stressors in their adaptation to refugee experiences and acculturation processes.

Chronic Alcohol Use

The chronic consumption of three to five drinks per day over a prolonged period of time (years) has been linked to an increase in mortality rate. Consumption of six or more drinks per day significantly increases the health risk even more. Paradoxically, one drink per day may be beneficial in reducing the risk of coronary artery disease, since consumption of alcohol at this level has been associated with an increase in the plasma concentration of high-density lipoproteins (HDL). HDL are felt to be important in the prevention of atherosclerosis.

Medical problems associated with chronic alcohol use include liver disease, gastrointestinal problems, and damage to the nervous system. Some of these problems are of particular concern to those providing care to the elderly. Fatty degeneration of the liver, progressing in severe cases to cirrhosis, must be a consideration in a population in which liver function is already decreased. Although poor nutritional status seems to increase the incidence of liver disease, there is no indication that adequate nutrition can prevent liver damage. Alcoholic gastritis is caused by the direct caustic effects of alcohol on the tissues of the gastrointestinal tract. In addition to the pain and the damage to the tissues, one must recognize that gastritis carries with it the possibility of bleeding (aggravated by aspirin, coffee, and tea), anemia, diarrhea, weight loss, and multiple vitamin deficiencies. Diarrhea and consequent volume depletion can be disastrous in the elderly because compensatory mechanisms are not able to cope adequately with the situation. Changes in nervous system function include impairment of motor function, emotional liability, reduced perceptual acuity (particularly visual acuity), and amnesia, all of which may be confused with the effects of normal aging.

Drinking patterns, such as morbidity and mortality related to alcohol abuse, vary among ethnic groups. The incidence of alcohol-related medical problems, especially liver cirrhosis and cancer of the esophagus, is high among African Americans. Alcohol-related mortality from cirrhosis is very high for African Americans, Latinos, and Native Americans, and is especially problematic for men in these ethnic groups.[77]

Alcoholics can be divided into long-term and reactive problem drinkers. Long-term drinkers who live to old age can be called survivors because life expectancy is lower for alcoholics than for reactive problem drinkers and nonalcoholics. Survivors are probably endowed with a hardier constitution than most alcoholics. This group could be at risk for serious medical problems and alienation from their families. They may be withdrawn or depressed, paranoid and hostile, manipulative, or demonstrative of sociopathic behavior.[78]

Between one fourth and one third of problem drinkers have a relatively recent onset of problems with alcohol. This reactive problem drinker is reacting to some event, such as the loss of a loved one, or to more general negative feelings, such as helplessness or depression stemming from role losses in later life.[77,78]

In a recent review article, Maddox[79] concluded that, although neither alcohol use nor abuse is high among older adults, alcohol abuse poses special risks for older people. Virtually every organ system is adversely affected by alcohol. Alcoholic patients show more signs of mental aging at every chronologic age than those who don't abuse alcohol. Alcohol abuse is associated with an increased susceptibility to infectious disease. It can have adverse effects on the endocrine system. Alcohol abuse leads to serious health problems.[40] Alcohol-related risks include certain diseases, interaction of alcohol with drugs, higher incidence of falls and accidents, and trouble with social relationships while in a drunken state.

Willenbring and Spring[81] suggest that health professionals, especially physicians, fail to screen their older patients for alcohol use because of their professional attitudes and not because they lack reliable screening techniques. These are some professional attitudes that help explain the failure to screen older patients for alcohol abuse.

1. Inadequate medical education about alcoholism and its many stages.
2. Lack of training, which places treatment of alcoholism outside their realm of competence. Alcohol abuse is seen as a problem that should be treated by mental health professionals, not by health professionals.
3. Ambivalent cultural feelings about alcohol use and inquiry and treatment of a "drinking problem." Health professionals are hesitant to treat alcoholism as a health problem until the patient is a late-stage alcoholic or the problem is revealed in a crisis situation such as a DUI arrest.
4. Denial may be more intense among the elderly due to the cohort's stigmatization of alcoholics (as alcoholic street bums).
5. Other medical problems may mask alcohol dependence.

Willenbring and Spring[81] suggest that elderly patients should be screened for alcohol use problems routinely. The authors suggest that health professionals use the HEAT screening method.[82] HEAT is a mnemonic for four open-ended questions. A positive response on any one item is a reason to obtain a fuller history.

1. **How** do you use alcohol?
2. Have you ever thought you used alcohol to **excess?**
3. Has **anyone** else ever thought you used too much?
4. Have you ever had any **trouble** resulting from your use?

Health care professionals, including physical therapists, can become more sensitive to early warning signs of alcohol misuse among their elderly clients. Denial of a drug or alcohol problem is the most common response among the elderly. Family and friends are often the key in assisting health professionals in identifying problem drinking and getting the person to treatment.

The use of elderly peers who are former alcoholics as outreach and social supports for other elderly alcoholics has been demonstrated to be a key element in effective treatment strategies. Family dynamics are a critical component of the alcoholic's treatment regimen because family members can assist the older person on the road to sobriety or can erect barriers along that road.[82]

Disulfiram (Antabuse) to prevent alcohol intake is not recommended for older persons because they do not have the reserve capacity to cope with the adverse effects that may occur with inadvertent or deliberate use of alcohol while receiving Antabuse. Treatment of alcohol withdrawal symptoms in the elderly is the same as in younger people, but overhydration is a serious health risk.[83]

Enjoyment of alcoholic beverages in later life can be pleasurable if such beverages are used in moderation. Small amounts of alcohol even provide some health benefits, such as stimulation of appetite and digestion or relaxation and analgesic effects;[84] improvements in morale, concentration, memory, self-confidence, and cognitive functioning in intact elderly.[85] Kastenbaum[86] suggests some general guidelines for moderate use of alcohol. Use beverages with lower alcohol content and slower absorption rates, such as wine and beer. Include these beverages as part of a meal, and enjoy them in the company of other people. Enjoy the beverage in a leisurely manner. Limit the consumption to one beer or glass of wine per occasion.

Obstacles to Rehabilitation

The major goal of rehabilitation is the restoration or arrest of further decline in functional capacity. Many obstacles may affect the patient's response to rehabilitation, such as motivation level, drug side effects or interactions, and inappropriate alcohol use. For example, problem drinking can increase the number of falls and accidents experienced by the older person. Certain drugs may produce side effects that are of particular concern to therapists. They include symptomatic postural hypotension, fatigue and weakness, depression, confusion, involuntary movements, dizziness and vertigo, ataxia, and urinary incontinence.[87] All these side effects of drugs and alcohol may interfere with the effectiveness of medical and health regimens prescribed for elderly patients.

Rehabilitation specialists must therefore become increasingly familiar with the medication and alcohol history of their clients because this history may contain critical factors in the patient's response or compliance with his or her treatment regimen. Rehabilitation specialists who see clients on a semi-long-term basis can spot behavioral indicators of negative side effects that drugs or alcohol may have on elderly people, and do so before hospitalization or permanent damage results. Any unusual behavioral changes should be reported to the physician to determine their cause.[88,89]

REFERENCES

1. Cooper, JW: Drug-related problems in the elderly patient. Generations 18(2):19, 1994.
2. Baum, C, Kennedy, DL, Forbes, MB, and Jones, JK: Drug use in the United States in 1981. JAMA 251:1293, 1984.

3. Beizer JL: Medications and the aging body: Alteration as a function of age. Generations 18(2):13, 1994.
4. Everitt, DE and Avorn, J: Drug prescribing for the elderly. Arch Intern Med 146:1185, 1986.
5. American Association of Retired Persons: Prescription Drugs: A Survey of Consumer Use, Attitudes, and Behavior. Washington, DC, 1984.
6. Special Committee on Aging, U.S. Senate: Developments in Aging: 1992, vol. 1. U.S. Government Printing Office, Washington DC, 1993.
7. Nelson, CR: Drug utilization in office practice: National Ambulatory Medical Care Survey, 1990. Advance Data 232:1, 1993.
8. Simonson, W: Geriatric drug therapy: Who are the stakeholders? Generations 18(20):7, 1994.
9. Schernitzki, P, Bootman, JL, Byers, J, Likes, K, and Hughes, JH: Demographic characteristics of elderly drug overdose patients admitted to a hospital emergency department. J Am Geriatr Soc 28:544, 1980.
10. Vestal, RE (ed): Drug treatment in the elderly. ADIS Health Science Press, Sydney, 1984.
11. Jarvik, L (ed): Clinical Pharmacology and the Aged Patient. Raven Press, New York, 1981.
12. Pagliaro, LA and Pagliaro, AM (eds): Pharmacologic Aspects of Aging. CV Mosby, St. Louis, 1983.
13. Roe, DA: Drugs and Nutrition in the Elderly Patient. Churchill Livingstone, New York, 1984.
14. Sullivan, GM and Korman, LB: Drug-associated confusional states in older persons. Top Geriatri Rehabil 8(4):14, 1993.
15. U.S. Health Care Financing Administration: Medicare: Use of Prescription Drugs by Aged Persons Enrolled for Supplemental Medical Insurance, 1967–1977. U.S. Government Printing Office, Washington, DC, 1981.
16. Lamy, PP: Prescribing for the Elderly. PSG Publishing, Littleton, MA, 1980.
17. Krondl, A: Present understanding of the interaction of drugs and food during absorption. Can Med Assoc J 10:360, 1970.
18. D'Arcy, PF and Merkus, FWHM: Alcohol and drug interactions. Pharm Interna 2:273, 1981.
19. Reilly, MJ: Folic acid USP, Drug information digest. Am J Hosp Pharm 27:494, 1970.
20. Pierpaoli, P, Coarse, J, and Tilton, R: Antibiotic use control: An institutional model. Drug Intell Clin Pharm 10:258, 1976.
21. Prestwood, KM: Medication use and mineral metabolism in older adults. Top Geriatr Rehabil 8(4):52, 1993.
22. Stewart, RB: Drug use in the elderly. In Delafuente, JC and Stewart, RB (eds): Therapeutics in the Elderly. Williams & Wilkins, Baltimore, 1988.
23. Hale, WE, Perkins, LL, May, FE, Marks, RG, and Stewart, RB: Symptom prevalence in the elderly: An evaluation of age, sex, disease and medication use. J Am Geriatr Soc 34:333, 1986.
24. Sharpe, TR and Smith, MC: Final Report: Barriers to and Determinants of Medication Use among the Elderly. Submitted to the American Association of Retired Persons-Andrus Foundation, Washington DC, June, 1983.
25. Guttman, D: Patterns of legal drug use by older Americans. Addiction Dis 3:337, 1978.
26. Gibson, RJ and Waldo, DR: National health expenditures, 1980. Health Care Financing Review 3:1, 1981.
27. Stewart, RB, Hale, WE, and Marks, G: Analgesic drug use in an ambulatory elderly population. Drug Intell Clin Pharm 16:833, 1982.
28. Cummings, JH: Progress report: Laxative abuse. Gut 15:758, 1975.
29. Kofoed, LL: Abuse and misuse of over-the-counter drugs by the elderly. In Atkinson, RM (ed): Alcohol and Drug Abuse in Old Age. American Pyschiatric Press, Washington, DC, 1984.
30. Coons, SJ, Hendricks, J, and Sheehan, SL: Self-medication with non-prescription drugs. Generations 12(4):22, 1988.

31. Finchman, JE: Over-the-counter drug use and misuse by the ambulatory elderly: A review of the literature. Journal of Geriatric Drug Therapy 1(2):3, 1986.

32. Atkinson, RM and Kofoed, LL: Alcohol and drug abuse. In Cassel, CK and Walsh, JR (eds): Geriatric Medicine: Fundamentals of Geriatric Care, vol 2. Springer-Verlag, New York, 1984.

33. Miller, RR: Prescribing habits of physicians. Drug Intell Clin Pharm 7:557, 1973.

34. Office of Technology Assessment, U.S. Congress: Achieving Safer, More Effective, Less Costly Utilization of Therapeutic Drugs. Washington, DC, 1976.

35. Simonson, W: Medications and the Elderly: A Guide for Promoting Proper Use. Aspen Systems Corporation, Rockville, MD, 1984.

36. Muller, C: The overmedicated society: Forces in the marketplace for medical care. Science 176:488, 1972.

37. U.S. Senate: Developments in Aging: A Report of the Special Committee on Aging. Part 4: Health. U.S. Government Printing Office, Washington, DC, 1982.

38. Kane, RL and Garrard, J: Changing physician prescribing practices. J Am Med Assoc 271:393, 1994.

39. Thompson, TL, Moran, MG, and Nies, AS: Psychotropic drug use in the elderly. New Engl J Med 308:134, 1983.

40. Lipton, H and Lee, P: Inappropriate drug use by the elderly: The problem of noncompliance and some potential solutions. In Lipton, HL and Lee, PR (eds): Drugs and the Eldery: Clinical, Social, and Policy Perspectives. Stanford University Press, Stanford, 1988.

41. Cooper, JW: Community and nursing home drug monitoring guidelines. Consultant Press, Watkinsville, GA, 1993.

42. Goyan, JE: Foreword. In Lipton, HL and Lee, PR (eds): Drugs and the Elderly, op cit.

43. U.S. PDI: National Academy of Sciences/Drug Review Council Report. Mack Printing, Easton, PA, 1994.

44. Chapron, DJ: Drug-drug interactions in the elderly: An update. Top Geriatr Rehabil 8(4):67, 1993.

45. Sherman, DS: Geriatric psychopharmacotherapy: Issues and concerns. Generations 18(2):34, 1994.

46. Harper, MS: Survey of drug use and mental disorders in nursing homes. In Moore, SR and Teal, TW (eds): Geriatric Drug Use: Clinical and Social Perspectives. Pergamon Press, New York, 1985.

47. Shorr, RI, Fought, RL, and Ray, WA: Changes in antipsychotic drug use in nursing homes during implementation of the OBRA 87 Regulations. J Am Med Assoc 271:358, 1994.

48. Blazer, DG: The epidemiology of depression in late life. J Geriatr Psychiatr Neurol 22:35, 1990.

49. Blazer, DG, George, L, and Hughes, D: The epidemiology of anxiety disorders: An age comparison. In Salzman, C and Leibowitz, B (eds): Anxiety Disorders in the Elderly. Springer, New York, 1991.

50. Green, L, Mullen, P, and Stainbrook, G: Programs to reduce drug errors in the elderly: Direct and indirect evidence from patient education. J Geriatr Drug Therapy 1(1):3, 1986.

51. Weintraub, M: A different view of patient compliance in the elderly. In Vestal, RE (ed): Drug Treatment in the Elderly. ADIS Health Science Press, New York, 1984.

52. Bergman, U and Wilholm, B: Drug-related problem causing admission to a medical clinic. Eur J Clin Pharmacol 20:193, 1981.

53. Finchman, J and Wertheimer, A: Identifying the initial drug therapy defaulter. Patient Counseling in Community Pharmacy 3(3):12, 1985.

54. Eraker, S, Kirscht, J, and Becker, M: Understanding and improving patient compliance. Ann Intern Med 100:258, 1984.

55. Kendrick, P and Bayne, J: Compliance with prescribed medications by elderly patients. J Can Med Assoc 127(1):961, 1982.

56. Ascione, F: Medication compliance in the elderly. Generations 18(2):28, 1994.

57. Wolfe, SM, Hope, RE and Public Citizen Health Research Group: Worst Pills, Best Pills. Public Citizens Health Research Group, Washington, DC, 1993.

58. Miller, R: Doctors, patients don't communicate. FDA Consumer 17:6, July/August 1983.
59. Lundin, D: Medication taking behavior of the elderly: A pilot study. Drug Intell Clin Pharm 12:518, 1978.
60. Shimp, LA and Ascione, FJ: Causes of medication misuse and error. Generations 12(4):17, 1988.
61. Haynes, R, Sackett, D, and Taylor, D: How to detect and manage low patient compliance in chronic illness. Geriatr 355:91, 1980.
62. Brand, F, Smith, R, and Brand, PG: Effect of economic barriers to medical care on patients' noncompliance. Public Health Rep 92:72, 1977.
63. Sullivan, SD, Gardner, LB, and Strandberg, LR: The economics of outpatient prescriptions drug coverage for the elderly: Implications for health care reform. Generations 18(2):55, 1994.
64. Haynes, R, Haynes, RB, Wang, E, and Gomes, MD: Process versus outcome in hypertension: A positive result. Circulation 65:28, 1982.
65. Rice, D and Estes, CL: Health of the elderly: Policy issues and challenges. Health Affairs 3:25, 1984.
66. Rupp, RR: Understanding the problems of presbycusis. Geriatrics 32:63, 1970.
67. Marmor, MF: The eye and vision in the elderly. Geriatrics 32:63, 1977.
68. Knapp, DE, Biard, JT, and Winter, WJ: How consumers view drugs. Apothecary 88:8, 1976.
69. Hurd, PD and Blevins, J: Aging and color of pills. New Engl J Med 30:202, 1984.
70. National Center for Health Statistics: Current Estimates from the National Health Interview Survey: United States, 1982. Vital and Health Statistics, Series 10, DHHS Publication No. (PHS)85-1578. U.S. Government Printing Office, Washington, DC, 1985.
71. Ebersole, P and Hess, P: Toward Healthy Aging: Human Needs and Nursing Response. CV Mosby, St Louis, 1981.
72. Odenheimer, JL and Busby, J: Common disorders of the nervous system. In Delafuente, JC and Stewart, RB (eds): Therapeutics in the Elderly. Williams & Wilkins, Baltimore, 1988, p 57.
73. Lamy, PP: Introduction to the aging process. In Delafuente, JC and Stewart, RB (eds): Therapeutics in the Elderly, op cit.
74. Hibgee, MD: Consumer guidelines for using medications wisely. Generations 18(2):43, 1994.
75. National Institute of Alcohol Abuse and Alcoholism: Alcohol and Health. DHHS Pub. No. (ADM) 87-1519, U.S. Department of Health and Human Services, Rockville, MD, 1987.
76. Moos, RH, Brennan, PL, Fondacaro, MR, and Moos, BS: Approach and avoidance coping responses among older problem and non-problem drinkers. Psychology and Aging 5(1):31, 1990.
77. Yee, BWK and Thu, ND: Correlates of drug use and abuse among Indochinese refugees: Mental health implications. Journal of Psychoactive Drugs 19:77, 1987.
78. Gomberg, E: Overview: Issues of alcohol use and abuse in the elderly population. Pride Institute Journal Long-term Home Health Care 4:4, 1988.
79. Maddox, GL: Aging, drinking and alcohol abuse. Generations 12(4):14, 1988.
80. Lamy, PP: Actions of alcohol and drug in older people. Generations 12(4):9, 1988b.
81. Willenbring, M and Spring, WD: Evaluating alcohol use in elders. Generations 12(4):27, 1988.
82. Rathbone-McCuan, E: Promoting help-seeking behavior among elders with chemical dependencies. Generations 12(4):37, 1988.
83. Walker, JI and Covington, TR: Psychiatric disorders. In Covington, TR and Walker, JI (eds): Current Geriatric Therapy. WB Saunders, Philadelphia, 1984.
84. Usdin, E: Anxiolytics: An overview. In Malick, JB, Enna, SJ and Yamamura, HI (eds): Anxiolytics: Neurochemical, Behavioral and Clinical Perspectives. Raven Press, New York, 1983.
85. Mishara, BL and Kastenbaum, R: Alcohol and Old Age. Grune & Stratton, New York, 1980.
86. Kastenbaum, R: In moderation. Generations 12(4):68, 1988.
87. Chapron, DJ and Besdine, RW: Drugs as an obstacle to rehabilitation of the elderly: A primer for therapists. Top Geriatr Rehabil 2(3):63, 1987.

88. Gurwitz, JH, Noonan, JP, and Soumerai, SB: Reducing the use of Hs-receptor antagonists in the long-term care setting. J Am Geriatr Soc 40:359, 1992.
89. Tobias, DE: Ensuring and documenting the quality of drug therapy in the elderly. Generations 18(2):40, 1994.

BIBLIOGRAPHY

Ascione, FJ, Brown, GH, and Kirking, DM: Evaluation of a medication refill reminder system for a community pharmacy. Patient Education and Counseling 7:157, 1985.
Conrad, KA and Bressler, R (eds): Drug Therapy for the Elderly. CV Mosby, St Louis, 1982.
Craig, CR and Stitzel, RE (eds): Modern Pharmacology, ed 4. Little, Brown, Boston, 1994.
Gilman, AG, Rall, TW, Nies, AS, and Taylor, P: (eds): Goodman and Gilman's The Pharmacological Basis of Therapeutics, ed 8. Macmillan, New York, 1990.
Hansten, PD: Drug Interactions, ed 5. Lea & Febiger, Philadelphia, 1985.
Katzung, BG (ed): Basic and Clinical Pharmacology, ed 5. Appleton & Lange, Norwalk, 1992.
Korman, LB and James, JA: Medical management of Parkinson's disease in the elderly. Top Geriatr Rehabil 8(4):1, 1993.
Lipton, HL and Lee, PR: Drugs and the Elderly: Clinical, Social and Policy Perspectives. Stanford University Press, Stanford, 1988.
Ouslander, JG: Drug therapy in the elderly. Ann Intern Med 95:711, 1981.
Rowland, FN and Fallon, B: Chronic pain in the elderly: The use of opioids and selected adjuvants. Top Geriatr Rehabil 8(4):27, 1993.
Shimp, LA et al: Potential medical-related problems in non-institutionalized elderly. Drug Intell Clin Pharm 16:833, 1985.
Shinn, AF and Shrewsbury, R (eds): Evaluations of Drug Interactions, ed 3. CV Mosby, St. Louis, 1985.

Appendix 14–1

Checklist for Elderly Consumers and Their Caregivers

1. Know critical drug therapy information.
   a. Name of drug
   b. Dose
   c. Appearance (brand or generic)
   d. Reason for use
   e. Expected action
   f. Quantity to be taken
   g. Frequency of administration
   h. Duration of therapy
   i. Adverse effects and what to do if there are side effects
   j. Precautions
   k. Special instructions (foods, drinks, or other medicines)
   l. What to do if a dose is missed
   m. Refill information
   n. Storage requirements

o. Cost of medication

p. Physician-ordered changes in drug regimen

q. Expiration dates

2. Develop an effective strategy to organize medicines so that you can follow your doctor's orders regarding medication usage:

   a. Use pill boxes.

   b. Use pill calendars.

   c. List pill taken, time, and date.

   d. Develop pill-taking routines during the day.

   e. Have someone else give you the medicines if you are unable to do so.

3. Drug therapy review:

   a. All prescription drugs and OTC drugs used regularly should be reviewed by physician or pharmacist on an annual basis (bring drugs in brown bag or list all drugs used).

   b. Whenever a new drug is introduced, patient should indicate which drugs are currently being taken. Include OTC drugs in list.

   c. Outdated drugs should be flushed down the toilet.

   d. Hard-to-identify or unknown medications should be examined by your pharmacist.

4. Request that all medications be put in non-child-proof containers if desired.

5. Review doctor's instructions with pharmacist to ensure that you understand his or her instructions and ask additional questions regarding any unanswered questions in item 1 above.

6. Your doctor needs your help in evaluating the effectiveness of the prescribed drug therapy. Let the doctor know what other medications you are currently taking, including over-the-counter drugs. Even when taken as directed, some medications may produce adverse effects. Call your doctor immediately to obtain further instructions about drug usage when you have any side effects or are having a problem taking your medication.

Appendix 14–2

Resources

FOR THE HEALTH PROFESSIONAL

1. *Preventing Geriatric Medication Misuse: A Manual for Developing a Model Program*

   K. Eng
   SRx Regional Program
   1182 Market St, Rm. 204,
   San Francisco, CA 94102

2. *Wise Use of Drugs—A Program for Older Americans* (film)

   National Institute on Drug Abuse
   RHR Filmedia (lends film free nationwide)
   1212 Avenue of the Americas
   New York, NY 10035

3. *NIDA Resource Center Film Library* (lends Elder-Ed Film free nation-wide through interlibrary loan)

   Rockville, MD 10857
   (301) 443-6614

4. *Drugs and the Elderly* and *A Resource Guide for Drug Management for Older Persons*, 1985

   M.Bogaert-Tullis
   Institute for Health and Aging
   University of California—San Francisco
   San Francisco, CA 94143-0612

5. *Priorities and Approaches for Improving Prescription Medicine Use by Older Americans*, 1987, $10.00
   Community Brown Bag Medicine Review "starter kits," $45.00
   Let's Talk About Prescriptions Posters ($1.00) and Brochures ($20,00/100)

   National Council on Patient Information and Education
   666 11th St NW, Suite 810
   Washington, DC 20001
   (202) 347-6711

6. *Alcohol and the Elderly* Order No. MS306

   Alcohol and Black Americans Order No. MS319
   Alcohol and Hispanics Order No. MS309, RP0253
   Alcohol and Native Americans Order No. RP0307
   Alcohol and Safety Order No. MS311
   Prevention of Alcohol Problems Order No. MS247
   Health Insurance and Alcoholism Order No. MS307

   The National Clearinghouse for Alcohol and Drug Information
   P.O. Box 2345
   Rockville, MD 20847-2345
   (800) 729-6686 (English, Spanish)
   (800) 487-4889 (TDD, for hearing-impaired callers)
   (301) 468-2600

7. *Older Americans: CSAP Prevention Resource Guide.* Oct. 1992

   Center for Substance Abuse Prevention National Clearing House
   for Alcohol and Drug Information
   PO Box 2345
   Rockville, MD 20847-2345

(301) 468-2600

(800) 729-6686

8. CSAP's Drug-Free Workplace Helpline (for employers)

(800) 843-4971

9. Department of Labor's Substance Abuse Information Database (SAID)

(800) 775-7243

10. Health Promotion Team, Health Advocacy Services

American Association of Retired Persons
601 E St NW, Fifth Floor-B
Washington, DC, 20049
(202) 434-2240

FOR ELDERLY CONSUMERS OR THEIR CAREGIVERS

1. *Worst Pills, Best Pills, II.* 1993 ($15)

Sidney M. Wolfe, MD and Rose-Ellen Hope, RPh
Public Citizens Health Research Group
2000 P St NW, Suite 600
Washington, DC 20036

2. *Aging and Health: The Role of Self-Medication,* ed 3. 1991
Connie J. Evashwick, ScD
Nonprescription Drugs Modern Medicines for Mature Americans
Nonprescription Drug Manufacturers Association
(202) 429-9260 fax: (202) 223-6835

3. *You and Your Medicines*
Your Personal Medication Record
Medicines without Prescriptions
Everything You Ever Wanted to Know about Generic Drugs
Caregivers' Medication Guidelines

Elder-Ed
University of Maryland School of Pharmacy
636 W Lombard St
Baltimore, MD 21201

4. *USP Dispensing Information: Advice for the Patient,* (vol 2), 1994 About
Your Medicines Newsletter

U.S. Pharmacopeia DI, Publications Dept.
12601 Twinbrook Parkway
Rockville, MD 20852
(301) 816-8351

5. *The Smart Consumer's Guide to Prescription Drugs,* brochure, D 13579 AARP Pharmacy Service from Retired Persons Services, Inc. (mail prescription pharmacy service to AARP members)

   American Association of Retired Persons
   601 E Street, NW
   Washington, DC 20049

6. *Medication Is No Mystery* (Medication education program)
   National Council on Aging
   Publications Department
   5087
   Washington, DC 20041-5087
   (202) 479-1200

7. *Age Pages.* Fact Sheets (Selected titles in Spanish and Chinese)
   Arthritis Medicines
   Safe Use of Medicines by Older People
   Safe Use of Tranquilizers
   "Shots" for Safety
   Should You Take Estrogen?

   National Institute on Aging Information Center
   PO Box 8057
   Gaithersburg, MD 20898-8057
   (301) 495-3455

8. National Clearinghouse for Alcohol and Drug Information
   P.O. Box 2345
   Rockville, MD 20852
   (800) 729-6686

9. National Drug Information Treatment and Referral Hotline
   (800) 662-HELP (4357)
   (800) 662-9832 (Español)
   (800) 228-0427 (TDD, hearing impaired callers)

10. *Aging and Alcohol Abuse* (Fact sheet)
    National Institute on Aging
    National Clearinghouse for Alcohol and Drug Information
    PO Box 2345
    Rockville, MD 20847-2345
    (301) 468-2600
    (800) 729-6686

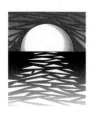

CHAPTER 15

Sexuality and the Elderly

Molly Laflin, PhD

BEHAVIORAL OBJECTIVES

Upon completion of this chapter, the reader will be able to:

1 Describe the normal age-related changes in the human sexual response cycle.
2 List the barriers to sexual expression among the elderly.
3 Discuss techniques that enhance sexual participation among older persons.
4 Recognize the sexual implications of certain illnesses and treatments.
5 List possible sexual implications attributable to prescription drug use.
6 Recognize the complications associated with sexual expression among nursing home patients.

Sexuality exists, in one form or another, throughout life. Contrary to popular humor, sex after 60 is not the province of so-called dirty old men, nor is it the wishful invention of sexologists. Age affects the strength of one's sexual response, but there is certainly no uniform chronologic age at which sexual interest, ability, and activity cease. According to Kaplan,[1] "sexuality is among the last of our faculties to decline with maturity . . . most of us are still sexually active long after we have begun to use hearing aids and eyeglasses, and some . . . are still enjoying good sex, although they cannot always remember the name of their partner" (p 186).

Many elderly people maintain a lively interest in sex. In fact, a study of men averaging 71 years of age found that 75 percent had sexual desires.[2] A longitudinal study of men over age 60, begun in 1954 by the Duke University Center for the Study of Aging and Human Development, found a gradual decline in the reported frequency of sexual intercourse with advancing age. Yet 40 to 65 percent of the subjects between the ages of 60 and 71 still reported having sexual intercourse with some frequency. An interesting finding was that about 15 percent of the subjects showed increasing patterns of sexual interest and activity,[3] most likely attributable to increased privacy (children no longer living in the home), increased leisure time due to retirement, elimination of the fear of pregnancy, or a new partner.

Most studies have found that, although sexual activity persists in later life, it generally declines with age. Nevertheless, sexual satisfaction and enjoyment generally do not show a decline with increasing age.[4,5] A closer examination of the research reveals that few studies have been designed in a way that will distinguish between an age effect and a cohort effect. For example, although cross-sectional studies reveal that older people have sex less often than younger people today, we cannot determine whether the reason for the difference in sexual activity is age or the different socialization and value orientation of the cohorts. Hudson and others[6] and Keller and associates[7] have found that today's elderly have a higher degree of sexual guilt, more conservative sexual attitudes, and more restricted sexual behaviors than today's youth. It is entirely possible that, even in their youth, today's elderly were never as sexually active as the youth of today.

Because their values tend to preclude divorce as an option, some older people feel trapped in marriages characterized by poor communication and low marital satisfaction. These factors can lead to low levels of sexual activity. Other explanations for decline in sexual vigor include a general decline in physical and physiologic capacity,[8] boredom and overfamiliarity, illness, fatigue, preoccupation with competing interests, loss of confidence in potency,[9] high rates of marital problems,[10] overeating, and heavy use of alcohol.[11] Despite all these explanations, longitudinal data from the second Duke longitudinal study on aging reveal that the level of sexual activity is more stable over time than previously suggested.[12] Although some slowing down is evident,[13] differences among individuals regarding sexual interest and frequency tend to be greater than the differences that individuals experience over time.

Some studies of sexuality and aging do not take marital status into account. Given the fact that 15 percent of men and 48 percent of women age 65 and over are widowed,[14] it seems clear that lack of a suitable partner is a major reason for reduced sexual activity among the elderly. After losing a spouse, many elderly persons have difficulty in creating permanent and intimate connections, thereby limiting their ability to develop satisfactory sexual relationships. A study by Weizman and Hart[15] found that there was a decline in frequency of sexual intercourse in elderly men ages 66 to 71 compared with men ages 60 to 65; however, men aged 66 to 71 masturbated more often.

Another problem with many sex and aging studies is that they operationally define *sexually active* as having intercourse. To do so is heterosexist and limiting for any age group, but this narrow perspective is particularly inaccurate and misleading when studying the elderly. The Starr and Weiner[16] report, *On Sex and Sexuality in the Mature Years,* reveals that among older people there is less emphasis on goal orientation and more on pleasuring, cuddling, and touching. This difference is not viewed as a loss to be regretted any more than most elderly people regret their loss of interest in carnival rides or loud music. As one older woman explains:[17]

> Sex isn't as powerful a need as when you're young, but the whole feeling is there: it's as nice as it ever was. He puts his arms around you, kisses you, and it comes to you—satisfaction and orgasm—just like it always did . . . don't let anybody tell you different. Maybe it only happens once every two weeks, but as you get older, it's such a release from tensions. I'm an old dog who's even learned a few new tricks. . . . Like oral sex, for instance. . . . I know I'm getting old, and my skin could use an ironing, but we love each other—so sex is beautiful. (p 43)

The age-related trend toward using quality of sexual experience over quantity as a measure of sexual experience is true for homosexuals as well as heterosexuals.[18] Cole and Rothblum state that one of the participants in their research on sexuality among menopausal lesbians expressed the feelings of many of the women in the study when she wrote:[19]

> Sex at menopause is great. It helps me feel good about myself—an opportunity to celebrate life. It's fun. I love the playful times; they're terrific for little aches and pains. Releases tension, makes me feel connected to my physical being, to all of humanity and to the universe. I love it. (p 38)

Contrary to popular myth, older homosexuals are not more lonely and unhappy than heterosexuals. In fact, homosexuals tend to be better prepared for coping with the adjustments of aging than heterosexual men and women because they have planned for their own financial support and have deliberately created a network of supportive friends.[20, 21] One study found that elderly homosexual men equaled or exceeded comparable groups in the general population on a measure of life satisfaction. Their frequency of sexual activity remained stable, but there was a change over time toward fewer sexual partners. Seventy-five percent were satisfied with their current sex life.[22]

ROLE OF REHABILITATION SPECIALISTS

The rehabilitation specialist should take on the job of helping people learn to function at their optimal levels despite physical setbacks. Generally, patients seek care out of a need to reduce pain and/or increase mobility. Although the focus of your treatment plan is the presenting symptoms, it is the patient as a whole person who must be treated. It is important to be sensitive to the social and emotional, as well as the physical, implications of treatment, disease, and injury. If sexual behavior is integral to a person's lifestyle, then part of rehabilitation is enabling the patient to adapt sexually.

Sexual dysfunction can reduce quality of life. It may cause marital problems, diminish self-esteem, or be clinically manifested in the form of anxiety, depression, tension, and hypochondrial complaints. Old age in and of itself is no barrier to sexual activity and sexual satisfaction; therefore, careful attention is required in the administration of drugs and medical treatments that may cause sexual impairment. When sexual dysfunction does exist in an older person, it should not be dismissed lightly. Masters and Johnson have found high rates of success in treating sexual dysfunction in clients 50 years old and older—a 75 percent success rate in treating impotence and 59 percent in helping women achieve orgasm in sexual relations.[23] Older people should not be denied all the necessary therapy given to young people suffering from sexual dysfunction, including appropriate referrals to sex counseling.

In treating a woman with an arthritic hip, for example, if you overlook the sexual implications of the patient's condition, either because of personal embarrassment or an assumption that elderly people are not interested in sex, then you are not treating the whole person. You need to be open to discuss the sexual implications of illness and treatment with your elderly patients without pushing them to deal with areas in which they are uncomfortable. An appropriate place to initiate a discussion of sexual issues is to address them in the context of normal life activities in the Activities of Daily Living (ADL) portion of an evaluation. Goldstein and Runyon[24] suggest asking, "Do you have any questions/concerns about your current medical condition and how it may influence sexual function?" You have to walk the fine line between conveying a negative attitude about sex through silence or embarrassment and being too confrontational and shocking. Your primary concern is to treat patients as individuals, with dignity, and with the realization that sexuality—although it is generally not as vigorous among the elderly as among young people—is still part of the total person at any age.

Rehabilitation therapists are in an excellent position to deliver educational programs to the community and to assist their sexually trouble patients with levels 1 to 3 of the PLISSIT model.[25] The four levels are **P**ermission, **L**imited **I**nformation, **S**pecific **S**uggestions, and **I**ntensive **T**herapy. Each level of approach requires higher degrees of knowledge, training, and skills on the part of the therapist. It is important to know when to refer and to whom one can confidently refer.

MENOPAUSE AND ESTROGEN REPLACEMENT THERAPY

The life expectancy for women has increased to the point where today more than one third of a woman's life is postmenopausal. Menopause refers to the cessation of menstruation that occurs to women over a period of several months to a few years as a result of physiologic changes that occur generally between the ages of 45 and 50. The cessation of menstruation and fertility does not eradicate sexual desire or response. One study found that, in women at least 1 year past menopause, 21 percent felt that menopause (or a hysterectomy) had had a negative effect on their sexuality; 30 percent felt it had a positive effect.[26]

Most women go through menopause without major physical difficulties. However, 25 percent of menopausal women seek consultation for problems related to menopause.[27] The major medical concerns are vasomotor syndrome (primarily hot flashes), atrophic vaginitis, and osteoporosis.[28]

About 10 to 20 percent of women report extreme discomfort from hot flashes.[29] Hot flashes occur sporadically during the day and at night. They generally cease within 2 years without hormone therapy. The physiologic cause of hot flashes is the fluctuating hormone levels occurring during menopause. Fluctuation in the hormones affecting the nerves that control the diameter of blood vessels can cause rapid dilation of the vessels, resulting in a momentary rush of heat, typically in the face. Hot flashes can be so intense that within a matter of seconds, a woman can perspire profusely and require a change of clothing. These vasomotor changes are also related to headaches and insomnia.

Atrophy of the genital epithelium may result in "vaginitis with symptoms of irritation, burning, pruritus, leukorrhea, dyspareunia, and occasionally, even vaginal bleeding."[30] Because the integrity of the lower urinary tract mucosa depends on estrogen, symptoms of irritation such as dysuria and burning on urination may occur, and episodes of cystitis (which can be exacerbated by prolonged periods of intercourse when a male partner has a delayed ejaculatory response[31]) become more frequent. These changes occasionally lead to decreased libido.

More than 20 million older Americans, of whom 90 percent are postmenopausal women, suffer from osteoporosis. Indeed, it is estimated that 25 percent of postmenopausal women suffer bone fractures resulting from osteoporosis. Genetically determined risk factors include phenotype shortness in stature and blond hair. Lifestyle habits such as lack of moderate weight-bearing exercise, inadequate intake of calcium, high intake of fiber (which interferes with the absorption of calcium), and excessive use of "bone robbers" (caffeine, tobacco, and alcohol) greatly increase the risk of osteoporosis.[32]

Estrogen replacement therapy (ERT) may alleviate some of the problems associated with the significant reduction in estrogen after menopause. The benefits include cessation of hot flashes; return of normal vaginal elasticity, integrity, and lubrication; and, of great significance, prevention and in some cases reversal of osteoporosis.[33-35] According to the National Institute of Health Consensus Development Conference on Osteoporosis,[33] (1) estrogen therapy is the best means of preventing osteoporosis; (2) calcium supplementation should be started at about age 40 (approximately 10 years prior to menopause) in daily dosages of 1000 mg of elemental calcium; and (3) weight-bearing exercise is the best activity to prevent osteoporosis. Higher doses of estrogen, from 1.25 to 2.5 mg, are required if osteoporosis is already present.[30]

Early research indicated an increased risk of endometrial cancer associated with ERT. However, the current practice of adding cyclic progestogens to the estrogen regimen for 10 to 14 days has almost eliminated the risk of endometrial cancer with ERT. Progestin causes the lining of the uterus to shed each month. As a result, it is highly unlikely that the lining will develop cancer from estrogen stimulation. Despite fears of an association between breast cancer (a disease that strikes 1 in 11 women) and estrogen therapy, numerous long-term studies of large groups of women have failed to incriminate ERT for any significant increased risk of breast cancer. In fact, there is increasing evidence that when progestogen is added to ERT, the risk of breast cancer is reduced in some women.

Small doses of estrogen may provide some protection against heart disease, but when progestin is added to prevent endometrial cancer, there may be an increased risk of stroke and heart attacks by altering the type of fats in the bloodstream. Smokers, diabetics, very obese women, women who do not exercise, and women with high blood pressure and high cholesterol levels are at greatest risk for complications associated with ERT.[36] Women considering hormone replacement should consult their health care practitioners and thoroughly discuss the potential benefits and risks of ERT against the symptoms of estrogen deficiency. Good nutrition, food supplements, and physical exercise (walking is highly recommended) can sometimes alleviate some menopausal symptoms.[37]

Hormonal replacement therapy, so useful in dealing with the reduction in vaginal lubrication commonly experienced by postmenopausal women, is contraindicated for some women. Currently, a nonsteroidal moisturizing cream that coats the vagina and enhances pliability and moisturizing (such as Replens or Gyne-Moistrin) is available and appears promising based on early research findings.[38] Various low-dose topical estrogen creams (Premarin Cream, Estrace, Ogen) have proven efficacious as well for those women who are appropriate candidates. Over-the-counter creams and lubricants such as Astroglide, Lubrin, Today, or Transilube are readily available as well.[39] Some women prefer vegetable oil (which is compatible with the mucous membrane) over water-soluble lubricants that may evaporate too quickly.

Somewhat in keeping with the "use it or lose it" admonition, research has found that age-related genital changes (eg, decreased lubrication in elastic and thin vaginal tissues) are less pronounced in women who are sexually active (masturbation as well as intercourse). It generally requires several weeks or months for women to engage in sexual intercourse comfortably after an extended period of abstinence (eg, a widow remarries and reactivates her sex life). Masters and Johnson use the term "widower's syndrome" when referring to men experiencing partial or incomplete impotence due to an extended period of abstinence caused by illness or lack of partner. When a man resumes sexual activity, it generally takes some time and an understanding and helpful partner to reverse or avert the widower's syndrome.[40]

AGE AND SEXUAL RESPONSE

Although there is no age-related end point for sexual functioning, there is an age-related general slowing of the human body, which in turn slows the sexual response cycle. The general effects of aging are listed below.

Men

1. Circulating testosterone is decreased but rarely contributes to erectile disorders in healthy aging men (a 20-year-old has 600 to 1200 ng/dL of serum testosterone; a 60-year-old has 200 to 600 ng/dL).
2. Penile erection takes more time and may not be as hard as before (full turgidity and girth seconds before ejaculation); direct, continuous penile stimulation is usually required.
3. Testicles do not increase in size; they elevate later and to a lesser degree.
4. Nipple erection becomes less discernible.
5. Ejaculatory control increases; ejaculation may take place every third sexual episode, owing to less preoccupation with orgasm. (Lack of ejaculation decreases the refractory period).
6. Sex flush is rare in men over 50.
7. Sense of ejaculatory inevitability is diminished or absent.
8. Ejaculation is less powerful and orgasm is often less intense.

9. Ejaculation during orgasm consists of one or two expulsive contractions instead of the four major contractions followed by minor contractions over several seconds typical of younger men.
10. Ejaculate is expelled with less force and contains less seminal plasma. Although fertility levels are reduced, men do not become sterile.
11. Decreased myotonia makes extragenital spasms uncommon; rectal sphincter contractions during orgasm occur less frequently.
12. Loss of erection after ejaculation and testicular descent occur rapidly.
13. Refractory period between ejaculations is longer; it generally takes 12 to 48 hours after ejaculation to redevelop an erection, in contrast to several minutes for adolescents.
14. Climax still provides extreme sensate pleasure.

Women

Most sexual changes in women are associated with a decline in female hormones.

1. Vaginal lubrication takes longer.
2. The expansion of the vaginal barrel is reduced in length and width.
3. The lining of the vagina begins to thin and becomes easily irritated.
4. The bladder and urethra may become irritated during intercourse.
5. Vaginal secretion becomes less acid, increasing the possibility of vaginal infection.
6. The uterus does not elevate as high.
7. There is a reduction in pubic hair, the labia majora loses fullness, the clitoral size decreases, and the clitoral hood atrophies, as does the fat pad over the mons veneris.
8. Orgasmic phase is shorter.
9. Resolution phase occurs more rapidly.
10. Capability for multiple orgasm remains.

Despite steroid insufficiency, many women who maintain active sex lives continue unimpaired vaginal lubrication capacity, and the regular contractions during intercourse and orgasm retain vaginal muscle tone. Contact with the penis helps preserve the shape and size of the vaginal space.[41]

Knowledge of the normal physiologic changes associated with aging can greatly enhance adjustment and enjoyment of sexual expression. For example, women suffering sexual dysfunction or other problems associated with loss of female hormones may wish to discuss the advisability of estrogen replacement therapy with their physicians. An elderly couple who understand that it is normal for an older man not to ejaculate every time he has sex can relax and enjoy the advantage of more frequent erections, the side effect of decreased refractory periods resulting from less frequent ejaculations.

LACK OF PARTNER

Not everyone has the opportunity to maintain a sexually active life despite an interest in doing so. There are now 3.5 unmarried women over the age of 65 for each unmarried man in the same age range.[14] If all the unmarried men over the age of 65 married women over the age of 65, there would still be over 7.5 million women without husbands. Sheer numbers indicate a great deal of unmet sexual need among elderly heterosexual women.

Grown children of widows and widowers often actively discourage their parents from seeking new partners or behaving as sexual beings.[42] Sometimes these "children" are fearful of loss of inheritance, but more often they are fearful of a change that seems uncomfortable and perhaps, in their eyes, morally reprehensible.

In a society that associates sexual attractiveness with youthful bodies and sexual activity with marriage, it is difficult for many older people to overcome their own prejudices without having to deal with such overwhelming societal pressure. The folkloristic view of the elderly as impotent, uninterested in sexuality, and sexually nonfunctional becomes, for many older people, a self-fulfilling prophesy. Homosexuality and masturbation are only a couple of the options open to the elderly who are without partners, but more often than not, societal pressure eliminates these choices from active consideration.[43]

SEX AND ILLNESS

Lack of a partner probably accounts for discontinuance of sexual activity in many of the elderly, but illness also steals the sex lives of many. According to the U.S. National Center for Health Statistics, 40 percent of Americans age 65 and older have activity limitation, and 24 percent have major activity limitation.[44]

Sexual activity may be limited by specific disabilities, but fortunately sexuality and the expression of love and caring do not have the same limitations. Rather than focusing on the losses associated with illness, more attention should be paid to what is possible. The psychosocial impact of disability generally has a greater negative impact on sexuality than the physical limitations of the disability itself. An emphasis on confidence building and new forms of sexual expression can be a great help to people suffering from debilitating illnesses.

Arthritis, with its joint deformities, possible contractures, and pain; cancer, with its pain and devastating treatments of surgery, chemotherapy, and radiation; and neuromuscular diseases with their muscle atrophy, abnormal muscle tone, and movements can cause a person to feel unattractive and sexually unappealing. These negative feelings impede the development of

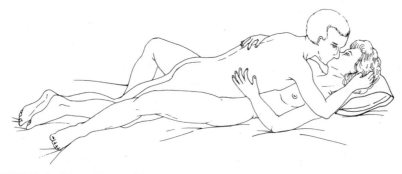

FIGURE 15–1. This position enables the woman to participate fully in intercourse without expending a great deal of energy supporting her weight on her arms.

emotional and physical intimacy. Any illness associated with decreased endurance or pain can be expected to limit sexual desire and activity. Even transient ill health is likely to produce enough anxiety to deter libido and sexual expression. These anxieties and negative self-perceptions must be dealt with so that patients can begin to take pleasure in what is left rather than dwelling on what has been lost.

For many people, the key to maintaining personal sexual fulfillment is the ability to adjust old patterns to meet ongoing changes successfully. Intercourse in the traditional man-on-top position may have been very satisfactory for a person in his or her youth, but gradual experimentation over time is likely to uncover a variety of positions and practices that are equally, if not more, enjoyable. Attitudes and practices that have increased sexual participation for many elderly people are listed below.

1. Understand normal changes associated with aging.
2. Increase communication on nonsexual topics as well as improve communication of sexual feelings and preferences.
3. Enjoy each moment. Don't hurry. Decrease performance anxiety.
4. Use sexual positions (such as side-lying or sitting) that do not require support of the body on isometrically contracted arm muscles (Figs. 15–1 through 15–7).

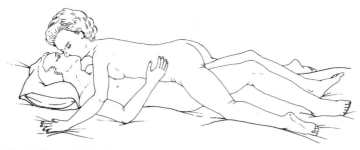

FIGURE 15–2. Lying on his back, the man does not expend energy supporting his weight on his arms.

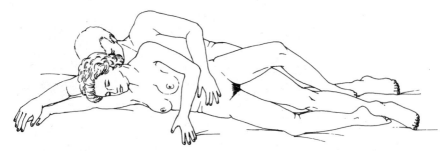

FIGURE 15–3. Here, neither partner overworks muscles to support weight.

5. Use sexual positions that do not put pressure on joints or areas of the body prone to pain or muscle strain (Figs. 15–8 through 15–10).
6. Use Kegel exercises to improve muscle tone and to achieve more vigorous vaginal contractions during sexual activity. (Men and women can benefit from Kegel exercises because they improve bladder and rectal sphincter strength). Kegel exercises should be performed several times a day by contracting the pubococcygeal muscles 20 to 30 times. Kegel exercises can best be described as pretending to hold back from urinating and defecating.
7. Practice oral-genital stimulation (Fig. 15–11).
8. Stimulate partner's genital area digitally (Figs. 15–12 and 15–13).
9. Use a vibrator alone or with a partner.
10. Masturbate alone or with a partner.
11. Consult a physician concerning treatment for impotence. Treatment options include inflatable, flexible, and semirigid prostheses ($5,000–$12,000); injection therapy ("pharmacological erection"—$900–$1,200 annually); or a vacuum constriction device (simple to use, effective, nonpermanent—$295–$400).

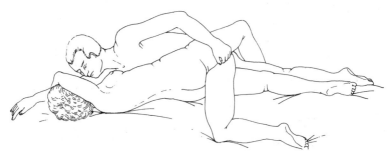

FIGURE 15–4. Use of this position alleviates prolonged pressure on joints for both partners.

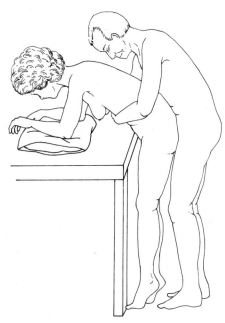

FIGURE 15–5. To increase comfort for someone with limited joint motion, rear entry by the man is supported by the woman.

12. Use a technique called "stuffing," in which the penis is stuffed into the vagina before a full erection is obtained. The penis will often become more erect as a result of the stimulation of being inside the vagina.
13. Explore the pleasures of touch and massage. Use of creams and massage oil can be fun. A deemphasis on intercourse can be pleasurable for both men and women and can decrease performance anxiety for men.
14. Use a water-soluble lubricant such as K-Y jelly during intercourse or masturbation. Some women prefer vegetable oil because it lasts longer.

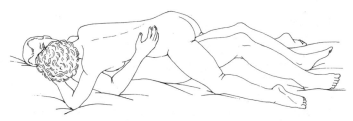

FIGURE 15–6. In this position, the man does not experience prolonged pressure on his joints.

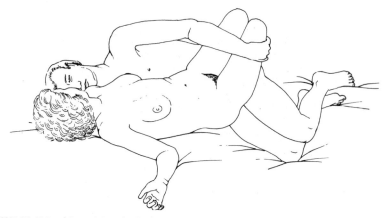

FIGURE 15–7. In this position, both partners are well-supported.

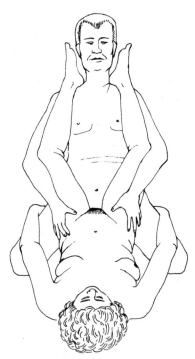

FIGURE 15–8. This position may be comfortable for a woman who is not able to straighten her hips.

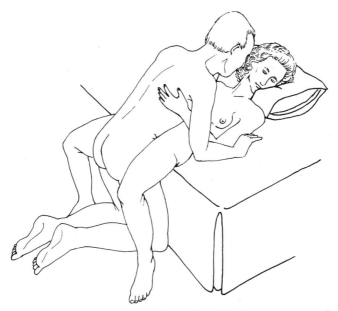

FIGURE 15–9. This position allows greater comfort and participation to a woman who is unable to bend her hips and/or straighten her knees.

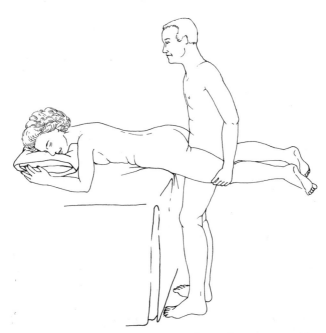

FIGURE 15–10. A woman who is not able to bend her hips or knees can use this rear-entry position.

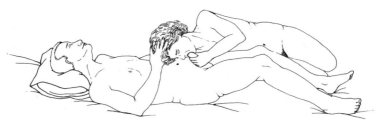

FIGURE 15–11. Older couples usually require more direct genital contact to stimulate and to maintain sexual excitement. Fellatio (oral stimulation of a man's genitals) may be used as a prelude to intercourse or as an independent activity. Cunnilingus (oral stimulation of a woman's genitals) is a sensual experience used as part of foreplay or as an alternative to intercourse.

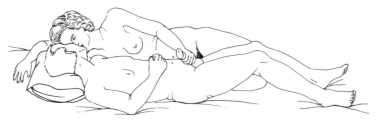

FIGURE 15–12. Fondling and stroking the genitals often helps stimulate and maintain erections.

15. Engage in hugging, kissing, stroking, talking, and laughing (Fig. 15–14).
16. Live a healthy lifestyle: get plenty of rest, exercise moderately, don't smoke, don't eat or drink excessively.
17. Be imaginative and romantic (lighting, clothing, flowers, locations, music, travel, compliments). Purchase and use a book offering romantic tips (*A Husband's Little Black Book* by Robert J. Ackerman, *1001 Ways to Be Romantic* by Gregory J.P. Godek).
18. Show respect by paying attention to personal hygiene and grooming (bathing, shaving, etc.) and taking care to make the partner feel attractive.

Making specific recommendations that patients can use to successfully adjust their sexual activity to the effects of aging or illness can be embarrassing for rehabilitation therapists. Accurately describing some of the recommended positions can prove difficult and awkward. To minimize their discomfort and still provide necessary information, many therapists have found it useful to make copies of the figures and suggestions in this chapter for use as handouts to patients needing specific techniques that will assist them in avoiding "sexual retirement."

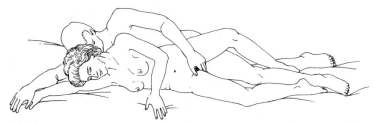

FIGURE 15–13. Rhythmic stroking of the female genital area is helpful in stimulating vaginal lubrication. Some women prefer it to intercourse, others prefer it as a prelude to intercourse or as a means of reaching orgasm after intercourse.

It is not feasible in this chapter to detail the sexual implications of all the major diseases and to give specific suggestions for sexual adjustment. Nonetheless, several disabilities warrant brief discussion because they are so prevalent among the elderly.

Arthritis

More than 30 percent of people age 65 and older are limited by arthritis and rheumatism.[44] Although arthritis may limit some forms of sexual behavior, there is evidence that regular sexual activity helps people with rheumatoid arthritis, probably because of adrenal gland production of cortisone and because sexual activity tends to lessen stress.[41] Arthritis patients have reported that, as a result of sexual stimulation and/or orgasm, they experienced less pain, discomfort, and depression.

Sore joints can impede sexual performance, but rarely reduce the desire for loving contact and sexual exchange between caring partners. However, steroid treatment may decrease sexual drive. The assault on body image re-

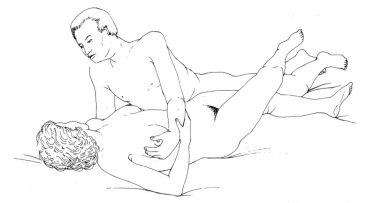

FIGURE 15–14. Sexual expression is not limited to genital stimulation. Hugging, kissing, stroking, talking, and laughing are all part of sexual communication.

sulting from progressive disfigurement may lead to feelings of sexual unattractiveness. Possible functional problems include contractions, joint degeneration, pain, and loss of mobility. A list of suggestions for dealing with these problems follows:

1. Exercise to increase or maintain joint mobility.
2. Use heat (hot shower or bath or paraffin bath, hot-water bottle, or heating pad) prior to sexual activity.
3. Use aspirin prophylactically for pain prior to sexual activity or after sexual activity (with permission of personal physician).
4. Communicate with partner about feelings of unattractiveness (partner may not share such feelings) and communicate about position limitations (alleviates partner's fear of causing pain and patient's fear of being hurt).
5. Avoid positions that put prolonged pressure on the involved joints.
6. Experiment with adaptive positions and/or alternatives to intercourse, such as mutual masturbation or oral sex.
7. Use a waterbed.
8. Set aside a rest period before engaging in sexual activity to help prevent fatigue (one of the hallmarks of rheumatoid disease). Try sexual activity in the morning or after a nap.
9. Place a pillow under painful limbs.
10. Empty the bladder to facilitate more comfortable love play and sexual exchange.
11. Report diminished sex drive to the personal physician. It may be a complication of drug therapy.

Hysterectomy

It is estimated that 1 in 4 women will reach menopause through hysterectomy,[45] the second most common surgical procedure performed in the United States. Reports vary concerning sexual interest and behavior following hysterectomy. Many of the women who suffered from pain and excessive bleeding prior to surgery report that their sexuality is much improved postsurgery. Complaints of sexual dysfunction range from a high of 46 percent[45] to a low of 10 percent.[46] Problems include painful intercourse, reduced sexual sensations, negative changes in orgasmic quality, and reduction or cessation of sexual desire. Much of the variance in sexual comfort is accounted for by type of surgery, whether supravaginal or abdominal hysterectomy, total (ovaries plus uterus removed), or partial (uterus only), and the woman's preoperative distress and expectations.[47]

Cancer

One of the three leading causes of death in the United States, cancer elicits fear and horror in most people. A diagnosis of cancer can cause severe depression and anxiety. The psychological turmoil associated with coming to terms with the disease must be dealt with before intimate sexual relations can be achieved. Physical closeness and affection, sexual or nonsexual, can be very beneficial to cancer patients, who are often feeling anxious, insecure, and depressed. Sexual activity can demonstrate love and support, and it offers normalcy to a life that has been thrown into disorder.

Possible functional problems include deformity caused by surgery, nausea, low endurance, pain, and changes in overall physical appearance owing to weight and hair loss. A list of suggestions for dealing with these problems follows:

1. Explore mutual masturbation or oral sex.
2. Time sexual activity around a pain-medication schedule so that pain is not a limiting factor.
3. Take a less active role. Change the sexual script.
4. Use non-weight-bearing positions to avoid fatigue.
5. Avoid positions in which the partner looks directly at a scar if nudity causes self-consciousness or discomfort for the cancer survivor. Mastectomy patients may feel more comfortable at first if they use positions other than woman-on-top.
6. Try sex in a sitting position, propped up on pillows, or in a large comfortable chair if breathing is difficult when lying down.
7. Incorporate massage or deep breathing into sex play to help relax and to relieve pain.
8. Reassure partner that he or she is still sexually desirable.

Heart Disease

Coronary attacks lead many people to give up sex altogether under the assumption that it will endanger their lives. However, the truth is that the oxygen usage (or "energy cost") for sex (average couple taking 10 to 16 minutes for the sex act) approximates climbing one or two flights of stairs, walking rapidly at a rate of 2 to 2½ miles per hour, or completing many common activities, such as driving a car.[41] Therefore, a patient who can comfortably climb one or two flights of stairs or take a brisk walk around the block is ready to resume sexual activity—usually 4 to 5 weeks after the coronary attack, provided that there are no complications. Other sexual activities, involving stroking, touching, and embracing, are possible in any event.[48] Nevertheless, numerous studies of men who had heart attacks have shown that sexual difficulties are common 6 to 12 months past recovery. The reasons for this are usually not physical but mental—anxiety, misinformation, and avoidance create most of the sexual difficulties. Interestingly, women who have suffered heart attacks are less likely to develop subsequent sexual problems than men.

Health care professionals should discuss sexuality with heart patients in a direct manner, explaining what the patient can and cannot do. Professionals should not wait for patients to ask sexual questions because patients are often too embarrassed, baffled, or resigned to the situation to initiate a discussion about sexual problems that have developed during the illness. Some questions, or gentle prompting by the physician, may therefore be necessary to bring these matters out into the open.[49,50]

Possible functional problems include fear of sudden death during sex, low endurance, and erectile problems caused by medication. Here is a list of suggestions for patients for dealing with these problems.

1. Learn that the likelihood of a heart attack during sex is very small. Deaths during coitus account for 0.6 percent of all sudden deaths; of these, 80 percent occurred during intercourse with an extramarital partner.[51]
2. Masturbate (cardiac cost is less than that of intercourse).
3. Decrease performance anxiety (take a less active role).
4. Begin sex play gradually. Allow the heart to warm up slowly.
5. Use energy-conserving, non-weight-bearing sexual positions (sitting, side-lying, and so forth).
6. Improve overall fitness and endurance through a medically supervised conditioning program.
7. Avoid sexual activity when anxious or fatigued.
8. Avoid sexual activity in extremely cold, hot, or humid settings (to eliminate the energy expenditure involved in maintaining body temperature).
9. Learn and use relaxation techniques.
10. Consult physician if medication affects libido, lubrication, or erectile capacity. (Medication should not be discontinued without medical consultation.)

Stroke

In the United States, it is estimated that 550,000 cerebrovascular accidents occur each year; more than 200,000 survivors are added to the stroke population annually. One study of 35 stroke survivors found that most experience some form of sexual dysfunction after the stroke, despite the fact that the majority of stroke survivors maintain consistent levels of sexual desire and believe that sexual function is important.[52] The dysfunction is occasionally related to fear of causing another stroke, even though it is extremely unlikely that further strokes can be produced through sexual exertion.[41]

Possible functional problems include sensation loss, communication problems, perceptual problems, contractures, loss of mobility, tremors, and visual problems. Here is a list of suggestions for dealing with these problems.

1. Use nonverbal communication.
2. Emphasize stimulation of areas that are still sensitive to touch.

3. Experiment with comfortable positions.
4. Ask partner to stay on the seeing side if vision is impaired on only one side.
5. Use a waterbed.
6. Explore through touch and smell rather than depending on vision.
7. Use a vibrator if hands are weak or uncoordinated (vibrator may be strapped to hand).
8. Share fantasies in writing.

Prostatitis

As men age, the prostate gland tends to increase in size, a condition known as benign prostatic hypertrophy. The enlarged prostate tends to constrict the urethra, thereby decreasing urine flow.[53] Approximately half of middle-aged and older men experience prostate problems such as inflammation and painful swelling against the bladder. Half of these will require surgery. The operation (prostatectomy) need not affect sexual functioning even though it may alter ejaculatory sensations. Most men are sterile after surgery but fully capable of sexual activity through retrograde ejaculation, in which the semen is ejaculated into the bladder. Most prostatectomy patients recover from surgery within a couple of months and are fully able to resume sexual activity. If serious readjustment problems persist, a sex counseling referral should be offered.

Diabetes

Diabetes mellitus is common in later life. Many diabetic men are not impotent, but it is one of the few illnesses that can cause chronic impotence. Although sexual interest and desire may continue, about 50 to 60 percent of diabetic men have erectile dysfunction, which can occur as an early symptom of the disease or may not develop until years after the diagnosis of diabetes. Most cases of diabetes-produced impotence are reversible. If the disease has been poorly controlled, there is a fair chance that proper regulation thereafter will improve potency. Unfortunately, when impotence occurs in well-controlled diabetes, it may be permanent.[41] In women, one study found that 35 percent of the diabetic persons interviewed, versus 6 percent of the nondiabetic persons interviewed, reported complete absence of orgasmic response during the year preceding the inquiry. Orgasmic dysfunction developed gradually and was directly correlated with the duration of diabetes.[54] The primary cause of these sexual problems is nerve damage, a complication of diabetes. In a smaller number of cases, these dysfunctions are caused by circulatory problems.

Possible functional problems include impotence, sensation loss, and visual problems. A list of suggestions for dealing with these problems follows:

1. Reduce anxiety.
2. Communicate through touch, smell, and imagination to make up for vision loss.
3. Ask partner to emphasize stimulation of areas still sensitive to touch.
4. Use a hard doughnut-shaped rubber device slipped over the partially erect penis to help maintain an erection; these are available in shops dealing with sexual materials. (Rubber bands are sometimes used for this purpose, though not recommended.)
5. Seek pragmatic counseling if impotence is psychogenic.
6. Consult a physician concerning treatment for impotence.
7. Consult a physician about possible problems associated with use of medications.

SEX AND DRUG USE

Although elderly persons currently make up 13 percent of the population, because of increased incidence of illness, they consume 35 percent of all prescription drugs. All too often, elderly patients are not informed of the sexual implications associated with the use of certain prescription drugs. Many physicians are uncomfortable discussing sexual issues, and many erroneously assume that there is no need to discuss such things with their elderly patients. The consequences of not discussing sexual implications of drug use can be quite serious. For example, a man who does not know that some medications for hypertension can produce erectile problems or decrease libido may blame himself and become very depressed or attribute the dysfunction to problems in the relationship with his partner.

The generic drugs listed in Table 15–1 are capable of affecting some aspects of sexuality.[55] As would be expected, the principal therapeutic effect of each of these is on the nervous or circulatory system. As with any drug effect, the nature and degree of altered sexual function vary greatly from one individual to another. Although such effects may occur at any age, they are usually more frequent and more troublesome after age 50. Suspicion of the possibility of such a drug response should result in consultation with the attending physician regarding the advisability of modifying treatment. Drug use should not be discontinued without physician consultation.

SEX IN NURSING HOMES

Although the vast majority of the elderly in this country live in homes or apartments, approximately 5 percent of people over 65 live in nursing homes or other long-term care institutions. Cole's study of elderly patients in nursing homes found that at least 50 percent wanted sexual activity.[56] The

Table 15–1. **Drugs and Sexuality**

POSSIBLE DRUG EFFECTS ON MALE SEXUALITY

Increased Libido

androgens (replacement therapy in deficiency states)
baclofen (Lioresal)
chlordiazepoxide (Librium): antianxiety effect
diazepam (Valium): antianxiety effect
haloperidol (Haldol)
levodopa (Larodopa, Sinemet): may be an indirect effect due to improved sense of well-being

Decreased Libido

antihistamines
barbiturates
chlorpromazine (Thorazine): 10–20% of users
cimetidine (Tagamet)
clofibrate (Atromid-S)
clonidine (Catapres): 10–20% of users
danazol (Danocrine)
diazepam (Valium): sedative effect
disulfiram (Antabuse)
estrogens: therapy for prostatic cancer
fenfluramine (Pondimin)
licorice
medeoxyprogesterone (Provera)
methyldopa (Aldomet): 10–15% of users
perhexilene (Pexid)
prazosin (Minipres): 15% of users
propranolol (Inderal): rarely
reserpine (Serpasil, Ser-Ap-Es)
spironolactone (Aldactone)
tricyclic antidepressants (TADs)

Impaired Erection (Impotence)

anticholinergics
antihistamines
baclofen (Lioresal)
barbiturates: when abused
beta blockers
chlordiazepoxide (Librium): in high dosage
chlorpromazine (Thorazine)
cimetidine (Tagamet)
clofibrate (Atromid-S)
clonidine (Catapres): 10–20% of users
cocaine
diazepam (Valium): in high dosage
digitalis and its glycosides
disopyramide (Norpace)
disulfiram (Antabuse): uncertain
estrogens: therapy for prostatic cancer
ethacrynic acid (Edecrin): 5% of users
ethionamide (Trecator-SC)
fenfluramine (Pondimin)
furosemide (Lasix): 5% of users
guanethidine (Ismelin)

haloperidol (Haldol): 10–20% of users
heroin
hydroxyprogesterone: therapy for prostatic cancer
licorice
lithium (Lithonate)
marijuana
mesoridazine (Serentil)
methantheline (Banthine)
metoclopramide (Reglan): 60% of users
monoamine oxidase inhibitors (MAOIs), Type A inhibitors
perhexilene (Pexid)
prazosin (Minipres): infrequently
reserpine (Serpasil, Ser-Ap-Es)
spironolactone (Aldactone)
thiazide diuretics: 5% of users
thioridazine (Mellaril)
tricyclic antidepressants (TADs)

Impaired Ejaculation

anticholinergics
barbiturates: when abused
chlorpromazine (Thorazine)
clonidine (Catapres)
estrogens: therapy for prostatic cancer
guanethidine (Ismelin)
heroin
mesoridazine (Serentil)
methyldopa (Aldomet)
monoamine oxidase inhibitors (MAOIs)
phenoxybenzamine (Dibenzyline)
phentolamine (Regitine)
reserpine (Serpasil, Ser-Ap-Es)
thiazide diuretics
thioridazine (Mellaril)
tricyclic antidepressants (TADs)

Swelling of Testicles

tricyclic antidepressants (TADs)

Inflammation of Testicles

oxyphenbutazone (Tandearil)

Atrophy of Testicles

androgens: moderate to high dosage, extended use
chlorpromazine (Thorazine)
cyclophosphamide (Cytoxan): in prepubescent boys
spironolactone (Aldactone)

Priapism

anabolic steroids (male hormonelike drugs)
chlorpromazine (Thorazine)
cocaine

guanethidine (Ismelin)
haloperidol (Haldol)
heparin
levodopa (Sinemet)
molindone (Moban)
prazosin (Minipres)
prochlorperazine (Compazine)
trazodone (Desyrel)
trifluoperazine (Stelazine)
warfarin (Coumadin)

Peyronie's Disease

beta blocker drugs (see Drug Class, Section Four)
phenytoin (Dilantin, etc.)

Gynecomastia (Excessive Development of the Male Breast)

androgens: partial conversion to estrogen
BCNU
busulfan (Myleran)
chlormadinone
chlorpromazine (thorazine)
chlortetracycline (Aureomycin)
cimetidine (Tagament)

clonidine (Catapres): infrequently
diethylstilbestrol (DES)
digitalis and its glycosides
estrogens: therapy for prostatic cancer
ethionamide (Trecator-SC)
griseofulvin (Fulvicin, etc.)
haloperidol (Haldol)
heroin
human chorionic gonadotropin
isoniazid (IHN), (Nydrazid)
marijuana
mestranol
methyldopa (Aldomet)
metoclopromide (Reglan)
phenelzine (Nardil)
reserpine (Serpasil, Ser-Ap-Es)
spironolactone (Aldactone)
thioridazine (Mellaril)
tricyclic antidepressants (TADs)
vincristine (Oncovin)

Feminization (Loss of Libido, Impotence, Gynecomastia, Testicular Atrophy)

conjugated estrogens (Premarin, etc.)

POSSIBLE DRUG EFFECTS ON FEMALE SEXUALITY

Increased Libido

androgens
chlordiazepoxide (Librium): antianxiety effect
diazepam (Valium): antianxiety effect
mazindol (Sanorex)

Decreased Libido

See list of drug effects on male sexuality. Some of these may have potential for reducing libido in the female. The literature is sparse on this subject.

Impaired Arousal and Orgasm

Alcohol (delayed orgasm)
anticholinergics
clonidine (Catapres)
methyldopa (Aldomet)
monoamine oxidase inhibitors (MAOIs)
tricyclic antidepressants (TADs)

Breast Enlargement

penicillamine
tricyclic antidepressants (TADs)

Galactorrhea (Spontaneous Flow of Milk)

amphetamine
chlorpromazine (Thorazine)
cimetidine (Tagamet)
haloperidol (Haldol)
heroin
methyldopa (Aldomet)
metoclopramide (Reglan)
oral contraceptives
phenothiazines
reserpine (Serpasil, Ser-Ap-Es)
sulpirid (Equilid)
tricyclic antidepressants (TADs)

Source: Adapted from Long and Ryback[55] with permission.

percentage who engage in sexual acts is much less, though, because most nursing home patients are treated like children with no option for the privacy necessary for conjugal visits, masturbation, or even kissing or holding hands. ADL evaluations, which assess everything from patients' bowel movements to dental hygiene, rarely include information about sexual adjustment. The goal of the skilled nursing care staff is generally to encourage and to facilitate optimal functioning of residents physically, emotionally, and socially. Avoiding the topic of sexuality tends to perpetuate the myth that sexual expression among the elderly is perverted, sick, or nonexistent. In reality, sex can be an expression of pleasure, love, joy, intimacy, and a continuing reaffirmation of life. The healing quality of being touched, held, and caressed does not diminish with age.

A 1974 federal regulation[57] concerning skilled nursing facilities states, "A married patient in a long-term care facility shall be assured privacy for visits by his or her spouse and married inpatients may share a room unless medically contraindicated and so documented by the attending physician in the medical record." The regulation states further that "the patient may associate and communicate privately with persons of his choice" (p 193). States are required to implement these federal regulations in their health codes if they receive federal funds. Administrators of long-term care institutions are having to come to grips with the increasing emphasis on patients' rights, including rights to privacy with regard to sexual expression. This is not an easy task.

Specific policies regarding sexual expression may pose administrative problems, including the answers to the following questions:

1. How is privacy ensured for the roommate of a sexually active person living in a semiprivate room?
2. How is privacy ensured without allowing doors to be locked?
3. How are patients who do not want sex protected from those who do?
4. Should the facility provide "sex therapy rooms" or waiting rooms for roommates or a specifically designated unit to patients interested in sexual activity?
5. Should visitors be allowed to spend the night?
6. Should extra wide beds be available?
7. Who is liable if a patient doesn't use siderails during sex, falls out of bed, and breaks a hip?
8. Should intellectually impaired patients be allowed sexual activity?
9. Should the wishes of the family or the patient come first?

Here are some recommendations for promotion of healthy sexual expression in nursing homes:

1. Recommend books to patients, have them available in the institution, and make provisions for books to be read to those patients unable to read. Examples of such books are *The Joy of Sex* by Comfort, *Love and Sex after Sixty* by Butler and Lewis, *Sexuality and Aging* by Solnick, and *Love, Sex and Aging: A Consumer's Union Report* by Brecher and the editors of Consumer Reports Books.
2. Include sexual history in the ADL assessments.
3. Institute a patient education program outlining sexual activity related to medical problems of the elderly.
4. Listen for verbal and nonverbal cues of sexual concerns.
5. Ensure confidentiality.
6. Avoid personal shyness about the subject; although sex is a very personal and private matter, it does not need to be a taboo topic.

7. Be aware of the nonverbal message sent by the staff.
8. Emphasize what is left rather than what has been lost.
9. Redirect inappropriate sexual expression to more healthy outlets, instead of using punishment to change residents' behavior.

SUMMARY

Sexuality is not just genital stimulation. It encompasses the entire realm of human contact and communication; it is the way people define and present themselves. Sexual expression can enhance both self-esteem and a positive self-image. Health care providers can enhance quality sexual adjustment to aging and illness by conveying a humanistic, pleasure-oriented view. Discussion of aspects of health, illness, and treatment that affect sexuality conveys an understanding of sex as an expression of self, not a segment of the self used up in youth.

As a rehabilitation specialist, you have the opportunity, without proselytizing, to foster a view of sexual expression as an enriching experience that can open communication and increase intimacy and self-esteem. A little reassurance against their own false expectations and the hostility of society can go a long way toward promoting healthy sexual adjustment for elderly patients.

It is worthwhile to keep in mind that, despite the decreased speed and agility associated with growing older, the elderly generally have a great deal of free time, as well as life experience to bring to sexual expression. For some, old age is a cold winter with no refuge, but for others it is the harvest of a life's learning and loving.

REFERENCES

1. Kaplan, HS: Sex, intimacy, and the aging process. J Am Academy Psychoanalysis 18(2):185–205, 1990.
2. Kaplan, HS: The New Sex Therapy. Brunner/Mazel, New York, 1974, p. 104.
3. Pfeiffer, E, Verwoedt, A, and Wang, HS: Sexual behavior in aged men and women. Arch Gen Psychiatry 19:753, 1968.
4. Schiavi, RC, Schreiner-Engle, P, Mandeli, J, Schanzer, H, and Cohen, E: Healthy aging and male sexual function. Am J Psychiatry 147(6):766–771, 1990.
5. Schiavi, RC, Mandeli, J, and Schreiner-Engle, P: Sexual satisfaction in healthy aging men. J Sex Marital Ther 20(1):3–13, 1994.
6. Hudson, WH, Murphy, GJ, and Nurius, PS: A short-form scale to measure liberal vs. conservative orientations toward sexual expression. J Sex Res 19:258–272, 1983.
7. Keller, JF, Eakes, E, Hinkle, D, and Hughston, GA: Sexual behavior and guilt among women: A cross-generational comparison. J Sex Marital Ther 4:259–165, 1978.
8. Kinsey, AC, Pomeroy, WB, and Martin, CE: Sexual Behavior in the Human Male. WB Saunders, Philadelphia, 1948.
9. Masters, WH and Johnson, VE: Human Sexual Response. Little, Brown, Boston, 1966.
10. Shamoian, CA and Thurston, FD: Marital discord and divorce among the elderly. Med Aspects Hum Sex 20:25–34, 1986.
11. Masters, WH. Sex and aging: Expectations and reality. Hosp Pract 21:175–198, 1986.

12. George, LK and Weiler, SJ: Sexuality in middle and late life. Arch Gen Psychiatry 38:919–923, 1981.

13. Persson, G and Svanborg, A: Marital coital activity in men at the age of 75: Relation to somatic, psychiatric, and social factors at the age of 75. J Am Ger Soc 40:439–444, 1992.

14. U.S. Department of Commerce, Bureau of the Census: Marital Status and Living Arrangements: March 1993. U.S. Government Printing Office, Washington, DC, 1994.

15. Weizman, R and Hart, J: Sexual behavior in healthy married elderly men. Arch Sex Behav 16(1):39–44, 1987.

16. Starr, B and Weiner, MB: On Sex and Sexuality in the Mature Years. Stein & Day, New York, 1981.

17. Wax, J: Sex and the single grandparent. New Times 5:43, 1975.

18. Kimmel, D: Adult development and aging: A gay perspective. J of Social Issues 34:113–130, 1978.

19. Cole, E and Rothblum, E: Commentary on sexuality and the midlife woman. Psychology of Women Quarterly 14(4):509–512, 1990.

20. Dawson, K: Serving the older gay community. SIECUS Report 11:5–6, 1982.

21. Friend, RA: Older lesbian and gay people: A theory of successful aging. J Homosexuality 20(3/4):99–118, 1990.

22. Berger, RM: The unseen majority: Older gays and lesbians. Social Work 27(3):236–241, 1982.

23. Masters, WH. Sex and aging: Expectations and reality. Hosp Pract 21:175–198, 1986.

24. Goldstein, H and Runyon, C: An occupational therapy education module to increase sensitivity about geriatric sexuality. Physical & Occupational Therapy in Geriatrics 11(2):57–76, 1993.

25. Anon, JS: The Behavioral Treatment of Sexual Problems: Brief Therapy. Harper & Row, New York, 1976.

26. Purifoy, FE, Martin, CE, and Tobin, JD: Age-related variations in female sexual arousal and orgasmic response. Paper presented at the 26th Annual Meeting of the Society for the Scientific Study of Sex. Chicago, IL, November 19–20, 1983.

27. Perlmutter, J: A gynecological approach to menopause. In Notman, M and Nadelson, C (eds): The Woman Patient. Plenum, New York, 1978.

28. Notelovitz, M and Lewis, AP: Keeping menopausal women healthy. Medical Aspects of Human Sexuality 20:70–76, 1986.

29. Seaman, B and Seaman, G: Women and the Crisis in Sex Hormones. Bantam Books, New York, 1978.

30. Gambrell, RD: Estrogen replacement therapy for the elderly woman. Medical Aspects of Human Sexuality 21:8–93, 1987.

31. Mooradian, AD and Greiff, V: Sexuality in older women. Arch of Internal Medicine 150:1033–1038, 1990.

32. Notelovitz, M and Lewis, AP: Keeping menopausal women healthy. Medical Aspects of Human Sexuality 20:70–76, 1986.

33. Peck, WA, Barrett-Conner, E, Buckwalter, JA, Gambrell, RD, Jr., et al: Consensus conference: Osteoporosis. JAMA 252–799, 1984.

34. Gordan, GS: Drug treatment of the osteoporoses. Ann Rev Pharmacol Toxicol 18:253. 1978.

35. Nachtigall, LE, Nachtigall, RH, Nachtigall, RD, et al: Estrogen replacement therapy. vol 1: A 10-year prospective study in the realtionship to osteoporosis. Obstet Gynecol 53:277, 1979.

36. Greenwood, S and Margolis, A: Outercourse. Advances in Planned Parenthood 15:4, 1981.

37. Ritz, S: Growing through menopause. Medical Self-Care Winter: 15–18, 1981.

38. Notelovitz, M: Noncontraceptive hormone therapy and breast cancer: A personal perspective of clinical guidelines. Menopause Management 2(3):5–8, 1989.

39. Lieblum, SR: Sexuality and the midlife woman. Psychology of Women Quarterly: 14(4): 495–508, 1990.

40. Masters, WH and Johnson, VE: Sex and the aging process. J Am Ger Soc 29:385–390, 1981.
41. Butler, RN and Lewis, MI: Sex after Sixty. Harper & Row, New York, 1976.
42. Pocs, O and Godow, AG: Can students view parents as sexual beings? The Family Coordinator 26:31, 1977.
43. Ludeman, K: The sexuality of the older postmarital woman. A phenomenological inquiry. Unpublished dissertation.
44. U.S. Department of Commerce, Bureau of the Census: Statistical Abstract of the US 1988, ed 208. U.S. Government Printing Office, Washington, DC, 1988.
45. Zussman, L, Zussman, S, Sunley, R, and Bjornson, E: Sexual response after hysterectomy-oophorectomy: Recent studies and reconsideration of psychogenesis. Am J of Obstetrics and Gynecology 140:725–729, 1981.
46. Huffman, J: The effect of gynecologic surgery on sexual reactions. Am J of Obstetrics and Gynecology 59:915–917, 1950.
47. Lieblum, SR: Sexuality and the midlife woman. Psychology of Women Quarterly: 14(4): 495–508, 1990.
48. Steffl, BM: Sexuality and aging: Implications for nurses and other helping professionals. In Solnick, RL (ed): Sexuality and Aging. University of Southern California Press, 1978, p. 139.
49. Crenshaw, TL: In consultation: Sexual problem case of the month: Painful intercourse caused by extensive arthritis of the hip. Medical Aspects of Human Sexuality 10:45, 1986.
50. Hobson, KG: The effects of aging on sexuality. Health and Social Work 9(1):25–35, 1984.
51. Dagon, EM: Sexuality and sexual dysfunction in the elderly. In Lazarus, LW, Jarvik, LF, Foster, JR, Lieff, JD, and Mershon, SR (eds): Essentials of Geriatric Psychiatry: A Guide for Health Professionals. Springer, New York, 1988.
52. Broy, GP, et al: Sexual functioning in stroke survivors. Arch Phys Med Rehabil 62:286, 1981.
53. Ritz, S: Growing through menopause. Medical Self-Care 15–18, Winter, 1981.
54. Schiavi, R: Sexuality and medical illness. Specific references to diabetes mellitus. In Greene, R (ed): Human Sexuality: A Health Practitioner's Test. William & Wilkins, Baltimore, 1979, p. 203.
55. Long, JW and Rybacki, JJ: The essential guide to prescription drugs: What you need to know for safe drug use. Harper & Row, New York, 1994, pp. 1120–1126.
56. Ledebur, J and Strax, TE: Geriatric sexuality manual for patients, spouses, and family. Department of Physical Medicine and Rehabilitation, Philadelphia Geriatric Center, Philadelphia.
57. Medicaid and Medicare—HEW issues additional standards for skilled nursing facilities, and establishes requirements for discharge of patients. Department of Health, Education and Welfare 39:193, Part 2, October 3, 1974.
58. Goldstein, H and Runyon, C: An occupational therapy educational module to increase sensitivity about geriatric sexuality. Physical & Occupational Therapy in Geriatrics 11(2):57–76, 1993.
59. Crose, R and Drake, LK: Older women's sexuality. Clinical Gerontologist 12(4):51–56, 1993.

Appendix

Student Assignments and Experiential Classroom Exercises

Students of geriatric rehabilitation should be encouraged to examine their own attitudes, misconceptions, countertransferences, and comfort level regarding sexuality and the elderly. Development of a mature, nonjudgmental attitude in this highly sensitive area is essential for clinicians in practice. Role-playing activities and homework assignments can assist students in this effort and facilitate their patient interaction skills while desensitizing them to discussions of sexual issues.

Role-Playing Exercises[58]

1. A patient with a cardiac problem who expresses fears about becoming sexually active.
2. A woman with rheumatoid arthritis who complains of increased joint pain and decreased vaginal lubrication causing pain and discomfort during sexual activity.
3. Post-CVA patient residing in a nursing home who expresses anger because everyone thinks she should be asexual.

Homework Assignments

1. Interview one or more elderly persons concerning their personal definitions of sexuality, their earliest memories of sexual experience, their perceptions of when and why any changes had occurred as they aged, what they need for a satisfying sexual relationship, and how their attitudes about sex have changed from 40 years ago and from 20 years ago.[59]
2. Interview one or more elderly persons concerning incidence of sexual activity, interest in sexual activity, frequency of orgasms, feelings of sexual desire, feelings of pleasure with sex, and satisfaction with sex life.[59]
3. *Sexual Values Generational Inventory*[58]*:* Explore how attitudes and values could influence treatment. Survey several people in the 18-to-30-year-old generation and several from the 65 and older generation about their agreement with the following:
   a. It is appropriate to openly discuss your sexual needs and concerns.
   b. Sexual activity is acceptable in a nonmarriage situation.
   c. Sexual activity is appropriate if it is done for physical pleasure.
   d. Sexual activity is only for procreation.
   e. The naked body is very private. Nudity is unacceptable.
   f. Women should discuss their sexual needs with their partners.
   g. It is appropriate for women to initiate sex.
   h. Masturbation is a normal sexual act.
4. *Written reflections:* How do I feel about my parents or grandparents having sex? Do I consider sexual activity among older persons to be shameful, perverse, funny, or embarrassing? How do I react when I see two elderly people kissing and fondling each other? Is sexual activity in a nursing home acceptable? Is it OK for unmarried elderly persons to engage in sexual activity? Can I comfortably discuss sexuality with my patients? Can I treat my homosexual patients with the same care and respect I show my heterosexual patients? When I think about sexual expression between older people, how do I feel? How will my attitudes affect my ability to do my job effectively?

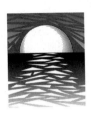

CHAPTER 16

Working with the Dying Older Patient

Linda C. Campanelli, PhD

Dedicated to the memory of Richard Kalish (1930–1988), gerontologist, thanatologist, teacher.

BEHAVIORAL OBJECTIVES

Upon completion of this chapter, the reader will be able to:

1 Discuss major factors affecting the dying older patient.
2 Describe the process of dying.
3 Discuss the process of grieving.
4 Communicate effectively with the dying person and his or her family.
5 Describe alternative health care settings.

Loss is a universal theme. Throughout life we experience losses in different degrees. For example, as children we may lose a pet or a friend; as teenagers we may experience the loss of a romance; as young adults, possibly the loss of grandparents, parents, or our so-called innocent view of the world. In midlife, losses become more central to ourselves. The status of our health may become unpredictable and poorly developed stress management skills may exacerbate or aggravate preexisting conditions. Also, aging relatives or friends remind us of both the hardiness and frailty of being human.

In our later years, for some, loss may include the deterioration of functioning in various limbs, actual paralysis, or, in the extreme, amputation. For others, slowed motor functions or cognitive impairment may appear. Generally, it can be said that loss becomes a way of life for everyone who lives long enough. Accepting, coping with, or understanding loss is a lifetime task dependent on several factors.

OVERVIEW

Sex Roles, Death Attitudes, and the Older Adult

It has been reported that fear of death diminishes with advancing age.[1] One can surmise this to be so because older persons have had more experience with the deaths of others, which often includes the deaths of one's parents or one's child or children. Still, although death is expected when a person is older, it is questionable whether the person becomes fully resigned to its timing and place.

In her book on the role of sex differential in death and death-related concerns, Stillion[2] states that evidence seems to be growing that elderly people, compared with younger people, fear death less. Also, most studies indicate that men and women show different reactions to death and death-related concerns. Men are less expressive about their anxiety or fears, whereas women continue to seem freer to discuss and admit their fears. Factors such as religiosity, place of residence, socioeconomic status, race, and intelligence are also important in determining an elderly person's response to death.[2]

Psychologic and Cognitive Changes

In 1961, Kleemier[3] observed intellectual changes in older adults 2 years prior to their deaths. Since that time, researchers[4–6] have observed similar results based on both IQ and behavioral tests. The concept of a decrease in intellectual functioning prior to death is called "terminal drop." In one study in which terminal drop was supported, researchers[7] found that the percentage of female deaths for those who scored in the lower range in IQ measures was significantly higher than for those who scored in the middle and higher ranges. The percentage of deaths among the lower IQ ranges was not statistically significant for men, however.[2] This may indicate sex differences in cognitive changes before death, with the most severe drop in IQ affecting women.

WHEN AN OLDER ADULT IS DYING

What is different about working with older patients as opposed to young or middle-aged patients? In terms of the quality of clinical care demanded by various diseases, nothing is different. However, within the larger scheme of things, subtleties abound, serving to distinguish terminal older patients from their younger counterparts.

Kalish[1] found six matters that affect the elderly more than any other age group:

1. The social value of the remaining life of the older person is perceived by others to be diminished. By comparison, the loss of a younger life is perceived by most people to be more tragic than the loss of an older life. Therefore, less attention may be paid to the older person.
2. Motivation for providing optimum care to the older person may be dulled by the belief that older people will die soon anyway.
3. Less than 10 percent of the elderly population is in chronic care or long-term care facilities before being hospitalized. Family contact is sometimes diminished for these dying elderly patients, isolating them further.
4. Older people are more likely to be confused or comatose during the period leading to death. As a result of this condition, communication between patient and care provider is, at best, difficult. Kalish[1] expresses it well when he says that this lack of communication "may even engender resentment from those who are required to care for them, because the demanding nature of their illness is not compensated for by a reciprocal human relationship" (p. 204).
5. Many older persons, particularly women, often have no surviving spouses or mates and no remaining siblings. For example, if an older adult is childless, there are no sons, daughters, or grandchildren to provide attention, comfort, love, or affection. Moreover, the individual is also less likely to have an advocate to intercede on his or her behalf.
6. An older adult often engages in reminiscence. This process is also known as the "life review." Reviewing one's life, according to Butler,[8] helps to integrate a person's entire life. Butler is of the opinion that reminiscing may make death more acceptable. He explains, "I do not intend to imply that a 'severe and dignified acceptance of death' is necessarily appropriate, noble, or to be valued. Those who die

screaming may be expressing a rage that is as fitting as dignity" (p. 494).

THE PROCESS OF DYING

Dying has its privileges. Many institutions relax their visitation rules, family comes flocking to say good-bye, and friends make an effort to visit. Passions for certain pleasures are honored, such as offering the dying person an occasional sip of wine, bits of chocolate, or a piece of fried chicken.

Dying also has its disadvantages. If the dying person takes too long to die, family members, as well as friends, tend to stay away; doctors or nurses sometimes begin to disengage; and the dying person, who may still perceive himself or herself to be merely sick (as opposed to actually dying), becomes anxious at the obvious changes in behavior around him or her.[9]

Kalish[1] has noted that the major factor in dying is not the age of the person but, rather, the condition causing death. He reminds us that, for most older adults, dying is most often more lonely and isolated than for younger persons. Weisman[10] explains, "The terminally ill aged may be as helpless as children, but they seldom arouse tenderness" (p. 144). As stated earlier, perhaps it is because we expect an older person to die; the cycle of life is completed on death's arrival.

For many, the most revealing analysis of the terminally ill person's reactions to death is that of Elizabeth Kübler-Ross,[11] a psychiatrist, who created a framework based on interviews with, and observations of, both dying patients and those who worked with them.

According to Kübler-Ross, the five stages of dying are:

1. Denial and isolation
2. Anger
3. Bargaining
4. Depression
5. Acceptance

Although this hierarchy provides us with a framework in which to operate, by no means have these stages been proven to be serial, experienced by all or most dying persons, and self-contained.[12–14] Kastenbaum[14] noted that the existence of stages has not been demonstrated, that no evidence is presented that people do move from stages 1 through 5, and that the available evidence—although not definitive—fails to provide support for a stage theory of aging. However, society has latched onto these stages as though knowing and understanding them would facilitate the dying process.

He observed that even efforts by Kübler-Ross to discourage a rigid adherence to stage theory were unsuccessful. Allied health practitioners should bear in mind the alternative viewpoint of thanatologist Mansell Pattison,[15] who dissents from the Kübler-Ross stage theory. He writes:

I find no evidence . . . to support specific stages of dying. Rather, dying patients demonstrate a wide variety of emotions that ebb and flow throughout our entire life as we face conflicts and crisis. It does seem misleading, then, to search for and determine stages of dying. Rather I suggest that our task is to determine the stresses and crisis at a specific time, to respond to the emotions generated by that issue, and, in essence, to respond to where the patient is at in his or her living-dying. We do not make the patient conform to our idealized concept of dying but respond to the patient's actual dying experience. (p. 141)

The dying trajectory, the pattern and rate of decline toward death, is also a part of the process of dying. As common wisdom dictates, the chronically ill elderly patient has a longer trajectory than someone who dies suddenly because of an accident or an acute illness. Unfortunately, due to modern medical technology, the dying trajectory is often viewed as endless. The ramifications are such that social and family support tend to decrease with time, thus contributing to increased social isolation in the final stage of life.[16] Greater emotional demands are then placed on health care providers.

GRIEVING

The price a person pays for loving and commitment is pain. In other words, the cost of knowing and caring for the dying person is grieving.[8] If the process of grieving is not recognized for what it is, it may be misunderstood and, consequently, mishandled.

The first statement in this chapter was, "Loss is a universal theme." We have all lost someone or something important to us at one time or another. Loss of control over a situation, loss of a job, retirement, quitting smoking, surgery, and burglary are everyday examples. However, some losses are more critical than others. Losing someone in our immediate family will render us more grief-stricken than losing a tooth or a favorite pen.

Generally, grieving for a loss follows a very simple pattern. We grieve profoundly for someone or something that we perceive to be central to our lives, and less intensely for someone or something that is not. More specifically, the trauma produced by loss is related to the degree of emotional bond made with the lost person, place, or thing; the type of loss; an individual's personality and reaction to past losses; and the timing and prior knowledge of the loss.[17]

These four factors imply that the grief response is both highly individualistic and highly complex. Stephenson[18] has identified a set of stages to assist us in determining where we are in relation to stages of development as we progress through our grief period. These include the stages of reaction, disorganization and reorganization, and reorientation and recovery. However, not everyone experiences the grieving process, per se. These stages may be interrupted, anticipatory grieving may lessen the length of certain stages, or grieving may be prolonged, leaving the bereaved "stuck" within a stage. The key is to recognize that reorientation and recovery are the end points of a grieving process. For example, Parkes[19] has described the grieving process in four stages: numbness, pining, depression, and recovery. Although more descriptive in nature, particularly regarding the emotional intensity of grieving, the end point of Parkes's stages parallels those of Stephenson and Kübler-Ross.

It has been said that it takes at least 1 year for a *reasonable* recovery from a death, with 2 years being the most frequently quoted norm. Actually, the duration of grief varies and depends on particular factors influencing the grief response. As with any loss, periodic reminders bring feelings of sadness. These feelings are normal and are to be expected, particularly around an anniversary date such as a birthday, death day, or family holiday.

Observations of older married couples have led thanatologists to discover that differences exist between the sexes with regard to the grieving process. In a review of the literature, Stroebe and Stroebe[16] concluded that, on a physiologic and psychologic level, widowers suffered more than widows. This can be seen in the higher morbidity and mortality rates exhibited by widowers soon after the death of their spouses.

DETERMINING THE GRIEVING PROCESS

According to Rando,[20] psychologic, sociologic, and physiologic factors all influence how and when we grieve. Among the psychologic factors, three are noted: (1) the characteristics and meaning of the lost relationship (for example, the role and function filled by the deceased; the amount of unfinished business between the deceased and the survivor; (2) personal characteristics (for example, coping behaviors, personality, and mental health; past experience with loss); and (3) specific circumstances of the death (for example, sudden versus expected death, timeliness of the death).

Sociologic factors, such as one's social support system; funerary ritual; sociocultural, ethnic, and religious-philosophical background; and educational, economic, and occupational status, also play a role. Lastly, physiologic factors influencing one's reaction to the loss of a loved one include one's dependence on or use of drugs or sedatives, proper nutrition, exercise, adequate rest and sleep, and general health status.

In general, the duration of one's grief, as well as which aspects of grieving are more resolvable than others, will depend on all of the above-mentioned factors. It may be prudent to note that unresolved grief (the absence of normal grief), or the prolongation or distortion of normal grief, is considered unhealthy and may pose health-related risks.

COMMUNICATING WITH THE DYING PERSON

Providing health care to a dying person often gives us the opportunity to become a close confidant, sharing loneliness and fear, wisdom and lessons learned, or regrets and apologies. Below are a few guidelines to enable the health care provider to communicate effectively with dying persons and their families:

1. Be sincere. Follow your feelings rather than rules that commonly dictate behavior.
2. Remember that dying people are still alive and need to be treated as living people.
3. Don't avoid the reality of imminent death; let the dying person set the pace in communications about dying and related matters.
4. Be aware that crying is a natural reaction to loss and is understood as an expression of caring. It is okay to cry in front of and with the patient.
5. Offer support and assistance when needed, but don't try to assume control. The dying person needs to have as much control of the situation as possible in order to maintain self-esteem.
6. Don't confuse the dying person's needs and values with your own. There is no single *right way* to die. Each person must deal with death individually, according to his or her own needs and desires.

COPING WITH THE STRESS OF GIVING CARE

The emotions confronting the health care provider who works with dying patients may range from calmness to outright despair. For the novice health professional, this emotional roller coaster may contribute to physical exhaustion and emotional distress. An adaptation process for the health care provider new to the field of working with the dying patient must include positive stress-management practices and solid social support systems.

Harper[21] has conceptualized a five-stage process that health professionals experience over a 1- or 2-year period while working with the terminally ill. Understanding this multistage process may help the provider to know what to expect and how to handle unexpected feelings. Harper's stages are discussed below.

1. **Intellectualization.** Health care providers who are just beginning to work with the dying are usually very intellectual regarding their clinical duties. Generally, the health professional is concerned for the patient but is unable to discuss anything relating to death or dying with the patient.
2. **Emotional survival.** This is the most difficult stage, because it is here that the health care provider understands that pain, suffering,

and death are unavoidable. It is in this stage that the health care provider may be too emotional to face the patient or may question his or her own mortality.

3. **Depression.** This stage is often referred to as the "grow or go" stage. The health professional either quits or learns to accept the reality of death. Feelings of grieving begin to be expressed here.

4. **Emotional arrival.** In this stage, more appropriate responses to the patient are developed. The health care professional becomes more aware of and sensitive to the needs of the dying.

5. **Deep compassion.** In this stage, the health professional has matured fully. Personal feelings are now channeled into activities that are constructive for the patient and the patient's family. There are no mixed emotions about one's own mortality or the death of the patient.

Caring for the dying is a tremendous investment of personal energy and time. Essentially, health care providers need to develop skills to work with dying patients and their families. Time and experience, as well as a supportive professional environment, help the novice develop these skills.

It should be pointed out that sometimes health care services provided to the dying patient are erratic because of changes in the patient's physical condition. When one member of the health care team provides consistent care, that person is most likely to be the one who will provide the patient with continuous information about his or her condition and will establish a trusted and supportive relationship with the patient. That is not to say that other staff do not; however, as human relations go, the health care provider who is most familiar to and recognized by the patient will bear a different responsibility to the patient and the patient's family.

The health care provider, through active listening, can help the patient share feelings, perceptions, and final thoughts. Both verbal and nonverbal cues should be acted upon. Also, in communicating with the family, reassurance that the loved one is not suffering from physical pain or discomfort is almost always gratefully received by the family. Above all, when death is close at hand, regardless of the state of the patient (unresponsive versus responsive), the provider should continue to treat the patient with care and concern, involving and informing the family whenever possible.

When a patient dies, the health care providers who contributed to his or her care are often the only source of "family." Some medical institutions provide a release policy that permits staff to arrange and/or attend funeral services. Staff may also be responsible for informing other interested patients of a recent death.

ALTERNATIVE TERMINAL CARE SETTINGS

Briefly, care for the terminally ill, which is mostly determined by the patient's condition, may be both acute and long term. It has been stated that

80 percent of all terminal care is provided by hospitals and nursing homes. However, hospice care is becoming increasingly popular because of its philosophy and diversity of care.

Generally speaking, hospitals provide short-term acute care aimed primarily at rehabilitation. In the hospital setting, aggressive techniques are employed to diagnose symptoms, provide treatment, and sustain life.[22] Although nursing homes may provide less aggressive treatment than hospitals, they also strive to discharge the patient back into the community.

On the other hand, hospice care is designed strictly for the terminally ill. The goal of hospice care, both in the patient's home and within the hospice itself, is to provide freedom from physical pain in a caring and homelike environment. Dying, therefore, is experienced in a homelike setting, where friends and relatives are encouraged to become an integral part of the patient's health care. And, because medical interventions to resuscitate the patient are not part of the hospice plan, family and friends are spared the emotional trauma such measures often bring.

Hospice care requires a higher staff-to-patient ratio than that provided by other health care facilities; however, because the vast majority of patients often remain in the home throughout their illness, this type of health care is deemed more cost effective.

If hospice care is not a suitable choice for a loved one, palliative care units within hospital settings (such as that at the Royal Victoria Hospital in Montreal) or separate hospital wards for the terminally ill may be alternative choices. Whatever the choice, more health care systems are incorporating a human approach to caring for the dying, and more rigorous assessments of available health care settings provide us with additional opportunities to improve upon existing services.

SUPPORT FOR THE HEALTH PROFESSIONAL

Caring for a terminally ill patient is extremely demanding on one's psyche and one's body. Proper steps should be taken to ensure adequate interventions that provide support and relief for the health care provider.

Most often, a health care team has already provided a formal or informal support network. If such a system is not available, initiate steps to implement policies that will help mitigate the stresses experienced by all who are involved in the patient's care. An opportunity should be provided for all members of the health care team to discuss their feelings and to talk about the quality of care being provided to the patient.

SUMMARY

Providing health care to individuals in their last stages of life requires skill combined with a genuine concern and appreciation for the constraints experienced by the individual. These constraints include a lack of control over the environment, a need to retain a sense of self-worth and dignity, and freedom from pain and suffering. Skill in coping with the psychologically taxing aspects of losing a patient once cared for, and the grieving process that ensues, will be acquired over time, provided that there is a supportive environment in which to work and learn. Caring for the dying is a privilege, for the last individuals to minister to their needs are usually the health care team, especially when family is unavailable to lend support.

In an introspective first-person account of his father's death, Leviton[23] shares one of many lessons he learned as a professor and thanatologist caring for his dying father: Be respectful of individual differences and human variation. He cautions, "Research is helpful and necessary to understand the meaning and attitudes towards death and dying, but one can err and do harm in striving toward the typical or average dying behavior" (p. 142). Every patient is a special individual and every dying process unique to that individual.

REFERENCES

1. Kalish, R: Death, Grief, and Caring Relationships. Brooks/Cole, Monterey, CA, 1981.
2. Stillion, J: Death and the Sexes. Hemisphere, Washington, DC, 1985.
3. Kleemier, R: Intellectual changes in the serium, or death and IQ. Presidential address, Division 20, American Psychological Association, New York, September 1961.
4. Jarvik, L and Folek, A: Intellectual stability and survival in the aged. J Gerontol 18:173–176, 1963.
5. Reigel, K: The predictors of death and longevity in longitudinal research. In Palmore, E and Jeffers, F (eds): Prediction of Lifespan. Heath, Lexington, MA, 1971.
6. Botwinick, J, West, R, and Storandt, M: Predicting death from behavioral test performance. J Gerontol 33:755–762, 1978.
7. Liebermann, M and Coplen, A: Distance from death as a variable in the study of aging. Devel Psych 2:71–84, 1969.
8. Butler, RN: The life review: An interpretation of reminiscence in the aged. Psychiatry 26:65–76, 1963. Cited in Newgarten, B (ed): Middle age and aging. University of Chicago Press, Chicago, 1968, p. 494.
9. Schultz, C: Death anxiety and the structuring of a death concerns cognitive domain. Essence 3:171–188, 1977.
10. Weisman, A: On Dying and Denying. Behavioral Publications, New York, 1972.
11. Kübler-Ross, E: On Death and Dying. Macmillan, New York, 1969.
12. Schultz, R and Anderson, D: Clinical research and the stages of dying. Omega 5:137–143, 1974.
13. Schneideman, ES: Deaths of Man. Quadrangle/New York Times, New York, 1973.
14. Kastenbaum, R: Death, Society, and Human Experience. CV Mosby, St. Louis, 1981.
15. Pattison, EM: The living-dying process. In Garfield, CA (ed): Psychosocial Care of the Dying Patient. McGraw-Hill, New York, 1978.
16. Stroebe, M and Stroebe, W: Who suffers more? Sex differences in health risks of the widowed. Psych Bull 93:279–301, 1983.
17. O'Connor, N: Letting Go with Love: The Grieving Process. La Mariposa Press, Apache Junction, AZ, 1985.
18. Stephenson, J: Death, Grief, and Mourning. The Free Press, New York, 1985.
19. Parkes, CM: Bereavement. International Universities Press, New York, 1972.

20. Rando, T: Grieving. Lexington Books, Lexington, MA, 1988.
21. Harper, B: Death: The Coping Mechanism of the Health Professional. Southeastern University Press, Greenville, NC, 1977.
22. Donatelle, R, Davis, L, and Hoover, C: Access to Health. Prentice-Hall, Englewood Cliffs, NJ, 1988.
23. Leviton, D: Thanatological theory and my dying father. Omega 17:127–144, 1986–1987.

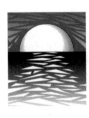

CHAPTER 17

Clinical Research in Geriatrics

Richard W. Bohannon, EdD, PT, NCS

BEHAVIORAL OBJECTIVES

Upon completion of this chapter, the reader will be able to:

1 Identify bibliographic information services that can be used to find journal articles relevant to geriatrics and rehabilitation.
2 Formulate a research question.
3 Differentiate between alternative research designs.
4 Discuss issues relevant to the selection of instrumentation or measures used in a research project.
5 Select an appropriate inferential test of difference based on the level of measurement of the dependent variable, the number of categories of the independent variable, and the presence or absence of repeated measures.
6 Outline the major issues to consider when communicating research findings.

The importance of research to rehabilitation has been emphasized in various ways for years. Leaders in the field of rehabilitation and physical therapy[1-3] have long exhorted therapists to be more involved in research activities. The American Physical Therapy Association (APTA) has made research an important priority for the profession.[4,5] Specifically, the APTA[5] has set goals to "expand the scientific base of physical therapy and achieve acceptance and support of that base by communities of interest" and to "achieve funding for and expand the scientific base of physical therapy" (pp. 63, 95).

Research focused on geriatrics should be of particular importance to rehabilitation professionals for three reasons. First, a growing proportion of the population of the United States is elderly. By the year 2020, about 17 percent of the nation's population will be 65 years or older.[6] Second, a number of pathologies and impairments either primarily affect the elderly or are related to age. For example, the annual incidence of stroke increases from 60 to 180 per 100,000 for people 45 to 54 years of age, to 600 to 1200 per 100,000 for people aged 65 to 74 years, to 4000 per 100,000 for people aged 85 years and over.[7] Standing balance[8] and muscle strength[9] decline with age. Third, the elderly make up a large percentage of the individuals within institutional settings who are referred for rehabilitation. For example, at one large metropolitan acute-care hospital, over 62 percent of the patients treated by physical therapy are over 60 years of age. Figure 17–1 illustrates clearly that older individuals predominate in that setting.

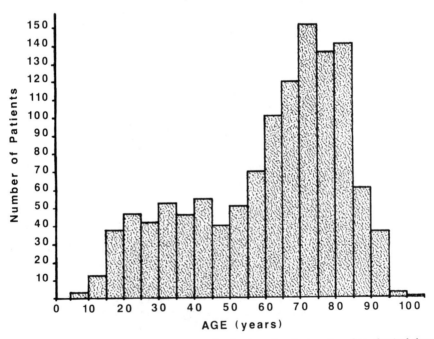

FIGURE 17–1. Histogram indicating the age distribution of patients referred to physical therapy in an acute-care hospital.

This chapter will provide an overview of research in geriatrics, with emphasis on rehabilitation. We will look at four issues relevant to the research process: previously published research, researchable questions, research methods, and research dissemination.

PREVIOUSLY PUBLISHED RESEARCH

Before undertaking research, it is important to find out what has already been researched. Along with the magnitude of the problem investigated and the theoretical rationale for the investigation, the accumulated findings of past research serve as the justifying foundation for further research. Therefore, it is important for researchers to know how to access the literature. This requires (1) a working knowledge of information sources and bibliographic information services and (2) a personal system for storing and retrieving relevant literature.

Information Sources

Although books and other individuals can be, and often are, consulted for information,[10,11] research articles published in peer-reviewed journals are generally considered a more legitimate foundation for practice and research. Thus, this section will focus on journal literature.

Lusardi and associates[12] have identified 86 journals with the words "gerontology," "geriatrics," and "aging" in their titles. Of these 86 journals, 20 were used most frequently as sources of information:

Age and Ageing
Annual Review of
  Gerontology and Geriatrics
Archives of Gerontology
  and Geriatrics
Clinics in Geriatric Medicine
Clinical Gerontologist
Experimental Aging Research
Experimental Gerontology
Geriatrics
Gerontologia
Gerontologist
Gerontology

Gerontologia Clinics
International Journal of Aging
  and Human Development
Journal of the American Geriatrics
  Society
Journal of Gerontology
Journal of Gerontological
  Nursing
Mechanisms of Ageing and
  Development
Psychology and Aging
Research in Aging
Topics in Geriatric Rehabilitation

Of the 92 core journals of gerontology identified by Lusardi and associates, only 16 included such words as "geriatrics," "gerontology" or "aging" in their titles.[12] The *Annals of Internal Medicine, British Medical Journal, Journal of the American Medical Association, The Lancet, New England Journal of Medicine, Neurology,* and *Science* were among the core journals.

There are many bibliographic information services available that can assist the rehabilitation researcher in identifying articles relevant to geriatric care. Five such services will be addressed here: the National Library of Medicine, Excerpta Medica, the Institute of Scientific Information, the Cumulative Index of Nursing and Allied Health, and the British Library.

National Library of Medicine

Physical therapists are probably most familiar with the National Library of Medicine information service.[11] The National Library of Medicine publishes *Index Medicus* and Medline. Medline is an on-line service that is now also available on CD-ROM. It includes about 3000 journals, but its coverage of the physical therapy and gerontology literature is somewhat limited.[13] Only two physical therapy journals—*Physical Therapy* and the *Journal of Orthopaedic and Sports Physical Therapy*—are included in the database. Lusardi et al found that 89.1 percent of the core journals of gerontology, and 24.4 percent of the gerontology journals identified, were included in the database of *Index Medicus*.[12]

To do a search in *Index Medicus*, researchers must use medical subject headings (MESH). The most useful to our readers are Aged, Age Factors, Geriatrics, and Geriatric—Assessment, Dentistry, Nursing, and Pyschiatry. However, a search based on these MESH terms alone will not retrieve all relevant articles from the database. Software programs such as Silver Platter used in conjunction with Medline on CD-ROM allow the user to select his or her own key terms, resulting in a more comprehensive listing of relevant research articles. For example, a search of Medline's 1993 database using the terms Geriatric and Rehabilitation resulted in a list of 48 articles. A key word search using Age or Elderly along with Rehabilitation produced a list of 1144 and 99 articles, respectively.

Excerpta Medica

Excerpta Medica produces 42 different abstract journals, including *Gerontology and Geriatrics* (Section 20), which is published eight times per year. Abstracts included in the index are obtained from a database of more than 3500 biomedical journals published in over 110 countries worldwide. Unfortunately, many rehabilitation professionals appear to be unaware of *Excerpta Medica*. None of the therapists interviewed by Bohannon mentioned this service spontaneously, and when asked specifically about it, only 1 of 29 interviewees acknowledged using the service since graduation.[11] Nevertheless, *Excerpta Medica*, particularly Sections 19 (Rehabilitation and Physical Medicine) and 20, can be very helpful to the physical therapy researcher in geriatrics. Lusardi et al found that 92 percent of the core journals of gerontology, and 27.9 percent of the gerontology journals identified, were included in the *Excerpta Medica* database.[12]

Institute for Scientific Information

The Institute for Scientific Information markets several products of potential value to the researcher in geriatrics. Only two, however, will be addressed here: the *Science Citation Index* and *Research Alerts*. Both are generated from a database of over 3000 journals.

The *Science Citation Index* is available as a printed index and on CD-ROM. The printed index is actually a series of indexes: *Citation, Corporate, Permuterm,* and *Source.* Both the *Citation* and *Source* indexes allow the researcher to find relevant information using author names.

The *Citation Index* lists works in which a particular author is cited. For example, if you are interested in functional capacity in the elderly and know that Amelie Aniansson[14] has published articles on the topic, you can look up her name in the *Citation Index.* In 1989, 12 of her articles published between 1980 and 1989 were cited in 31 different articles, many of which relate to physical functioning in the elderly.

The basis of the *Source Index* is that authors who write on topics of interest are likely to write on the topic again. Taking functional capacity in the elderly and Amelie Aniansson as our example again, we see that there were no listings in the 1989 index. That means either that she published no articles in 1989 or that she published in journals excluded from the Institute for Scientific Information database.

The CD-ROM version of *Science Citation Index* can be used to access information by author source or citation or by topic. Although the searcher is not bound to a thesaurus of search terms when looking for information on a topic, the program does not at this writing allow a search for a term of interest in article abstracts. Consequently, only a limited number of relevant articles can be found using the CD-ROM. A key word search using the term Rehabilitation with the terms Geriatric, Age, and Elderly produced one, zero, and five articles, respectively.

None of the practicing therapists interviewed by Bohannon[11] were familiar with *Science Citation Index.* Using the list of Lusardi et al, the database includes 75 percent of the core journals of gerontology, but only 15.1 percent of the gerontology journals were identified.

Research Alerts are mailed to subscribers on a weekly basis and list articles relevant to defined areas of investigation. In early 1994, each issue of the *Aging and Geriatrics Alert* identified more than 120 relevant articles. *Research Alerts* can also be custom-designed to access articles using subscriber-selected key terms, journal titles, and/or author names.

Cumulative Index of Nursing and Allied Health

The *Cumulative Index of Nursing and Allied Health (CINAHL)* has a very limited database (fewer than 400 journals). The index is available in printed form, with articles listed under a limited number of terms, and on CD-ROM, where a broad range of terms can be used to find relevant research. A key word search pairing Rehabilitation with Geriatric, Age, and Elderly produced 17, 143, and 15 articles, respectively, in the 1993 index.

None of the therapists interviewed by Bohannon claimed to have used the index since graduation. Because it includes in its database a large number of journals omitted from other databases, it may prove useful to geriatric researchers, despite its limited inclusion of core journals of gerontology (27.2 percent) and gerontology journals (15.1 percent).

The British Library

The Medical Information Service of the British Library publishes the *Rehabilitation Index, Physiotherapy Index,* and *Occupational Therapy Index.* These indexes, which are published monthly, are also available on line or on CD-ROM.

Personal Storage and Retrieval

Once the researcher has identified an article that is potentially relevant to an area of interest, he or she must decide if the information should be stored for future use. If the information in the article is deemed worth saving, several options can be exercised prior to storage: (1) the pertinent aspects of the article can be abstracted on an index card or piece of paper; (2) the page of the article that includes the abstract or summary can be copied; (3) the article can be copied in its entirety.

Whether saved in part or in its entirety, the information from relevant articles must be stored in a way that allows efficient retrieval. An indexed filing system is one such method of storage.[15] Although information can be organized in other ways, a topical system works well. One system involves the alphabetical filing of information by topic and subtopic. On the outside cover of each filing containing information on a topic are two additional aids to retrieval. The first is a list of specific topics (under the heading "Includes") that can be found in the file. The second is a list of other files to search (under the heading "See Also"). For the computer-oriented individual, programs are available to assist with the storage and retrieval of information by topic and author.

RESEARCHABLE QUESTIONS

Generating researchable questions may be second nature to the experienced researcher, but it may not be so obvious to everyone. New researchers may limit themselves to a rather narrow spectrum of research possibilities.

Beyond obvious questions like "What treatment works best?" there are a myriad of possible questions.

Framework One

Sackett and colleagues,[10] in outlining reasons for reading research, present four applications that can serve as a basis for research questions. First, research can be used to evaluate a new diagnostic test for such things as reliability, validity, sensitivity, and practicality. For example, Duncan and associates[16] evaluated a new balance test. More specifically, they examined functional reach in an anterior direction among individuals who were standing. Second, research can clarify the clinical course and prognosis of a disorder. With such information, clinicians, patients, and their families are in a position to make better decisions about therapeutic interventions and lifestyle options. A study by Reding and Potes[17] of recovery among patients with stroke is an example of an excellent study of this kind. Third, research can help to establish the etiology (cause) of a disease, making possible interventions of potential value. Thus, if bone density is shown to relate to muscle strength, exercises that strengthen muscle and stress the skeleton can be suggested for postmenopausal women with diminished bone density.[18] Although the relationship does not ensure that an exercise program will be efficacious, it does provide some direction as to potentially fruitful interventions. Fourth, research is able to examine the value of therapy. One such examination, recently published, was of the effect of resistance exercises on the muscle strength of the very old.[19] The study showed that such exercises did indeed have their intended effect.

Framework Two

Weiss and Bucuvalas[20] outlined a number of purposes of research that can serve as a foundation for research questions.

1. To clarify the relative advantages of alternative choices
2. To understand the background and context of program operations
3. To stimulate review of policy
4. To focus attention on neglected issues
5. To provide new understanding of problem or how things work
6. To clarify personal thinking
7. To reorder priorities
8. To make sense of or justify past or present actions
9. To reduce uncertainty
10. To question assumptions that are simply taken for granted

A research project may fulfill multiple purposes. For example, purposes 1 and 3 through 10 were addressed in part by research showing that, contrary to traditional teaching, the muscle strength of patients with stroke can be measured reliably, the measurements correlate with function, and such measures are better predictors of function than are measures of spasticity.[21,22]

Framework Three

Research questions can be categorized also in a traditional procedural and hierarchical manner that is strongly tied to research design: that is, as descriptive, correlational, and experimental.

Descriptive Studies

Descriptive studies seek to answer the question "What is the nature of this thing?" Whether cross-sectional (at one point in time) or longitudinal (across time), the value of descriptive research is not intrinsic. Its value is in the interpretation of its results relative to other known facts. For example, the walking speed of older individuals can be described, but is not intrinsically important. One fact that makes the speed important is the time allowed for the crossing of city streets.[23] Additionally, when the mean and standard deviation of walking speed is described for healthy individuals over 60 years of age, the described speed can be used to determine if an individual's speed is less than normal (≥2.0 standard deviations below the mean).

Correlational Studies

Correlational studies—that is, studies of the relationship or association between variables—seek to answer the question "What is important and how?" More specifically, correlational studies can help establish whether specific variables are possible determinants of or have implications for other variables. Correlational studies help to identify targets for clinical measurement and treatment. A recent study of stroke patients illustrates these uses of correlational research. The study showed significant correlations between knee extension strength on the paretic side, maximum weight-bearing through the paretic lower extremity, and gait speed.[24] By showing significant correlations, the study provided evidence that knee extension strength is a partial determinant of maximum weight-bearing, which in turn has implications for gait speed. Inherent in the results also is support for the measurement of and treatments aimed at increasing paretic knee extension strength and paretic lower-extremity weight bearing.

Beyond whether a significant correlation exists, correlational studies must answer three questions: What is the direction of the relationship (positive or negative)? How strong is the relationship? What is the nature of the relationship? Using the example just cited above, the relationship between paretic lower-extremity weight-bearing and gait speed was *positive* (as weight-bearing increased, so did gait speed), *strong,* (68.9 percent of the variance in gait speed could be explained by weight-bearing), and primarily *curvilinear,* as opposed to linear (see Figure 17–2). An often stated and important limitation of correlational research is that it does not prove cause and effect. In the context of the example above, therefore, the results do not prove that the ability to bear more weight through the paretic lower extremity *causes* faster walking. To strengthen the argument of causality between two variables, the researcher must determine the adequacy of four criteria: A theoretical rationale for causation exists. The independent variable (presumed cause) precedes the dependent variable (presumed effect). The association between the variables is strong. The relationship between the variables is not spurious.

Experimental Studies

Experimental studies focus on the effect of some intervention, treatment, or manipulation on outcome. The gold standard of experimental research is the randomized controlled trial, but other types of experiments will be described.

In the randomized controlled trial, a random sample is obtained from a population of subjects who meet specific criteria. Subjects of the sample are then randomly assigned to groups (one of which is a control group). Sub-

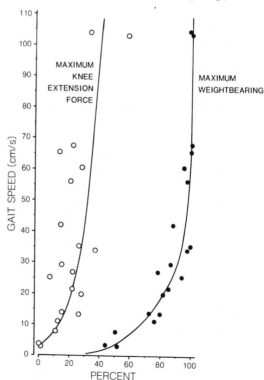

FIGURE 17–2. Scatterplot illustrating the curvilinear relationship between paretic lower-extremity weight bearing (as a percentage of body weight) and gait speed. (From Bohannon,[24] p 67, with permission)

jects in all groups are measured. An intervention is applied to experimental groups. Then, after a period of intervention, the subjects of all groups are measured again. Ideally, the individuals doing the measuring are "blind" to the group assignment of the subjects.

Alternatives to the randomized controlled trial include the quasi-experiment, which lacks a true control group and does not randomly assign subjects to groups. Although such experiments do not control internal threats to validity as well as a randomized controlled trial, they may be a necessary compromise if the researcher is ever to carry out the intended investigation and reach some conclusions. For example, you wonder whether there is a significant difference in the 6-month functional status of stroke patients who receive their postacute rehabilitation in a comprehensive inpatient rehabilitation facility versus a skilled nursing facility. As you are unable to randomly assign patients to receive care in one setting or another, you will have to compare the outcome of patients who ended up in each. Ideally, of course, important determinants of outcome (for example, admission functional scores) should be controlled statistically in any comparison of outcomes.

Another alternative to the randomized controlled trial is the ex post facto (after the fact) investigation. This type of research is not a true experiment because it lacks random allocation. Ex post factor experiments are, however, a necessary compromise if some questions are to be answered at all—for example, testing the relationship between smoking and stroke incidence. Given the potential harm in smoking, it is not advisable or possible to assign subjects to a smoking group. Therefore, in the ex post facto design, subjects who are smokers are identified, as are (case-control) subjects who have never smoked but are otherwise comparable on selected characteristics. Their respective incidences of stroke are compared after the actual "causal" events have already taken place.

A specific type of experiment distinguished by its relatively short duration is an explicatory experiment. Explicatory experiments are cross-sectional and involve the manipulation of an independent variable to see its immediate effects on a dependent variable.[25] An example of such an experiment is one in which the investigator sought to determine if head and neck position had an effect on elbow flexion force in patients with stroke.[26] The patients were simply directed to flex their elbows as forcefully as possible under two conditions—head turned toward and head turned away from the tested upper extremity. The forces under the two conditions were then compared and found not to differ significantly.

RESEARCH METHODS

Research Design

The design of a research project can be described in a number of ways. They can be retrospective or prospective, cross-sectional or longitudinal, quantitative or qualitative, or they can be based on individual cases or groups.

Retrospective research can be contrasted with *prospective research* in that it involves looking backward at data that was gathered in the past before a specific research plan was conceived, as compared to data gathered in the future after a specific research plan has been formulated. The study by Lusardi and associates[12] is an example of a retrospective study that employed document analysis. Retrospective research is sometimes easier and more expedient than prospective research and should not be disregarded as a viable research option. A retrospective endeavor, however, presupposes that the data that are available are of adequate quality and quantity to be useful. Unless data are recorded in a persistent and consistent manner, a database sufficient for later analysis is not likely to exist. Strategies that may help in the development of a potentially useful database include the use of specific patient-care protocols, data forms, and guidelines. Proper staff orientation and careful supervision may also improve the quality of recorded data. There is greater control and probably less bias inherent in prospective research. Fewer internal threats to validity, therefore, are likely to exist with prospective research. Such research can be carried out after testing the reliability of measurements and doing pilot work to refine the research procedure.

A design can be categorized as either *cross-sectional* or *longitudinal.* Cross-sectional research attempts to describe, correlate, or differentiate using data from one point in time. Examples of cross-sectional studies of age and muscle strength are those of Thorngren and Werner,[27] who showed a significant and negative correlation between age and strength, and Young and associates,[28] who showed a significant difference between the strength of a group of women subjects in their twenties and a group of subjects in their seventies. Because cross-sectional studies do not involve the repeated testing of subjects over time, they are not as likely to be accompanied by such problems as subject attrition. Nevertheless, some judgments made from cross-sectional research may be inappropriate[29] or inaccurate.[30] Longitudinal studies can be used to measure the nature of a variable over time in the same group and thus involve subjects being tested repeatedly. Although much more cumbersome than cross-sectional research, longitudinal research can provide a more accurate description of changes over time. Muscle strength, when measured longitudinally, has been shown to decrease at a different rate than is suggested by data from cross-sectional studies of the relationship between strength and age.[30] True experimental research presupposes longitudinal designs.

Although it has been argued eloquently that the *quantitative* versus *qualitative* distinction is a false one,[31] the categories provide yet another useful way of dichotomizing research endeavors. Quantitative research, which is the primary type of investigation employed in the biological and physical sciences, is objective and reductionistic. It usually involves many subjects and the use of statistical analysis. Qualitative research has been used primarily in the social and behavioral sciences. It might be characterized as subjective and naturalistic. Ideally, it allows the situations observed to dictate their description. A particular type of qualitative research, ethnography, involves the discovery and description of human behavior from the perspective of those examined in their own natural setting.[32] Bohannon and coworkers[33] used the qualitative approach to discover what patients with stroke hoped to achieve during rehabilitation. Rather than asking the patients about specific activities, the authors asked, "What are your goals? What do you hope to accomplish?" The authors were able, therefore, to find out from the patients' perspective what was important. The results of that study allowed Bohannon and colleagues[34] to refine the examination of patient preferences in a later quantitative study using closed-ended questions. Qualitative methods, I believe, are underused in research involving the elderly. Nevertheless, when performed, qualitative research should be carried out with adequate attention to validity. Too often, when clinicians describe what they see, they attribute causes to their observations. The identification of cause is usually beyond the scope of observation. For example, a therapist may observe that patients with left hemiparesis tend to fall toward their left side when sitting.[35] A therapist, however, cannot legitimately claim as a result of observation (as Bobath[21] has done) that spasticity of muscles of the left side is responsible for the leftward fall.

A fourth way of categorizing research is by whether it uses *individual cases* or *groups* to examine the question of interest. Of course, all research of human beings involves one or more cases. What is meant by the dichotomy here is to distinguish between research in which data are presented on a single individual or multiple individuals separately or on a group of individuals together. Although powerful generalizations cannot legitimately be made from single cases, there are a number of reasons for doing such research. If a therapist has an interest in a patient problem that he or she rarely sees, a single case design may be the only type of research possible. If a specific patient's response to therapy is of interest, it is best to examine that individual patient's response. Methods of examining clinical change among individual patients have been described in detail elsewhere.[36] Basically, they require the measurement and comparison of status between baseline periods and periods of intervention. Because individuals can vary in their response to treatment and because individual responses can cancel each other out when included in the data of a group, the reporting of multiple individual cases may be preferable sometimes to reporting the central tendency of groups. If low- and high-responding cases can be identified individually, explanations can be sought for the different responses. These can lead to more specifically directed interventions. In spite of the advantages of reporting individual cases, data from groups remains the primary method for reporting research results. What is important for the researcher in geriatrics is that he or she describe the group well enough for appropriate conclusions and generalizations to be made.

Methodology

Once general design issues have been addressed, the actual process of undertaking the research begins. That process involves selecting subjects, choosing instrumentation, collecting data, analyzing data, and drawing conclusions from the data.

Subject Selection

The testing of all subjects in a group (population) who possess a common characteristic of interest (for example, hip fracture) is not usually feasible, so a subset, or sample, of the population is usually tested. Samples can vary in size from one to thousands.

A *probability sample* is one in which there is an equal likelihood (probability) that any one individual will be selected as a subject. Random selection through use of a random-numbers table or generator is a means of obtaining a probability sample. When the researcher wants to ensure adequate representation of subjects with specific characteristics (for example, race), the population can be stratified first by that characteristic and a random sample obtained from each stratum.

The most common type of *nonprobability sample* and the kind of sample used often in geriatrics research is the convenience sample. Subjects in a convenience sample just happen to be in the right place at the right time: for example, all the patients with first strokes referred to physical therapy in 1990 in a specific institution. The researcher may not be able to use anything but a convenience sample. That is acceptable. Researchers must only be careful to acknowledge how convenience samples may differ from the population as a whole and temper their conclusions accordingly.

There is no absolute regarding appropriate sample size. Factors of relevance in identifying an adequate sample size are the representativeness of the sample, the type of study, the sensitivity and variability of the measurement, the number of variables measured, and the level of significance selected. Tables and/or equations can be used that take some of these factors into account when selecting a sample large enough to show a desired effect.[37] Such methods, however, do not take into account the researcher's resources or the number of subjects he or she can test with them.

Instrumentation

Instrumentation is the mechanism by which measurements are obtained. That mechanism can be a device that measures variables such as mass, force, time, distance, velocity, or acceleration. It can also be a standardized test such as the Barthel index,[38] which is used to measure independence in activities of daily living. Before developing a new instrument, the physical therapy researcher should familiarize himself or herself with available instruments that have been used by other investigators. If the instrumentation that is used traditionally is unavailable or prohibitively expensive, however, the researcher should not give up in despair. The use of novel instrumentation is permissible.

At least four other questions should be addressed in selecting instrumentation or measures to be used in research. The questions pertain to sensitivity, reliability, validity, and generalizability.

First, how sensitive is the instrument? Although immense sensitivity may not be required, an instrument needs to be sensitive enough to detect meaningful change. Thus, while a strength-measuring device need not be sensitive to changes in force of .01 newtons, it should be able to note a 20 percent change in force. Manual muscle testing may not detect such changes.[39] Instruments that are insensitive to differences in performance at low levels are said to suffer from floor effects. Instruments that are insensitive to differences in performance at high levels are said to be limited by ceiling effects.

Second, how reliable are measurements obtained with the instrument? Synonyms for reliability are reproducibility, consistency, and stability. Sources of inconsistency include the subjects themselves, the instrument, and the examiner applying the instrument to the subjects. Some inconsistency or variance in human behavior is to be expected and cannot be eliminated altogether. The accuracy of mechanical or electronic instruments should not be assumed.[40] The devices should be tested against known standards (that is, the instruments can be calibrated). Measurements that rely heavily on tester skill, capacity, experience, or judgment are more likely to suffer from unreliability because of the examiner. Such unreliability can be reduced by the agreement between testers on terms and procedures, practice, and comparison with standards.[41] A standard might be a more experienced individual with acknowledged skill. When acceptable consistency cannot be achieved using the aforementioned steps, substitution of instrumentation that is not so dependent on examiner performance is in order. Thus, if a tester cannot use a hand-held dynamometer reliably because of inadequate strength,[42] a fixed-force gauge or isokinetic dynamometer should be used instead. Reliability can be tested within (intra) or between (inter) sessions and within or between testers. Typically, intrasession reliability surpasses intersession reliability and intratester reliability exceeds intertester reliability.

Third, how valid is the measurement? Validity may be interpreted as accuracy or truthfulness, but a standard for comparison does not always exist. The two primary issues related to validity are what can be inferred from the test about what is being measured and what can be inferred from the test about other behavior. Reliability is a necessary component of validity. Evidence for validity can be derived from logic or expertise but may then reflect the biases or preconceptions of the experts. Several categories of validity are typically acknowledged. Face validity, which is insufficient alone to establish the validity of measurements, indicates the degree to which a measure gives the user the impression that it quantifies what it purports to measure. Content validity refers to the extent to which a measurement reflects a variable as defined. Thus, if spasticity is defined as a velocity-dependent response of muscle to passive stretch, the measurement of spasticity obtained with an instrument should vary with the velocity with which it stretches the muscle. Construct validity relates to the appraisal of a description, the existence of a situation, or the differentiation of conditions. A test can have convergent-construct validity or discriminant-construct validity. An example of the former would be the demonstration that scores for the motricity index and hand-grip strength, which are both supposed to measure motor loss following stroke, correlate significantly.[43] An example of the latter would be the demonstration that knee extension torque is decreased on the paretic relative to the nonparetic side in patients with stroke. Criterion validity has to do with the relationship or agreement of a measurement with a standard. If the issue is the relationship at the same time, concurrent validity is the concern. If the issue is the relationship across time, predictive validity is the concern. The demonstration of a significant relationship between hand-grip strength and total body protein supports the concurrent validity of the former as an indicator of the latter.[44] The demonstration of a significant relationship between preoperative hand-grip strength and postoperative complications among elderly female patients with hip fractures supports the predictive validity of grip strength measures.[45]

Fourth, how generalizable are the measurements? The generalizability of measurements depends partly on some of the issues already addressed in this section. Beyond those issues, however, are two that should be highlighted: the context of measurement and the context of application. If instrumentation, measurements, or treatments are used that are unavailable to or inapplicable by most practitioners, the breadth of their use will be restricted severely. If the findings are restricted to a specific environment, the results will not be generalizable either. An example of such findings would be walking capacity on a smooth tile floor that does not generalize to walking out of doors on unlevel terrain.

Collecting Data

With some notable exceptions, the collection of data should not begin until informed consent is obtained from the subjects to be tested. Such consent is usually in writing and involves the communication of the purposes of the research, associated risks and benefits, and an indication that the subject is free to withdraw at any time without prejudice. Prior to obtaining informed consent, approval of the project by an ethics committee or institutional review board is usually required.

Formal data collection should begin only after the researcher has developed an adequate familiarity with the instrumentation and procedures to be used. A knowledge of the relevant literature and pilot work are the foundation for such familiarity. The literature can alert the researcher to issues that should be addressed if flaws in the research are to be avoided. For example, the researcher who is planning to use isokinetic testing to examine knee extensor muscle function would find in the literature admonitions to correct measurements for the effects of gravity.[46] Pilot work can contribute to the refinement of testing procedures by revealing to the researcher some of the problems inherent in them. Pilot work, for example, revealed to me that the padding on the endpiece of a dynamometer I was using was not sufficient. As a consequence, subjects were prevented by discomfort from giving their best efforts. The problem was solved when the endpiece was modified.

Data collection can be facilitated by the use of well-designed data collection forms and computer databases. The forms, which should clearly link data with the subject from whom it was gathered, should be organized to facilitate the smooth transfer of data to a computer for statistical analysis.

Analyzing Data

With the advent of statistical analysis software for personal computers, the actual number-crunching component of statistical analysis is now relatively painless. Although some simple analyses (such as chi square) may be easier with a hand calculator and some very complex analyses of large data sets may require a mainframe, most analyses can be completed on a personal computer. Of the many available software packages, my preference is Systat.[47] However statistical analysis is performed, the researcher must still know which statistical procedures to perform.

Descriptive Statistics. The selection of descriptive statistics is rather straightforward. Nevertheless, there are some excellent papers on the selection and use of descriptive statistics that the researcher in geriatrics may wish to consult.[48] A common error in the descriptive summary of data is overreliance on the mean as a measure of central tendency. Although the mean has the advantage of being conceptually simple, it is not appropriate for ordinal data, even when a number of ordinal scores are gathered together into an index. Moreover, the mean is strongly influenced by outlying data points, particularly when the sample size is small. An example of such a strong influence is apparent in the following set of times since onset of stroke (4, 9, 6, 7, 14, 14, 13, 8, and 52 days). The mean, which is 14.1, is greater than all but one of the values in the set. Clearly, a better description of central tendency would be the median, which is 9 days.

Reliability Statistics. Descriptive statistics themselves can play an important role in characterizing the reliability of measurements. They may, in fact, be the most useful statistics for the clinician.[49] A clinician, for example, who is learning a new procedure and finds that her test-retest measurements differ by a mean 10%, range 6–25%, knows that her performance is in need of improvement if an experienced examiner's test-retest measurements differ by a mean 3.6%, range 0.2–13.7%. Beyond the descriptive summary of reliability, however, there are established statistics of choice (coefficients) for indicating the reliability of repeated measures. For nominal measurements, the statistic of choice is kappa.[50] It represents the agreement beyond that expected by chance in two raters' categorical judgments of observations (for example, shoulder subluxed, shoulder not subluxed). For ordinal measurements, the statistic of choice is weighted kappa.[51] It also represents the agreement beyond that expected by chance in two raters' categorical judgments of observations. Unlike kappa, though, it takes the magnitude of disagreement into account. Thus, disagreements spanning two categories (manual muscle test grades 3 versus 5) will depress the coefficient more than disagreements spanning one category (manual muscle test grade 4 versus 5). For interval or ratio measurements, which use real numbers and units for quantification, the reliability statistic of choice is the intraclass correlation coefficient (ICC).[52,53] A number of different ICC equations are available for use, but all utilize analysis of variance mean square values. ICC 1,1; ICC 2,1; and ICC 3,1 are most often reported in research by physical therapists. The two major issues relevant to equation selection are the nature of the selection of examiners and the generalizations that are intended from the ICC.

Inferential Statistics. Inferential statistics can be divided, albeit somewhat artificially, into those used to test for differences and those used to test for relationships. Once several basic questions are answered, the appropriate inferential statistic can be selected easily. For tests of difference the questions are these: What is the level or scale of measurement for the dependent variable? How many variables are there? Are there repeated measures? How many categories are there of the independent variable? Figure 17–3 shows how the answer to these questions can lead to the selection of an appropriate statistical test. For example, suppose you want to know if standing balance improves concomitant with an intervention to improve balance in a sample of geriatric individuals. You decide to grade balance with an ordinal scale where 0 represents an inability to stand and 6 represents the ability to stand on one lower extremity for 60 seconds. There are two variables—balance and time of measurement. Measurements are repeated because balance is graded twice, once preintervention and once postintervention. The independent variable is of two categories preintervention and postintervention. The statistic of choice, therefore, is the Wilcoxon matched-pairs signed-

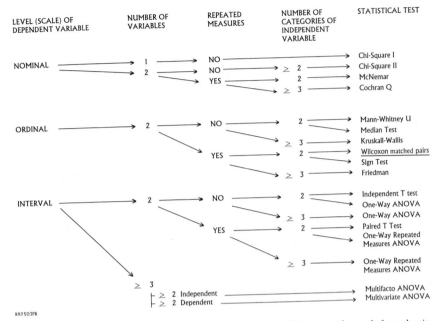

FIGURE 17–3. Diagram for selecting inferential statistics of difference. The path for selecting the Wilcoxon matched-pairs signed-ranks test is underlined.

ranks test. Tests of relationships (association) require the answering of some of the same questions, primarily those related to the level of measurement of the variables and the number of variables measured.

Drawing Conclusions from Data

Once statistical analysis is complete, the findings of a study should be clear. However, the interpretation of the findings involves some judgment, and not all researchers will draw the same conclusions. Nevertheless, guidelines exist for drawing conclusions: (1) Conclusions should be neither a mere restatement of findings nor inconsistent with the findings. (2) Conclusions should have a sound theoretical foundation. (3) Ideally, conclusions should have practical implications. (4) Statistical findings should be interpreted in light of precedent. Precedent holds, for example, that correlations in the 0.5 range should be considered of moderate magnitude.[54]

RESEARCH DISSEMINATION

Two primary issues are inherent in research dissemination. The first is related to the avenue selected for communication. The second has to do with rules of conduct.

Avenues of Communication

There are three primary avenues for communicating research findings. Research can be submitted as an article to a journal, presented orally at a meeting, or be shared via a poster.

Before submitting an article for publication, the writer should be familiar with appropriate target journals. For the researcher in geriatrics, such journals may focus on geriatrics or on some other aspect of the research (such as neuropsychology, muscle performance, physical therapy, or rehabilitation). The acceptance rates and priorities of different journals vary. There is nothing wrong with calling or writing the editor for information on such issues prior to paper submission. Journal styles also differ. The researcher, therefore, should carefully consult a journal's author guide and other articles published in a journal prior to submitting an article. Particularly variable among journals are reference formats. Although journal requirements differ in many respects, they have many features in common: organizational framework, necessary inclusions, and writing style.[55-57] Two issues relevant to style are a preference for the use of *Système International* (SI) units[58] and nonsexist language.[59]

Oral presentations at meetings of societies, such as the American Geriatrics Society, are usually accepted (or rejected) on the basis of abstracts submitted for review. It is important that abstract instructions are followed to the letter. Clear and uncluttered headings, slides, and illustrations are indispensable to an effective oral presentation. Slides can be created efficiently using a number of available computer programs.

Posters are also accepted (or rejected) on the basis of abstracts submitted to the society for review. They too should comply with guidelines to the letter. The letters of the headings and text should be large enough to read from several feet away. Photographs of testing procedures are an effective way of reducing the length of written descriptions of procedures. Graphs are similarly useful for summarizing findings.

Rules of Submission and Authorship

Although it is generally acceptable to submit a paper for publication that has been published before in abstract form or presented at a meeting, duplicate publication is unacceptable. Thus, it is not appropriate to submit a paper to more than one journal simultaneously. Neither is it considered ethical to rehash information that has been published elsewhere in another research paper submission. The necessary fragmentation of a work into multiple "least publishable units" is inappropriate. This does not prohibit, necessarily, the cautious dividing of a large study into manageable parts or the publication of different aspects of a larger study in different papers.

Authors should include only those who have made substantive contributions. Substantive contributions, however, can take place anywhere from idea conception, to data gathering, to the writing of the research paper.

SUMMARY

Before research on a topic is undertaken, the researcher should have a thorough knowledge of research already published. This requires a familiarity with information sources as well as their strengths and weaknesses. Thereafter the researcher must have a concrete understanding of what he or she wants to research. This should be reduced to a specific research question, and the design selected to answer the question must be practical if it is to be implemented. Only then can the research be performed, data analyzed, and results reported to others in an appropriate format.

REFERENCES

1. Basmajian, JV: Research or retrench: The rehabilitation professions challenged. Phys Ther 55:607–610, 1975.
2. Hislop, HJ: The not so impossible dream. Phys Ther 55:1069–1080, 1975.
3. Lehmkuhl, LD: Camelot revisited: Legacy of the physical therapy education program at Case Western Reserve University. Phys Ther 70:723–733, 1990.
4. Ballin, AJ, Breslin, WH, Wierenga, KAS, and Shepard, KF: Research in physical therapy: Philosophy, barriers to involvement, and use among California physical therapists. Phys Ther 60:888–895, 1980.
5. American Physical Therapy Association: *House of Delegates Handbook.* Alexandria, VA, 1991.
6. Kart, CS, Metress, EK, and Metress, SP (eds): Aging, Health, and Society. Jones & Bartlett, Boston, MA, 1988.
7. Aho, K, Harmsen, P, Hatano, S, Marquardsen, J, Smirnov, VE, and Strasser, T: Cerebrovascular disease in the community: Results of a WHO collaborative study. Bull WHO 58:113–130, 1980.
8. Bohannon, RW, Larkin, PA, Cook, AC, Gear, J, and Singer, J: Decrease in timed balance test scores with aging. Phys Ther 64:1067–1070, 1984.
9. Rice, CL, Cunningham, DA, Paterson, DH, and Rechnitzer, PA: Strength in an elderly population. Arch Phys Med Rehabil 70:391–397, 1989.
10. Sackett, DL, Haynes, RB, and Tugwell, P: Clinical Epidemiology: A Basic Science for Clinical Medicine. Little Brown, Boston, MA, 1984.
11. Bohannon, RW: Information accessing behavior of physical therapists. Physiother Theory Pract 6:215–225, 1990.
12. Lusardi, MM, Roberts, D, Bohannon, RW, and Seaton, PC: Journals publishing information relevant to gerontology and their coverage by four bibliographic indexes. Top Geriatric Rehabil 7(4):75–88, 1992.
13. Bohannon, RW and Tiberio, D: Physiotherapy literature in medical indexes: How comprehensive is index coverage of journals cited frequently by five physiotherapy journals? Physiother Pract 5:201–205, 1989.
14. Aniansson, A, Rundgren, Å, and Sperling, L: Evaluation of functional capacity in activities of daily living in 70-year-old men and women. Scand J Rehab Med 12:145–154, 1980.
15. Mater, DA: Managing your personal information files. Phys Occup Ther Pediatr 6:95–101, 1986.
16. Duncan, PW, Weiner, DK, Chandler, J, and Studenski, S: Functional reach: A new clinical measure of balance. J Gerontol 45:M192–M197, 1990.
17. Reding, MJ and Potes, E: Rehabilitation outcome following initial unilateral hemispheric stroke. Life table analysis approach. Stroke 19:1354–1358, 1988.
18. Sandler, RB, Cauley, JA, Sashin, D, Scialabba, MA, and Kriska, AM: The effect of grip strength on radial bone in postmenopausal women. J Orthop Res 7:440–444, 1989.

19. Fiatarone, MA, Marks, EC, Ryan, ND, Meredith, CN, Lipsitz, LA, and Evans, WJ: High intensity strength training in nonagenarians. Effects on skeletal muscle JAMA 263:3029–3034, 1990.

20. Weiss, CH and Bucuvalas, M: Truth tests and utility tests: Decision makers' frames of reference for social science research. Amer Soc Rev 45:302–313, 1990.

21. Bobath, B: Adult Hemiplegia. Evaluation and Treatment, ed 3. Heinemann Medical Books, London 1990.

22. Bohannon, RW and Andrews, AW: Correlation of knee extensor muscle torque and spasticity with gait speed in patients with stroke. Arch Phys Med Rehabil 71:330–333, 1990.

23. Robinett, CS and Vondvan, MA: Functional ambulation velocity and distance requirements in rural and urban communities. Phys Ther 68:1371–1373, 1988.

24. Bohannon, RW: Relationship among paretic knee extension strength, maximum weight-bearing, and gait speed in patients with stroke. J Stroke Cerebro Disl 1:65–69, 1991.

25. Feinstein, AR: Clinical Epidemiology: The Architecture of Clinical Research. WB Saunders, Philadelphia, 1985.

26. Bohannon, RW and Andrews, AW: Influence of head-neck rotation on static elbow flexion force on paretic side in patients with hemiparesis. Phys Ther 69:135–137, 1989.

27. Thorngren, KG and Werner, CO: Normal grip strength. Acta Orthop Scand 50:255–259, 1979.

28. Young, A, Stokes, M, and Crowe, M: Size and strength of the quadriceps muscles of old and young women. Eur J Clin Invest 14:282–287, 1984

29. Louis, TA, Robins, J, Dockery, DW, Spiro, A, and Ware, JH: Explaining discrepancies between longitudinal and cross-sectional models. J Chronic Dis 39:831–839, 1986.

30. Bassey, EJ and Harries, UJ. Normal values for handgrip strength in 920 men and women aged over 65 years, and longitudinal changes over 4 years in 620 survivors. Clinical Science 84:331–337, 1993.

31. Ratcliffe, JW. Notions of validity in qualitative research methdology. Knowledge: Creation, Diffusion, Utilization 5:147–167, 1983.

32. Schmoll, BJ. Ethnogaphic inquiry in clinical settings. Phys Ther 67:1895–1987, 1987.

33. Bohannon, RW, Andrews, AW, and Smith, MB. Rehabilitation goals of patients with hemiplegia. Int J Rehab Research 11:181–183, 1988.

34. Bohannon, RW, Horton, MG, and Wikholm, J: Importance of four variables of walking to patients with stroke. Int J Rehab Research 14:246–250, 1991.

35. Bohannon, RW, Cook, AC, Larkin, PA, Dubuc, WE, Smith, MB, Horton, HG, and Hypes, C: The listing phenomenon of hemiplegic patients. Neurology Report 10:43–44, 1986.

36. Ottenbacher, KJ: Evaluating Clinical Change. Strategies of Occupational and Physical Therapists. Baltimore, Williams & Wilkins, 1986.

37. Kraemer, HC and Thiemann, S: How Many Subjects? Sage, Newbury Park, CA, 1987.

38. Wade, DT and Collin, C: The Barthel ADL Index: A standard measure of physical disability? Int Disabil Studies 10:64–67, 1988.

39. Beasley, WC: Influence of method on estimates of normal knee extensor force among normal and postpolio children. Phys Ther Rev 36:21–41, 1956.

40. Bohannon, RW and Andrews, AW. Accuracy of spring and strain gauge hand-held dynamometers. J Orthop Sports Phys Ther 10:323–325, 1989.

41. Garraway, WM, Akhtar, AJ, Gore, SM, Prescott, RJ, and Smith, RG: Observer variation in clinical assessment of stroke. Age Aging 5:233–240, 1979.

42. Wikholm, JB and Bohannon, RW: Hand-held dynamometer measurements: Tester strength makes a difference. J Orthop Sports Phys Ther 13:191–198, 1991.

43. Sunderland, A, Tinson, D, Bradley, L, and Langton Hewer, R: Arm function after stroke: An evaluation of grip strength as a measure of recovery and a prognostic indicator. J Neurol Neurosurg Psychiatry 52:1267–1272, 1989.

44. Windsor, JA and Hill, GL: Grip strength: A measure of the proportion of protein loss in surgical patients. Br J Surg 75:880–882, 1988.

45. Davies, CWT, Jones, DM, and Shearer, JR: Handgrip: A simple test for morbidity after fracture of the neck of femur. J Royal Soc Med 77:833–836, 1984.

46. Winter, DA, Wells, RP, and Orr, GW: Errors in the use of isokinetic dynamometers. Eur J Appl Physiol 46:397–408, 1981.

47. Wilkinson, L: Systat: The system for statistics. Systat Inc, Evanston, IL, 1990.

48. Maxfield, M, Schweitzer, J, and Gouvier, WD: Measures of central tendency, variability, and relative standing in nonnormal distributions: Alternatives to the mean and standard score. Arch Phys Med Rehabil 69:406–409, 1988.

49. Engstrom, JL: Assessment of the reliability of physical measures. Research Nurs Health 11:383–389, 1988.

50. Cohen, J: A coeffecient of agreement for nominal scales. Educ Psychol Meas 20:37–46, 1960.

51. Fleiss, JL and Cohen, J. Large sample standard errors of kappa and weighted kappa. Psychol Bull 72:323–327, 1971.

52. Shrout, PE and Fleiss, JL. Intraclass correlation: Uses in assessing rater reliability. Psychol Bull 86:420–428, 1979.

53. Lahey, MA, Downey, RG, and Saal, FE: Intraclass correlations: There's more than meets the eye. Psychol Bull 93:586–595, 1983.

54. Okolo, EN. Health Research Design and Methodology. CRC Press, Boca Raton, 1990.

55. Daroff, RB, Rowland, LP, Rossi, A, and Ross, LS: Suggestions to authors. Neurology 40: 1907–1908, 1990.

56. Friedman, GD: Be kind to your reader. Am J Epidemiol 132:591–593, 1990.

57. Gardner, MJ, Michin, D, and Campbell, MJ: Use of check lists in assessing the statistical content of medical studies. Br Med J 292:810–812, 1986.

58. Lundberg, GD, Inverson, C, and Radulescu, G. Now read this. The SI units are here. Arch Neurol 43:547–557, 1986.

59. Guidelines for nonsexist use of language. Am Psychol 30:682–694, 1975.

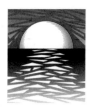

CHAPTER 18

Medicare Documentation: The Paperwork Challenge

Lynn M. Phillippi, MS, PT

BEHAVIORAL OBJECTIVES

Upon completion of this chapter, the reader will be able to:

1 Describe key points in the development of the Medicare program.
2 Identify the basic requirements for Medicare Part A and Part B.
3 Identify the basic covered and noncovered services.
4 Recognize the key components for successful documentation.
5 List common reasons for the denial of claims.
6 Identify the key components for a successful appeal.

THE DEVELOPMENT OF MEDICARE

As early as 1935, the U.S. Congress began investigating the establishment of a national health care insurance program. However, it was not until the Truman administration in 1949 that attention was focused on the issue of national health care coverage. Senators Wagner and Murray, along with Congressman Dengell, submitted a bill proposing universal health care that created an immediate controversy on Capitol Hill. As a consequence, numerous political squabbles developed, and competing lobbyists managed to stall the bill before any vote could take place. Avoiding total defeat, President Truman narrowed the scope of the health care proposal to only one target group.[1]

This target group was the elderly, who at that time in history were perceived to be an unproductive work force and were often the object of public sympathy. Truman's revised proposal limited national health care coverage to those individuals who were over 65 and had contributed to Social Security. To avoid the stigma of welfare, this proposal was combined with Old Age and Survivor's Insurance. These proposals were defeated, and from 1958 until 1965, Congress was embroiled in controversy over the issues of health care. Congress was the target of intense lobbying by various proponents of health care, such as organized labor, professional organizations, nonphysician health care providers, special-interest groups for the aging, and the political left. Groups opposed to the expansion of health care coverage included the American Medical Association, American Hospital Association, insurance representatives, management special-interest groups, and the political right.

In 1965, the House Ways and Means Committee, under the leadership of Wilbur Mills, spearheaded the passage of two amendments to the Social Security Act. These amendments consisted of Title 18 and Title 19—the two components of today's Medicare program. Title 18 provided two-part coverage: Part A for hospital insurance and Part B for medical insurance for a variety of outpatient services. Title 19 provided coverage for the poor.[1]

BASICS OF THE MEDICARE PROGRAM

Medicare is a Federal health insurance program providing hospital and medical coverage to anyone 65 years or older who is eligible to receive Social Security, railroad retirement benefits, disability benefits for more than 24 months, or who has chronic renal disease.[1]

Application for Medicare is usually combined with filing for Social Security. There is no additional cost for hospital insurance under Part A; however, Part B is an optional program that requires a monthly premium. The premiums are usually deducted from the monthly Social Security benefit. If the participant does not receive Social Security, he or she is billed quarterly. Under Medicare Part B, the participant has a yearly deductible and is responsible for 20 percent of all covered charges; Medicare pays for 80 percent of the covered charges.

Services Provided

Under Medicare Part A, an individual is entitled to:

- Inpatient hospital care
- Inpatient skilled nursing facility care (provided specific requirements are met)
- Home health care
- Hospice care

Under Medicare Part B, participants are entitled to outpatient services (See Appendix).

Administration

Medicare is administered by the secretary of Health and Human Services. In 1977, the Health Care Financing Administration (HCFA) was established to consolidate the health care financing functions in the Department of Health and Human Services. The central office for HCFA is in Baltimore, Maryland, with additional offices located in 10 specific regions of the United States. Within each region, HCFA hires various insurance companies or fiscal intermediaries to review and pay Medicare claims. (Figure 18–1 illustrates the structure of the Medicare system.) The primary functions of HCFA are

- To establish policies on coverage, eligibility, and reimbursement.
- To establish standards for providers.
- To provide program administration.
- To secure agreements with contractors.
- To monitor the performance of contractors and states.[2]

Medicare Part A

Basic Requirements

The patient must be eligible for Social Security and pay an annual deductible prior to Medicare payment. Services cover inpatient hospital, inpatient skilled nursing facility, home health care, and hospice care. The Code of Federal Regulations, Title 42, Parts 400 to 429 and 430 to the end[3] outline these rehabilitation services. These guidelines are an excellent resource for health care professionals.

Congress

Health Care Financing
Administration

HCFA develops interpretive guidelines
of the regulations

HCFA REGIONS

1	2	3	4	5	6	7	8	9	10

INTERMEDIARIES   (Insurance Co.)

Aetna	BC/ BS	WPS	Bankers Life

Intermediaries develop/implement the
interpretations. Retrospectively
review and pay claims.

PROVIDERS

Providers determine if
care will be covered
--will they be paid?

Home Health Agencies	Certified Rehab. Agencies	Certified PT, OT ST Independent Providers--limited to $900 per year per patient for Medicare Part B	Certified Skilled Nursing Facilities (SNF)	Hospital

Patient	Patient	Patient	Patient	Patient

FIGURE 18–1. The structure of the Medicare system.

Hospital

Medicare Part A benefits are paid on the basis of benefit periods. A benefit period begins the first day one receives a Medicare-covered service in a hospital. It ends when one has been out of a hospital or skilled nursing facility for 60 consecutive days. It also ends when one remains in a skilled nursing facility but does not receive any skilled care for 60 days. If one enters a hospital again after 60 days, a new benefit period begins.

If one is hospitalized, Medicare will pay all charges for covered hospital services during the first 60 days of a benefit period minus the deductible (which changes each year). From the sixty-first through the ninetieth days, Part A pays for all covered charges minus a daily deductible amount, again adjusted each year. A patient is also eligible to use a lifetime reserve of 60 days, which once used cannot be renewed.[4] Coverage guidelines in the hospital are largely governed by the Diagnostic Regulatory Guidelines (DRGs), which specify the number of coverable days for a specific diagnosis.

Rehabilitation Unit

In a comprehensive inpatient rehabilitation unit, Part A will cover an individual patient if several criteria are met. One of six areas of functional limitations must apply if a patient is to qualify.

- Self-care
- Mobility
- Safety dependence
- Communication deficits
- Swallowing disorders
- Cognitive dysfunction

In addition, the patient must

- Be medically and neurologically stable
- Demonstrate a level of consciousness that allows for a response to a command
- Be physically capable of benefiting from and participating in at least 3 hours of physical, occupational, and/or speech therapy
- Not have been previously treated in an intensive rehabilitation program for the same functional deficits unless a significant change in condition or functional status warrants further intensive rehabilitation.[5]

Skilled Nursing Facilities

Qualifications specific to skilled nursing facilities include the following:

1. The patient has a Medicare hospital insurance/Medicare card (Fig. 18–2). Information on the Medicare card includes:

- Beneficiary (patient) name.
- Medicare health insurance claim number. This is commonly called the Medicare number, and usually is nine digits and one or two letters. It helps verify identity.

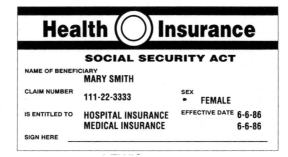

FIGURE 18–2. Sample Medicare Hospital Insurance/Medicare card.

- Sex: helps verify identity
- Entitlement and effective date. Entitlement is the type of benefits the beneficiary is entitled to including Medicare Part A and Medicare Part B, as well as the effective date when benefits were initiated.
- Beneficiary's signature

2. The patient is in a Medicare-certified facility in a Medicare-certified bed.
3. The patient meets the qualifications for a benefit period.
4. The patient requires and receives a daily skilled service. For example, skilled nursing care is needed and provided 7 days per week; skilled nursing care and another rehabilitative service are needed and provided 7 days per week; or a skilled therapy service is needed and provided a minimum of five times per week. Table 18–1 shows some of the qualified services.
5. The patient must have a qualifying acute hospital stay of at least 3 consecutive days, not including day of discharge.
6. The patient must transfer to a skilled nursing facility within 30 days of hospital discharge. The Medically Appropriate Exception or the on-off provision is the exception to the above rule and applies to patients who are medically unable to begin an active course of treatment within the 30 days following hospital discharge. However, it must be medically predictable at the time of hospital discharge that the patient will require covered skilled care in a predetermined time period. An example of this situation would be a patient with a hip fracture who is expected to be non-weight-bearing for 6 to 8 weeks. In this case, the provision allows the patient to receive the maximum

Table 18–1. **Medicare-Qualified Services**

Skilled Nursing and/or Rehabilitation Qualifiers	Patient Examples
NSG (nursing)	Patient receives daily (7 days per week) skilled nursing care.
NSG; PT/OT/SLP	Patient receives daily skilled nursing and any combination of skilled rehabilitation.
PT (physical therapy)	Patient receives skilled PT at least five times per week.
OT (occupational therapy)	Patient receives skilled OT at least five times per week.
SLP (speech-language pathology)	Patient receives skilled SLP at least five times per week.
Any combination of PT, OT, or SLP	Patient receives a combination of OT, PT, and SLP at least five times per week.

Source: Phillippi, L: Documentation: Write for Survival. LEARN Publications, Washington, D.C., 1994, with permission.

amount of his or her benefits by waiting until the weight bearing improves and he or she is able to tolerate a more vigorous rehabilitation program. While the patient is on the on-off provision, he or she may be discharged from therapy or continued on an alternative payer source.

7. The care in the skilled nursing facility must be for a condition that was treated in the hospital or for a condition that arose while receiving care in the skilled nursing facility for a condition that was treated in the hospital.

Home Health Care

Medicare Part A pays the full cost of medically necessary home health visits if the beneficiary is homebound and under the care of a physician. Coverage includes the intermittent services of a skilled nurse. A Medicare-certified home health agency can also furnish the services of a physical therapist and a speech pathologist. Other covered services include intermittent home health aide services, occupational therapy, medical social services, and medical supplies. Coverage is also provided for a portion of the cost of durable medical equipment provided under a plan of care established and overseen by a physician.

The same principles of coverage for a skilled nursing facility apply to rehabilitation therapies in home health. (See CFR 42, 410.80, pp. 239–241 for further requirements.)

Hospice Care

Under Medicare Part A, any Medicare beneficiary who is certified as terminally ill may choose to receive hospice care rather than hospitalization. Medicare Part A can pay for two 90-day hospice benefit periods, a subsequent period of 30 days, and a subsequent extension of unlimited duration. Hospice care is primarily a comprehensive program of care delivered in a patient's home. The emphasis of service delivery is on symptom management and pain relief. Coverage includes physician services, nursing care, medical appliances and supplies, short-term inpatient or respite care, counseling, rehabilitation therapies, and home health aide and homemaker services.[3]

Medicare Part B

Basic Requirements

Medicare Part B, considered an outpatient service (regardless of the location of the service), first requires that the patient has opted for the Part B premium. This information can be obtained from the Medicare card under "Entitled to: Medical Insurance."

To qualify for Medicare Part B rehabilitation services, a patient must demonstrate a decreased functional level secondary to a disease, condition, or injury; for which he or she may or may not have been hospitalized; and for which he or she is presently not covered under Medicare Part A. This decreased functional level can be secondary to (1) acute pain and/or involvement with resultant loss in functional abilities; (2) exacerbation of a chronic condition where there is a documented change in functional status; or (3) a patient who has exhausted benefits under Medicare Part A but still demonstrates continued potential for progress.

Skilled Rehabilitation Procedures Covered by Medicare

The following services are covered only if documentation supports the need for skilled intervention.[3] This list is a summary and is not totally inclusive.

1. Evaluation is covered if it is needed to provide baseline data for assessing expected rehabilitation potential, setting goals, establishing plan of treatment, and measuring functional progress. For an evaluation to be approved, it must show evidence of need of skilled intervention or it must show that it is reasonable and necessary for the therapist to evaluate the patient to determine the need for either a restorative or maintenance service appropriate for the patient's condition. A written treatment plan, established by the physician or therapist, must be reasonable and necessary for the diagnosis.
2. Reevaluations are covered when a patient exhibits a documentable decline in functional abilities, in order to re-establish appropriate treatment goals. Routine screenings are not covered.
3. Therapeutic exercises.
4. Gait training.
5. Range of motion tests and exercises.
6. Ultrasound, shortwave, and microwave diathermy.
7. Hot packs, infrared treatment, paraffin baths, and whirlpool treatments are covered if given prior to but as an integral part of a skilled physical therapy procedure. Generally, any of the above modalities given *alone* are not covered except for whirlpool. (See items 8 and 9.)
8. Hot packs, infrared, paraffin baths, and whirlpool treatments are covered when there are complications such as circulatory deficiency and areas of desensitization.
9. Whirlpool treatments are covered as a single modality when there are stage 3 or 4 open wounds.
10. Teaching transfer techniques
11. Establishment and design of a maintenance program to fit the patient's level of function.

12. Electrical nerve stimulation for the prevention of disuse atrophy where muscle innervation is intact.
13. Pool therapy when used with other modalities or procedures that require the skills or supervision of a qualified physical therapist.
14. Restraint evaluation.
15. Designing, fabricating, and fitting orthotic and self-help devices.
16. Vocational and prevocational assessment and training.
17. Teaching compensatory techniques to improve independence in ADLs.
18. Planning and implementing therapeutic tasks and activities to restore sensory-integrative function.
19. Selecting and teaching task-oriented therapeutic activities designed to restore physical function.
20. Patient and family training.
21. High-voltage pulsed current (HVPC) is covered for the control of muscle spasms, to increase circulation, for muscle reeducation, and for the prevention of disuse atrophy and thrombophlebitis. There are no HVPC units currently approved by Federal Drug Administration for use in wound healing.

Skilled Rehabilitative Procedures Not Covered by Medicare

1. Services to promote overall fitness and flexibility.
2. Services to provide diversion or general motivation.
3. Services related to activities for general good and welfare.
4. Repetitive services to maintain function.
5. Hot packs, infrared treatments, or paraffin baths when given alone.
6. Repetitious exercises to improve gait or maintain strength and endurance.
7. Cardiac rehabilitation.
8. Routine screening.
9. Electric nerve stimulation of motor function disorders, except for the prevention of disuse atrophy where muscle innervation is intact.
10. Electrical stimulation in (denervated) facial paralysis.
11. Ultraviolet, topical oxygen, or low-intensity direct current (LIDC) for treatment of skin ulcers.
12. Biofeedback for treatment of ordinary muscle tension or psychosomatic conditions.
13. Transcutaneous electrical nerve stimulation (TENS) beyond 30 days, or beyond a reasonable assessment period.[6]

Basic Criteria for Medicare Coverage of Rehabilitative Services

1. Services must be specific and effective treatments for the patient's condition. For example, this includes standards as reflected in state practice acts for individual rehabilitation disciplines.

2. Services must be of a level of complexity and sophistication or the condition of the patient must be such that services must be safely and effectively performed and supervised by a qualified therapist. For example, routine care or exercises that can be provided by a nursing assistant or other support staff would not be covered unless documentation reflected why the skills of a therapist were needed.
3. There must be an expectation that the condition will improve significantly in a reasonable (and generally predictable) length of time, or services must be necessary for the establishment of a safe and effective maintenance program. Again, there is a need to demonstrate progress, improvements in function, and why skilled intervention is needed.
4. Amount, frequency, and duration of services must be reasonable. For example, the services provided to an individual seen daily for 6 weeks who has demonstrated little progress in either functional level or pain control would not be viewed as reasonable or necessary.
5. If a patient is receiving rehabilitation for a chronic condition without documentation of a functional regression, the service could be questioned as to whether it is reasonable and necessary.
6. The physician needs to sign, not stamp, a certification at least every 30 days. With home health, the physician review and signature are required every 60 days.[3]

In all of these areas, documentation must reflect progress or the need for skilled intervention. It is important that rehabilitation professionals realize that there is an accountability factor in both the delivery and outcome of treatment intervention. The rehabilitation professional must reassess the patient during each treatment session to identify what gains have been achieved, what goals have been met, if training has been performed, and if carryover has been achieved in the home setting. An ongoing assessment of each patient's progress will help eliminate the possibility of services being denied.

COMPONENTS OF SUCCESSFUL DOCUMENTATION

The rehabilitation professional's ability to produce accurate, descriptive, and timely documentation for each patient is the most effective means at his or her disposal to prove the efficacy of rehabilitation intervention and to ensure reimbursement for that same intervention. The following components of documentation will be addressed: initial evaluation, daily treatment notes, bimonthly and monthly progress notes, and discharge notes.

Initial Evaluation

The primary purpose of the initial evaluation is to determine whether there is a reasonable expectation that the patient will improve if a rehabilitation service is provided.[3] The initial evaluation provides the baseline data for future comparisons reflecting progress achieved and the justification for skilled intervention. This is accomplished by addressing the medical history, primary and secondary diagnosis, date of onset, prior level of functioning, status of patient at time of evaluation in pertinent areas, development of a list of pertinent problems based on the evaluative findings, establishment of short- and long-term goals, rehabilitation potential, current functional level, and the specific rehabilitation treatment approach established in the plan of care. In the sample initial evaluation format (Fig. 18–3), all of these areas are addressed. Here is a step-by-step description of each numbered box.

In the upper right-hand corner are name, date of birth, facility (clinic,

```
       (STATE WHICH THERAPY) INITIAL EVALUATION    __/__/__

       Name:     PATIENT NAME;            MR # (if facility requires)
       D/O/B:    00/00/00                 1st Service: 00/00/00
       Facility: PUT IN NAME OF FACILITY  Room #:
       Physician:PHYSICIAN'S NAME         |  | OP          |  | IP

Primary Diagnosis (Onset Date):     1
Secondary Diagnoses:                2
Conditions/Communicative Disorders: 3
Precautionary Info:                 4
Physician Order (00/00/00):         5
Payor Source    6 :        A         B          Medicaid        Other

Prior Level of Function: 7


Initial Assessment:   8



Clinical Impressions:  9



Problem List:   10                    Short Term Goals:   10



Long Term Goal:   11                  Goal Potential:   12


Plan of Care:   13                    Frequency:    14
                                      Duration:     15

NURSING/ACTIVITY RECOMMENDATIONS:   16


   17                                      18


Therapist Signature      Date        Physician Signature     Date
```
FIGURE 18–3. Sample initial evaluation documentation form.

school, etc.) physician name, room number, inpatient or outpatient status, and initial date of service.

The medical history is summarized by completing points 1 to 7, as shown in Figure 18–3.

1. **Primary diagnosis:** This is the primary diagnosis established by the physician. This is the diagnosis either at the time of hospital admission or when a patient is referred to an outpatient clinic or skilled nursing facility.

2. **Secondary diagnoses:** These are additional diagnoses stated by the physician.

3. **Rehabilitation conditions and communication disorders:** These relate to the specific functional deficits each patient exhibits. Examples of these areas are decreased balance, decreased strength, decreased functional tolerance, limitations in activities of daily living, and increased pain. It is important to identify these rehabilitation conditions and communication disorders because the recording of these deficits can assist in justifying coverage, particularly if the primary diagnosis is considered questionable, for example, chronic heart failure or organic brain syndrome. Either the primary or the secondary diagnosis may relate directly to the focus of rehabilitation intervention. However, it is also possible that therapeutic intervention is required secondary to rehabilitation conditions and communication disorders. For example, a patient with a history of osteoarthritis may be seen by physical therapy for a condition such as decreased balance and ambulation.

4. **Precautionary information:** The clinician indicates any areas of precaution following review of the patient's chart. Examples of such areas are seizure status, heart arrhythmias, high blood pressure, altered weight-bearing status, combativeness, anxiety, and oxygen dependency. If, in reviewing the chart, there does not appear to be any record of precautionary areas, the clinician should note "none evident." This indicates that the clinician has reviewed the chart and has not identified any precautions. Avoid leaving this area blank.

5. **Physician order:** List the date and the specific wording of the physician's order.

6. **Payor source:** For ease of accessibility in billing and to record specific payor source, this area should delineate the financial party to be billed.

7. **Prior level of function:** This is the "before" picture of the patient's previous functional level. Some areas that are routinely addressed in this section include independence in mobility skills, use of assistive or adaptive devices, any previous therapy with dates and level of function at discharge, pertinent past medical history, and family and social history. It is particularly important to record recent losses, such as death of a family member.

8. **Initial assessment:** The initial assessment should provide objective baseline data in all areas pertinent to the patient's rehabilitation. Upon completion of this section, the reviewer should have a clear picture of the deficits and related functional disabilities exhibited by this patient.

9. **Clinical impressions:** Upon completion of the initial evaluation, the rehabilitation professional can assess the patient's overall potential based on the patient's responses during the evaluation.

10. **Problem list, short-term goals:** Each problem listed should correlate with a short-term goal. These goals need to be measurable, functional, and time-specific. *Measurable goals* include objective data reflecting such areas as pain rating, level of assistance required, range of motion and manual muscle test measurements, and percentage ratios. A *functional goal* is a statement that reflects what the patient is expected to achieve outside the therapeutic environment. In other words, it describes the ultimate benefit of therapeutic intervention for the patient. A goal must state a *time frame* that is realistic to the particular setting, diagnosis, and individual patient. For example:

PROBLEM	SHORT-TERM GOAL
PT: Decreased ambulation	Patient will stand in parallel bars with moderate assistance from one person in 2 weeks
OT: Decreased motor skills	Will increase ability to button shirt by 50 percent in 2 weeks

Short-term goals must reflect activities that build upon each other. For example, if a patient initially transfers with maximal assistance of one person, a short-term goal may be for the patient to weight-shift forward or pivot on one limb in 2 weeks with maximal assistance of one. Once this activity has been achieved, the next goal may be to perform single-limb stance and pivot with moderate assistance of one person in 2 weeks.

11. **Long-term goal:** This is a statement regarding the expected final outcome of therapeutic intervention. It should be specific to the functional outcomes expected. For example:

PT: Return home to community dwelling, ambulating independently with regular cane.

OT: Will live independently in apartment without adaptive equipment.

12. **Rehabilitation goal potential:** Rehabilitation potential is often expressed in simple terms: poor, fair, good, and excellent. Although these terms are very general, the categories are helpful in correlating other aspects of the initial assessment such as frequency and du-

ration of treatment, level of therapeutic interventions, focus of restorative training, and payor source willingness to reimburse over a period of time.

13. **Plan of care:** It is important to be specific when describing the treatment approach. In addition to stating the discipline and frequency, include the different types of approaches such as strengthening exercises, bed and mat mobility training, activities of daily living, caregiver and nursing training.

14. **Frequency:** It is important to address frequency of treatment and to note any subsequent changes in frequency (for example, two times per week, daily, etc.).

15. **Duration:** Duration of treatment should be reevaluated at the time each note is written. Lengthy and indefinite time periods (such as 6 months) are discouraged unless there is a specific reason to expect duration to be long (developmentally disabled patient, very complex neurologic disorder).

16. **Nursing and activity recommendations:** This area should describe (in easy-to-understand terminology) what activities will enhance the patient's care interventions. For example, a patient with a cerebral vascular accident may be suffering from severe hemianopsia on the right and instructions could include, "Encourage patient to turn head to right when turning a corner and eating."

17. **Therapist's signature:** These signatures must be written, not stamped. If a therapist is signing a note that was written by another therapist, it should be written:

Dictated by (Print name of the therapist who dictated note)

18. **Physician's signature:** The physician signature is particularly critical for Medicare reimbursement. This needs to be done every 30 days to reflect the physician's ongoing review of the claim.

This has been a basic overview of an initial evaluation. Once completed, the initial evaluation serves as the reference point for the remaining documentation. This documentation includes the daily note, the bimonthly and monthly progress reports, and the discharge summary. Each of the note types will be discussed individually with suggestions on how to document these notes most effectively.

Daily Treatment Notes

Daily treatment notes are often required or requested in multiple health care settings, such as hospital, outpatient clinics, home-care settings, and rehabilitation units. There are a number of possible formats. We will review two of them here: the SOAP and narrative formats. Both should focus on measurable progress that reflects functional improvement and the continued need for skilled intervention for an individual discipline.

SOAP Format

SOAP stands for subjective, objective, assessment, and plan.

Subjective: The patient's perception of his or her health status, pain level, and rehabilitation potential. A family or nursing perspective can be included if the patient is unable to communicate or additional information is required.

Objective: Specific measurable data on the patient's performance, status, or progress. This includes tests results of strength, range of motion, and balance and functional improvements.

Assessment: The clinician's perception of the patient's status, progress, and potential.

Plan: Immediate short-term goals, the specifics of the treatment plan, and long-term goals such as discharge planning.

Narrative Format

The narrative format is most effective when kept brief and succinct. Progress in specific areas of treatment needs to be highlighted, along with evidence of the need for skilled intervention. Frequently, a practitioner will repeat the treatment protocol such as number of repetitions or the amount of resistance used. Although this information is important, it is more relevant to discuss the functional improvements achieved and to describe the carryover into the nontherapeutic environment. The following are two samples of the narrative format that demonstrate this point.

> **Physical therapy:** The patient continues to be seen twice daily in physical therapy. Marked progress has been noted in the patient's ability to weight-shift to the right lower extremity. This is evidenced by patient's ability to initiate swing through 50 percent on the left lower extremity in the parallel bars. Transfers have improved as well from moderate assist of one to minimal of one with frequent verbal cues. Will continue on same program.

> **Occupational therapy:** The patient is demonstrating improved fine motor coordination skills in right hand, is now able to button and unbutton shirt independently. Patient exhibits improved ability to organize meal tray and to compensate for right hemianopsia by turning head to involved side. Will continue present program with increased focus on lower-extremity dressing (zippers) and improving visual tracking.

Bimonthly or Monthly Progress Report

The bimonthly (two times a month) or monthly progress note serves as the patient's report card. As in any report card, each subject must be addressed and performance evaluated. The progress notes must reflect each area of treatment and provide a detailed description of the patient's performance in each. Henri and Cornett[7] note:

> For Medicare claims, documentation includes a short narrative progress report and clear and concise objective information. Further, a statement is required regarding the patient's initial functional level at the present provider setting in contrast to the present level of function for each particular billing period. A statement regarding continued rehabilitation potential (that the patient is still expected to make significant practical improvement) is also required. Any changes in the treatment plan must be specifically noted. (p. 14)

The use of comparative data assists in reflecting the patient's performance and reflects significant progress.

> The term "significant" means that a generally measurable and substantial increase in the patient's present level of functioning has occurred during the treatment period covered in the progress note. (p. 14)

A comparative statement is a statement that describes clear before-and-after "pictures" of the patient's status in each particular treatment area. For example, a patient may be described as follows:

> The patient was able to sit unsupported on the mat for 30 seconds upon initial evaluation. The patient is now able to sit 2 minutes without balance loss and occasional minimal resistance to trunk.

It is also important to remember that the meaning of measurable and substantial significant progress can be qualified by addressing, if appropriate, variables of the patient's condition that should be considered in the treatment plan. For example, variables such as multiplicity of diagnoses, prolonged immobilization, malnutrition, severe emotional problems, change in medical condition or medication, and others can affect the patient's rehabilitation program. Along this same line of thinking, it is important to consider the patient who may not necessarily be expected to recover partially or fully from treatment. These patients may or may not still be eligible for coverage. Documentation in these cases must be written with emphasis on why skilled intervention is required to enhance the patient's level of care, present level of functioning, or the prevention of further deterioration. As an example, a patient who is terminally ill with cancer may require physical therapy to control pain.

The area of clinical impressions affords the therapist the opportunity to provide an overview of the patient's status, progress, and potential. This must be a simple yet clear reflection of the patient's response to therapeutic intervention. For example, "The patient appears to be an excellent candidate for physical therapy demonstrating marked improvement in transfers and bed and mat mobility. Patient has reported less fatigue and pain, progressing to ambulation in the parallel bars."

In addition, all progress notes need to exhibit an ongoing reevaluation of short-term goals. For instance, if the initial goal for transfers was to improve weight shifting to the right lower extremity in 2 weeks, then once this is achieved a revised goal must be established. For example, "Patient will perform pivot transfer on right lower extremity with minimal assist of one in 2 weeks." All too often, progress notes do not demonstrate any change in goals. Thus, when scrutinized under review, the reasonableness and necessity of the intervention come into question as the therapy appears to be repetitive and maintenance in nature.

Carryover into the home and on the nursing unit is expected to be an integral part of the rehabilitation intervention. Therefore, the progress note should reflect an updated summary of suggestions for the caregiver and nursing staff. For example, "Encourage the patient to turn his or her head to the right when eating meal."

Discharge Summary

Last, but certainly not least, is the discharge summary. Henri and Cornett[7] note that "for the primary clinician, the discharge summary does create an opportunity to bring closure to the entire intervention program and assess, if, in fact, the initially developed plan of care was adequate and appropriate" (p. 14). The discharge summary must define the plan of care and the treatment approaches used by comparing the patient's status at the time of admission and discharge. The reader should have a clear picture of the patient's overall progress and the degree to which specified goals have been met. In addition, a clear description of the patient's abilities and limitations (if any) is necessary to understand the patient's functional status. Included in the patient summary should be evidence of instruction in a home program, family and caregiver training, purchase of equipment, and any future goals for the patient.

The reason for discharge must be stated. For example, "Patient attained all goals," or "Patient refused further treatment at this time," or "Patient no longer appears to be a candidate."

The discharge summary should provide a forecast of the patient's potential functioning following discharge from therapy. This is required in reports submitted under rehabilitation guidelines. This can be as simple as stating whether the prognosis is poor, fair, good, or excellent; the report can use summary phrases such as "Patient reports she will continue home program," or "Patient has returned to work and is expected to be successful."

The preceding portion of this chapter has provided an overview of various documentation formats highlighting key areas of focus. In the concluding portion of this chapter, attention will be focused on the denial and appeal process, as all health care professionals will undergo the eye of scrutiny in claim review at some time during their practice.

THE DENIAL

There are numerous reasons why a particular claim is denied. For the purposes of this chapter, the seven most common reasons for denial will be addressed.

1. **"Technical denials" or errors in claim processing.** Data on an individual claim form are incomplete or inaccurate. Some of these errors or omissions include:

    - Omission of onset date
    - Omission of date of first service
    - Error in health insurance or social security number
    - Error in diagnosis code
    - Treatments in excess of allowed number of treatment units
    - Untimely submission of requested documentation
    - Use of incorrect forms

2. **Treatment is not considered "reasonable and necessary."** This type of denial is generally due to inadequate documentation of the need for skilled services and the lack of functional improvement. The clinician's documentation may state that a particular modality or portion of the treatment was ineffective.

3. **Treatment is considered unreasonable in amount, frequency, or duration.** The clinician's documentation may not reflect responsible decision making in these areas. Often a clinician's documentation may omit special considerations that affected treatment duration and frequency, such as complicating medical problems.

4. **Skills of a rehabilitation professional were not required.** In this instance, documentation does not reflect the need for skilled intervention. Furthermore, a lack of documented functional outcome may exist. For example:

    - Omission of comparative data to indicate functional progress
    - Lack of information of prior functional status
    - Lack of functional outcomes in goals
    - Activities sound repetitive and could easily be performed by non-skilled personnel

5. **Treatment or procedure is considered experimental.** A denial may occur secondary to the use of certain modalities or treatment because the equipment does not have prior approval of the payor source and/or has not been proven as an effective treatment method. Research plays a vital role in this area to educate the intermediaries involved.

6. **Treatment is of questionable medical necessity.** This denial presents itself as a practical matter. Could the service provided have been delivered in a more cost-effective manner? For instance, a Medicare intermediary may determine that it was not necessary for an indi-

vidual patient to be placed in a skilled nursing facility based on the availability and capability of family members in the home.

7. **Lack of documentation to justify professional skilled intervention and functional improvement.** The most important and most common reasons for denial of a rehabilitation claim result from insufficient documentation. For example:

- Lack of diagnosis and onset date
- Omission of prior history or status in relation to the specific discipline
- Lack of comparative data from the previous note or evaluation
- "Machine" printouts that show objective data but do not show the correlation to functional activities of daily living
- Data are subjective in nature and not objective or "real"
- Treatment does not match the diagnosis and plan of care
- The physician order and the established plan of care do not match
- The claim does not reflect the necessary data
- Terminology used is unique to a particular rehabilitative discipline, and not commonly understood
- Overgeneralization. For example, "In general all goals are met," yet treatment continues. A reviewer may focus on the statement of goal completion and not comprehend the need for revision of specific goals and continued skilled intervention.
- Lack of functional outcome showing how the patient's functional level is improved and enhanced as a result of therapeutic intervention.[8]

THE APPEAL

Once a claim is formally denied, it is in the best interests of the rehabilitation professional to appeal the claim. The appeal process can provide a positive learning experience for the clinician and at the same time be an educational tool for third-party payors.

The initial step is to formally review the claim and determine if the denial is based on a technical error, such as an incorrect diagnosis, or if the actual treatment plan and approach are in question.

If the denied claim is related to the treatment received, the clinician will need to review the case and thoroughly read the reason for the denial. He or she should then examine pertinent on-site documentation for the time period in question. Once this self-critique is performed, assessment of the need for further supportive documentation can be helpful in substantiating coverage on a claim. Examples of this supportive documentation can be written feedback from the referring physician, nurse, social services, other rehabilitation professionals, the patient, or the patient's family. Additional notes may include daily notes or specific tests, measurements, or training not previously noted. Be sure to submit all required forms and documentation for the time period in question as this will expedite the appeal process.

In addition to the above, a formal appeal letter (justifying coverage of the claim) can best summarize the key points to be conveyed to the reviewer. Make sure the appeal letter meets the following criteria:

1. List the intent of the letter. "This letter is to formally appeal the Medicare denial of Miranda Jones."
2. Include the patient's name, health insurance number, and dates of denied service.
3. Begin with an introductory paragraph summarizing the patient's diagnosis, hospitalizations, medical complications, if any, and prior level of function.
4. Summarize the functional gains that occurred during rehabilitation, provide specific comparative data.
5. Highlight any supportive documentation that was not previously reported and include with the letter.
6. Stress the need for the skilled intervention of a health care professional and include any home program instruction, family or caregiver training, and any other medical complications not previously noted.
7. Always identify the functional outcome achieved as a result of therapeutic intervention.
8. Conclude with a strong closing statement reinforcing the overall effects of therapy on the patient's long-term level of functioning.[9]

Figure 18–4 is an example of an appeal letter.

Dear Reviewer,

This letter is to formally appeal the Medicare Part B denial on Mr. X, health insurance claim number 123-45-6789A, from _____.

Mr. X has a complex history of chronic disease, including juvenile onset rheumatoid arthritis, degenerative joint disease, cervical spondylosis with myelopathy, peripheral neuropathy, Crohn's disease and anemia from chronic disease. He has severe multiple joint deformities and is confined to a power wheelchair, but alert, highly motivated and cognitively intact. He has had multiple hospitalizations, nursing home admissions and returns to community living within the past two years.

The Occupational Therapy treatment in question followed his _____ hospitalization at University Hospital and Clinics. Prior to admission he had lived in an apartment with an evening attendant. Progressive symptoms of gait deteriorations, impaired finger dexterity, and painful parethesias throughout his body prompted admission for a C2-3 laminectomy on _____. The neurologist documented these symptoms as above and beyond those associated with his arthritis.

Upon initial evaluation, Mr. X was found to be in possible nerve regeneration. Bilateral shoulder strength was 2- to 2+/5. Sensation was intact for light touch

FIGURE 18–4. Sample Medicare denial appeal letter.

localization and proprioception. Stereognosis, sharp/dull differentiation and temperature were impaired. He was maximal assist for activities of daily living (ADLs) and moderate assist for transfer. As nerve regeneration begins approximately one month after injury/surgery, Mr. X was anticipated to be a good candidate for 5 times per week occupational therapy treatment for strengthening, graded ADLs and coordination activities.

Mr. X made slow but steady gains in occupational therapy the first two weeks. When strength showed signs of plateauing in the third week, treatment shifted to compensatory ADL training. In week four, it was determined that the cost of adaptive and accessibility equipment was excessive and not fundable. Throughout this process, he had to accept the painful fact that he would not return to independent living.

Mr. X still resides within this facility but is within two months of discharge to an accessible apartment with 24 hour attendant care and a power wheelchair with power recliner. He has not lost his motivation and participates in daily independent exercises to maintain his skills.

I urge you to reconsider your decision to deny Medicare Part B benefits for 5 times per week treatment from _____. A legitimate attempt at rehabilitation was warranted following the C2-3 laminectomy to maximize any nerve return.

Thank you for this review.

Sincerely,

(Therapist's name), OTR

xx/jam

cc: file

FIGURE 18–4. Sample Medicare denial appeal letter, continued

Appealing a claim displays confidence on the part of the rehabilitation professional in the decision processes and efficacy of the treatment interventions. Further evidence of the confidence that a professional has in the therapeutic techniques is demonstrated when the claim is pursued at each level (appeal, hearing, and administrative law judge). Figure 18–5 is a diagram of the entire appeal process.

SUMMARY

Regardless of the format used for individual documentation, the content specificity of the patient's functional outcome remains a crucial factor in both timely and ongoing reimbursement for rehabilitation ser-

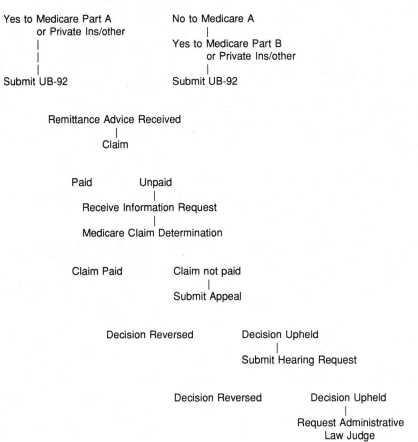

Determine eligibility for Medicare A or Medicare B

FIGURE 18–5. The Medicare appeal process.

vices. The relationship of therapeutic intervention and the final long-lasting functional outcome can be justified only by recording and comparing objective data. Correlation of this data with daily activities such as dressing, eating, bathing, transfers, and ambulating is paramount in demonstrating the efficacy of treatment. Survival in future health care reform will depend on the ability of rehabilitation professionals to paint a picture of multicolored outcomes—literally, a portrait of success for each patient.

REFERENCES

1. Lammers, WW: Public Policy and the Aging. CQ Press, 1983.
2. Rosenthal, G: The federal health structure. In Mechanic, D (ed): Handbook of Health, Health Care, and the Health Professions. Free Press, New York, 1983.
3. Code of Federal Regulations, 42, Public Health, Rev. Office of the Federal Register National Archives and Records Administrator, Washington, DC, Oct. 1, 1992.
4. U.S. Department of Health and Human Services: Guide to Health Insurance for People with Medicare. Washington, DC, 1992.
5. Understanding Observation Requirements. Medical Management Development Associates, Basic Requirements, p. 120.
6. U.S. Department of Health and Human Services: Outpatient Physical Therapy and Comprehensive Outpatient Rehabilitation Facility Manual (Medicare), rev. Washington, DC, January 1992.
7. Henri, BP and Cornett, BS: Planning and documentation: Essentials for quality and reimbursement. Journal of the Ohio Speech & Hearing Association 7(1):13, 1992.
8. Morris, BA: Speeding reimbursement and avoiding claims denials. Rehabilitation Today April 1992, p. 17.
9. Morris, BA: 19 tips for appealing claims denials. Rehabilitation Today March 1993, p. 23.
10. Abramson, B, Groom, M, and Spitzer-Resnick, J: Mastering the Medicare Maze. Center for Public Representation, Madison, WI, 1991.

BIBLIOGRAPHY

Foss, S: Utilization Review Coordinator, Extended Care Observations, Memo, March 9, 1994.
Gottschalk, Reesa, RRA, Health Informations Consultant, fe.rg/Gottschalk.1—March 13, 1993.
Mechanic, D. (ed): Handbook of Health, Health Care, and the Health Professions. Free Press, New York, 1983.
Peterson, H: From modest beginnings. Best's Review: Life Insurance Edition. 1991.
Rehabilitation, YYPRO Transmital, effective date December 1992, p. I–57.
Royer, J.D., Jeffrey T., "The Future of Observation Beds," Medicare Manage Series, Basic Regulation, Non-copyrighted hand-out, Fall 93.
Strum, J: Trends in rehab reimbursement. Rehab Management August/September, 1992.
U.S. Department of Health and Human Services, Health Care Financing Administration: Medicare Hospice Benefits. 312-146/60506. U.S. Government Printing Office, Washington, DC, 1992.

Appendix

Outpatient Services Covered under Medicare Part B

1. Physician services including diagnosis, therapy, surgery, consultation at home, office, or institutional visits. The term "physician" includes licensed MDs, osteopaths, dental surgeons, podiatrists, chiropractors,

and optometrists. It does not include Christian Science practitioners or naturopaths.

2. Second opinions regarding the decision to undergo elective surgery when the beneficiary feels the need for such an opinion. Peer review organizations (PROs) have the authority to require second opinions for certain elective surgical procedures. The cost of such a mandatory second opinion will be paid in full by Medicare. If the second opinion differs from the first, Medicare will also cover a third opinion.

3. Chiropractic services that relate to services and supplies incidental to treating a misalignment of the spine through manual manipulations. An x-ray must demonstrate that this misalignment exists.

4. Optometric services relating to the treatment of cataracts.

5. Dentist's services related to surgery of the jaw.

6. Services and supplies including drugs and biologicals that the beneficiary is unable to self-administer and that are furnished as part of a physician's professional services.

7. Outpatient hospital services and supplies as part of physician services to outpatients and drugs and biologicals that cannot be self-administered.

8. Diagnostic x-rays, laboratory, and other tests. Medicare covers Pap smears once every 3 years and more often for high-risk beneficiaries.

9. X-ray, radium, and radioactive isotope therapy, materials, and services.

10. Surgical dressings including bandages and devices for fractures and dislocations with a physician's prescription.

11. Ambulance services to and from a hospital or skilled nursing facility when use of other transportation is dangerous to the individual's health.

12. Prosthetic devices such pacemakers, hemodialysis equipment, colostomy bags, and other items that replace all or part of an internal body organ (see Item 21).

13. Leg, arm, back, and neck braces, artificial limbs and eyes, including necessary repairs, adjustment, and replacement (see Item 21).

14. Outpatient diagnostic services including drugs and biologicals furnished during the diagnostic study.

15. Physical and occupational therapy services furnished

   • On an outpatient basis by a participating clinic, rehabilitation agency, or public health clinic
   • By an independently practicing physical or occupational therapist in a therapist's office or patient's home
   • On an inpatient basis by a qualified provider to an inpatient of a hospital or skilled nursing facility

A doctor must write a treatment plan specifying the need for skilled services in order to receive the Medicare reimbursement.

16. Outpatient speech pathology.
17. Rural health clinic services.
18. Home and institutional dialysis equipment services and supplies.
19. Home health services, only if the beneficiary does not have Part A coverage.
20. Comprehensive outpatient rehabilitation facility (CORF) services.
21. Durable medical equipment (DME), such as wheelchairs, crutches, oxygen equipment, and hospital beds, are covered if the equipment

- Is long lasting
- Primarily serves a medical purpose
- Is appropriate for home use

For example, *Air conditioners* are not covered because they do not have a primarily medical purpose. *Wheelchairs* are covered because they are long lasting, primarily medical, and appropriate for use in the home. *Elastic stockings* are not covered because they are not long lasting.[10]

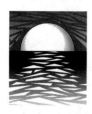

CHAPTER 19

The Frail Elderly and the Health Care Environment

Kathleen Kline, PhD, PT, GCS
Carole Bernstein Lewis, PT, GCS, MSG, MPA, PhD

BEHAVIORAL OBJECTIVES

Upon completion of this chapter, the reader will be able to:

1 List the pertinent components of a comprehensive assessment of the frail older patient.
2 Contrast the differences in assessment of the young versus the frail older patient.
3 Describe the importance and the implementation of the resident assessment instrument (RAI).
4 Design a motivational approach for working with the frail older patient.
5 Discuss strategies to enhance learning for the frail older patient.
6 Recognize the different type of rehabilitation care and living arrangements available to the frail older patient.
7 Confront the physical-restraint issue with a solid knowledge base and ideas for change.
8 Define the RUGS system and the role of rehabilitation in this system.
9 Refer the frail older patient to a variety of aging resources for information, support, or assistance.

Treatment of the frail elderly requires, first and foremost, special attention to comprehensive assessment in the changing health care environment. Additionally, however, it is essential to consider other factors throughout the treatment program. These factors include fostering patient motivation through understanding of the basis for treatment, looking at the long-term goals of treatment in view of progression through the health care venues (hospitals, rehabilitation centers, skilled nursing facilities), and the future of health care. In addition, this chapter explores a controversial and real problem for the aged: physical restraint. This chapter ends with a list of aging resources to assist the practitioner in recognizing areas for assistance and support in caring for the aged. By viewing the treatment program in its totality, the therapist can plan for the future and provide informed and well thought out care for the frail elderly.

COMPREHENSIVE ASSESSMENT OF THE ELDERLY AND THE MINIMUM DATA SET

Comprehensive Assessment

Comprehensive geriatric assessment is a necessary precursor to assisting patients in their attempt to return to their prior level of functioning. The twofold process involves careful clinical assessment to identify remedial problems and functional assessment to determine patient autonomy.[1] Clinical assessment can be difficult because the elderly often adapt to and compensate for illnesses or weakness, leading to underreporting of problems or difficulties. In addition, because of comorbidity (existence of two or more medical conditions), the assessment must be thorough. For example, the elderly patient may complain of back pain, which may be due to osteoarthritis, osteoporosis, compression fractures, or medical problems such as abdominal aortic aneurysms, retroperitoneal masses, or cancer. Careful clinical assessment and information gathering by all staff members lead to quality geriatric care.

The second process in comprehensive assessment is careful and competent functional assessment performed to ascertain how patient autonomy can be maximized by appropriate human and mechanical assistance and by environmental manipulations. To this end, functional assessment can be thought of in terms of an equation in which function equals the product of physical capabilities, medical management, and motivation divided by the patient's social and physical environment.

O'Neil and colleagues[2] have outlined desirable qualities of a physical therapy geriatric evaluation. It should be easy to administer, contain the necessary information for proper reimbursements, and be appropriate for patients with various diagnoses and functional levels. And it should measure a dimension of performance that is affected by age or age-related disease, important to ADL, and likely to respond to physical therapy intervention. To date, there is no "perfect" assessment tool for all frail geriatric patients; however, comprehensive assessment should include the evaluation procedures described below.

Evaluation Procedures

Assessment begins with descriptors of the patient's general behavior, mentation, and communication skills. General behavior includes descriptive words such as cooperative, agitated, friendly, depressed, flat affect, etc. Mentation is noted by orientation to person, place, and time and/or through the patient's ability to follow one-step, simple, or complex commands. Use of reliable and valid tests such as Folstein's Mini-Mental Status Test[3] or the Short Portable Mental Status Questionnaire[4] are recommended. The Folstein test is a 30-point, untimed test that concentrates only on the cognitive aspects of mental functions. Scores of less than 20 are found in patients with delirium or dementia.

Communication skills are reported for speech, vision, and hearing. The therapist notes if the patient is dysarthric or aphasic, has low voice volume, or uses jargon and word salad expressions. Visual impairments such as legal blindness, cataracts, or glaucoma can be obtained through the medical record. The therapist also notes hemianopia, visual neglect, and the need for and use of glasses. Hearing problems should be identified; the therapist should note the ear in which the patient wears a hearing aid and whether hearing is improved with the use of a biaural device. Effective communication with the frail elderly is essential if the rest of the evaluation is to be valid.

Clinical evaluation includes range of motion (ROM) assessment. Both active and passive assessments are performed. Limitations in movement are measured with a goniometer. Although the note "within functional limits" (WFL) is frequently used, it should be avoided because there is no standard or accepted definition of this term.

Muscle force can be measured by a variety of techniques. Manual muscle testing as described by Kendall and associates[5] or Daniels and Worthingham[6] are valid techniques. However, there are no accepted age-related changes in values. For example, one cannot give a "good or 4" grade to a 92-year-old woman who is able to make only minimal resistance against gravity because "It's good for a 92-year-old." Isokinetic dynamometers or hand-held muscle testers may also be used, but normative values have not been established for those in their eighties and nineties. If the patient is unable to follow commands, observation of functional activities may be the only gross indicator of muscle force. This type of assessment is limited to observation of spontaneous antigravity movements or performance during upright activities. In these circumstances, the statement for muscle force would be "Able to move arm against gravity for several repetitions consistent with fair to fair-plus strength," or "Lower-extremity buckle in upright position consistent with less than fair strength."

Pain is another area of clinical measurement. The therapist reports when pain is elicited or what brings it on; provides descriptive qualities such as sharp, dull, aching, or burning sensations; and notes objective measures of the pain using a visual analog scale (VAS) or numerical rating scale. There is some evidence that the elderly may have difficulty in comprehending the VAS, but this can be lessened with thorough instruction prior to use of the scale.[7]

Nervous system function is noted by assessment of muscle tone, reflex activity, sensation, involuntary movements, and coordination. Changes in any of these functions may be an indicator of neurologic improvement or deterioration. Excluding changes from a CVA, observed changes in tone can include clonus, Babinski, or rigidity (a prevalent side effect of psychotropic medication).[1] Sensation tests include light touch, superficial pain, and proprioception. Grading sensation is broad; it may range from absent, impaired, decreased, increased, to intact.

Involuntary movements include resting tremors, tarditive dyskinesia, or senile resting tremors; they may or may not be associated with functional changes. Coordination testing is essentially the same as that of a younger population. An upper-extremity test is the finger-to-nose movement and a lower-extremity test is the heel-to shin-movement. In both cases, past-pointing, dysmetria, or extreme slowness of movement is noted. Rapid alternating movements of supination-pronation or dorsiflexion-plantarflexion are also useful to elicit asymmetries in coordination.

Soft-tissue status is assessed by skin breakdown, swelling or edema, and skin appearance. Swelling and edema are recorded by circumferential measurements. In addition, the time of day and bilateral comparisons are documented. Senile purpura, the large persistent bruises from minimal trauma, are also noted.

In addition to reporting the size and location of pressure sores, it is necessary to report the stage of the sore. There are four general pressure sore stages. As defined in the Medicare guidelines,[8] a stage 1 sore is a persistent area of skin redness (without a break in the skin) that does not disappear when pressure is relieved or does not blanch when pressure is applied. Stage 2 manifestations includes the breakdown of epidermis and dermis, resulting in a shallow ulcer with distinct edges. The area may also present as blistering surrounded by an area of redness and/or induration. In stage 3, the wound extends into the subcutaneous tissue. The skin edges appear rolled and pigmented, and outline the wound. The sore may present as a shallow crater. In stage 4, the wound extends into the muscle and, occasionally, the bone. Drainage is present and sinus tracts with undermined areas may be present. The sore may be covered with an eschar or appear necrotic.

Functional assessment includes the gross motor skills of bed mobility and transfers. Grading is based on the amount of assistance needed by the patient; descriptors range from total assist, dependent, maximum assist, moderate assist, minimal assist, contact guarding, standby assist, supervision, and independent. Definitions of these terms are institution-specific. However, more concise descriptors of the activity are recommended for complete documentation. For example, in a bed-mobility activity, one can further define the action as rolling left or right, going from supine to sit, scooting left or right at the edge of the bed, etc. Similarly, with transfers, the therapist can document sit to stand, pivot to the right, pivot to toilet, etc. This further definition of gross motor skills allows more measurable and achievable goals to be set.

Posture assessment includes statements on forward head, kyphosis, scoliosis, and leg length discrepancies. A more objective measure is the REEDCO posture screen (see Chapter 7), which grades 10 posture domains on a scale from 1 to 10.

Balance assessment is complex, and there is a multitude of screening devices and assessment tools being developed to meet varying needs. Unfortunately, few have been validated with the frail or institutionalized population. However, more objective measures of dynamic balance than poor, fair, and good include the Berg Balance Test,[9] Functional Reach Test,[10] Tinetti's Functional Mobility Scale,[11] and Wolfson's Postural Stress Test.[12] Timed measures of static balance include standing on one leg, Romberg, and sharpened Romberg.

Locomotion assessment includes wheelchair propulsion and gait analysis. When assessing wheelchair propulsion, one notes the distance, time, and amount of assistance needed by the patient. Also included in the assessment is the ability to make turns, go on and off elevators, and propel across varied floor surfaces, as well as parts management of brakes, foot pedals, and arm boards. For gait analysis, distance, time, and amount of assistance are recorded along with gait deviations, appliances, and devices used. The functional ambulation profile[13] is an objective way to perform gait analysis. Endurance may be assessed during the locomotion assessment. Heart rate, respiration rate, and blood pressure should be monitored before and after the activity, and a timed walk of certain distance (for example, 6-minute walk test)[14,15] is an objective way to measure endurance.

Minimum Data Set

The resident assessment instrument (RAI) was devised to comply with sections 1819 and 1919 of the Social Security Act, which mandates nursing home facilities to conduct comprehensive, accurate, standardized, and reproducible assessments of each resident's functional capacity.[16] The RAI consists of the minimum data set (MDS) and the resident assessment protocols (RAPs). The purpose of these assessments is to develop a plan of care that will enable the resident to attain or maintain the highest practical physical, mental, and psychosocial functioning. Through standardized definitions and coding categories, the MDS provides information about residents' strengths, needs, and preferences. The RAPs are 18 "triggered" conditions that often affect nursing home residents. The RAPs are used to target particular problem areas for care plan review.

The timetables for completing the RAI are rigid. The MDS and RAPs must be completed by the end of the 14th day of residency for any new admission. Care plans that emanate from the RAPs must be completed by the 21st day of residency. Annual reassessments must be completed within 12 months of the most recent MDS. Quarterly review of selected MDS items are required no less than once every 3 months. RAPs are not required to be completed for quarterly reviews.

A full MDS and RAPs are completed when a significant, permanent change in resident status occurs. Guidelines for determining a significant, permanent change are clearly outlined. The first includes deterioration in two or more activities of daily living. Another change considered significant is the loss of ability to walk freely or to use one's hands to grasp small objects. If the resident exhibits a deterioration in behavior or mood to the point where daily problems arise or relationships have become problematic, a new RAI must be completed. Likewise, if there is a permanent deterioration in health status, or if the resident has not responded to treatment and the change involves onset of significant weight loss, threat to life, a serious clinical complication, or a new diagnosis of a condition likely to affect the resident's physical, mental, or psychosocial well-being over a prolonged period of time, a new RAI is needed. The last criterion for a significant change is when the resident exhibits improved behavior, mood, or functional health status to the extent that the established plan of care no longer matches what is needed.

Although a registered nurse is the coordinator of the RAI, each discipline can complete sections in its area of expertise. Physical and occupational therapists are often required to complete the sections on body control problems, contractures, mobility appliances and devices, and task segmentation. The section on body control problems helps to identify the presence of structural impairments that may affect the resident's ability to perform activities. This section questions whether residents are bedfast, hemiplegic, hemiparetic, or quadriplegic; if they have partial loss of voluntary leg or arm movement; or if they have had an amputation. The contracture section includes all body parts and is defined as any restriction of full range of motion of any joint due to deformity, disuse, or pain. The mobility appliances and devices sections determine which appliances, devices, or personal assistance protocols are used or followed when residents perform ADL or other activities. The task segmentation section queries whether the resident is able to perform a task independently if it is broken down into component parts.

An RAP commonly assigned to the therapies is the "fall" RAP. It is triggered if residents fell during the past 180 days, had a hip or other fracture during the past 180 days, use any psychoactive drugs, have an impaired sense of balance as defined in the body-control section of the MDS, or have a diagnosis of hemiplegia or quadriplegia. The "fall" RAP guides the therapist in the planning process so that both intrinsic and extrinsic factors contributing to falls are evaluated.

The RAI is an excellent tool for comprehensively screening a nursing home resident. Its completion requires that all members of the team review the resident's record thoroughly, communicate with and observe the resident closely, communicate with other direct-care staff, including the physician, and talk with the resident's family or next of kin. It assists in ensuring that the highest equality care for the resident is attained.

MAXIMIZING MOTIVATION AND LEARNING SKILLS

Misunderstandings of the motivation of the frail elderly and confusion regarding their ability to process new information has led to significant underachievement in the rehabilitation setting. This section attempts to present a better understanding of these two components in the treatment of the frail elderly.

Motivation

Motivation has been defined in psychological literature as the need, drive, or desire to act in a certain way to achieve a certain end.[17] The frail elderly are often mislabeled as poorly motivated, but frail elders do display motivation. Knowledge of certain psychological factors may enhance the therapist's perception of the elder's level of motivation.

One factor that affects motivation is the purpose of a given task. The task must have obvious meaning for the elderly to perform it well.[18] If the patient is left alone with the instructions to lift a weighted cane 30 times, it is highly probable that the task will not be performed because it is not obviously meaningful to the frail elder. Another factor that can affect the therapist's perception of motivation is that elders will do better at a given task if they are allowed to proceed at their own pace in a low-stress environment. Attempting to get through 10 new exercises in a 30-minute session is often a futile task for the therapist and frustrating for the patient. The third factor affecting motivation is risk. Elders tend to avoid an activity if they feel that they will fail. They avoid taking the risk (error of omission) versus trying (error of commission). It may appear that the elder does not want to perform a new activity, but in reality he or she may be avoiding the risk of failure.

The condition that therapists term "poor motivation" may actually be due to a variety of physical or pyschological changes that the frail elder is unable to control.[19] Decreased cognition is one major change that affects some frail elders' ability to appear motivated. Since motivation is a complex cognitive task, delirium or dementia can affect the ability to understand the rationale behind certain activities. Elders consequently do not perform an activity as recommended and are thus mislabeled "poorly motivated." Frail elders also may realize that despite rehabilitation, they have less function and more dependency than previously.[18] This reduced final outcome of rehabilitation may be misinterpreted as "poor motivation."

Additionally, frail elders may exhibit a reduced drive regulation. This means that, through a series of losses and compromises, the elder may be more comfortable with dependency and decreasing physical activity. Walking 500 feet outdoors may no longer be the personal goal of the frail elder; walking 50 feet from the bathroom to the living room is as much as they desire to do. Motivation may also appear decreased during times of stress.[18] Illness, functional losses, and anxiety related to the future can provide a deterrent to what therapists label as motivation.

Therapists can directly affect and improve perceived poor motivation. If it is viewed as a treatable problem, and not as an excuse to exclude someone, many more frail elders would receive appropriate care. Therapists may refer the elder to a physician for a psychological or medical workup to rule out depression, delirium, or dementia. Therapists should decide upon goals *with* their patients; many times discrepancies in patients' and therapists' goals are part of the cause of behavior that is labeled "poorly motivated." Therapists should also evaluate their own expectations of the patient's motivation. It is common for inexperienced therapists to transfer their level of motivation to the patient. In many cases, however, the patient is not a young, potentially employable person with one deficit, but rather someone who has multiple comorbid problems and may make only modest gains and return to a semi-dependent lifestyle. Therapists can also enhance the elder's performance by eliminating blocks in the rehabilitation setting. Creating a least-stressful setting and avoiding fast-paced activities are examples of enhancing performance.

Learning

The ability to learn depends on age-related changes in cognition and mental status.[17,18] Therapists can arrange successful learning situations by recognizing several age-related changes in learning. For example, free recall of information, acquisition of new information, solving complex and novel problems, and timed responses are all impaired with aging. There are no significant age-related changes in the elders' ability to retrieve information by category or in elders' crystallized intelligence (the intelligence needed for manipulation of previously learned information).[19,20]

Learning, like motivation, is affected by a series of physical and psychological factors[21,22] that must be taken into consideration for performance to be optimized. Of utmost importance is the visual and auditory acuity of the learner. The elder must be able to see and hear the information to be learned. The therapist should provide the elder with large-print material on high-contrast paper (preferably black print on white or ecru paper). Speech should be slow and lower than normal, and every syllable should be enunciated clearly. If necessary, speak in the "better" ear or use a biaural hearing device that amplifies the conversation.

Health status and level of anxiety will also affect learning. Just as in younger groups, illness affects the ability to concentrate. The frail elderly, who are often being treated because of some physical problem along with many other comorbid conditions, can generally be considered to have poor health status. Additionally, anxiety can often block other thoughts from entering into consciousness. These conditions can impede learning and hearing; extra time and patience are necessary to encourage learning under these circumstances.

Motivation, as stated before, is related to meaningfulness of the activity and the speed at which the activity is paced. If learning is the activity, the material presented must be meaningful to the patient and presented in an unrushed fashion. Both of these factors can be incorporated into the treatment program by the therapist to enhance motivation and learning.

Practice and feedback are two other therapist-dependent factors that can be used to augment learning. As with any activity, skill is developed after hours of practice. Whatever the particular exercise or task the elder needs to learn, practice sessions should be arranged to reinforce the learning process. Positive feedback, given in a timely fashion, has also been shown to facilitate learning.

Learning has also been shown to be affected by inherent characteristics of the elders themselves. Their intelligence level and past experiences contribute to what information will be perceived as novel and complex or as previously learned. Since impairment in novel, complex problem solving is an age-related cognitive change, elders who perceive the learning situation as such may take longer to learn the task at hand. Conversely, because of past experiences, another frail elder may perceive the same task as "commonplace" and learn it rather quickly. It becomes obvious that each elder must be viewed individually.

Elders also have individual learning styles. Learning styles vary from visual to auditory, passive to active, detail to main idea, and analytical to intuitive.[22] The person who is visually oriented will learn more easily if the material is presented in a visual format (handouts, slide presentation, books) versus lecture format (auditory). Active learners will learn more easily if allowed to participate in small-group discussions or experiential "lab stations." This is in contrast to the passive learner, who would prefer to be told all and not participate. The detail-oriented learner performs best when every step of a given process is completely dissected and presented as such. The main-idea learner, in contrast, would be overwhelmed with such details and prefers a simple task or purpose. Finally, the intuitive learner acquires information by "feel," whereas the analytical learner figures out a rationale and process for the task at hand.

Darkenwald and Merriam[23] have outlined principles for facilitating learning in the older adult. Several of these principles summarize the guidelines therapists should follow when treating the frail elder. The first principle is that the readiness of frail elders to learn or perform depends on their previous learning or performance. A patient who had unsuccessful therapy prior to this visit may not learn or perform as quickly now.

Another principle is that intrinsic motivation produces more pervasive and permanent learning. Tasks and material that are meaningful to the elder are more fully and easily learned. The key for therapists is to find out what the motivating factors are for the frail patient. Other principles include presenting the material in an organized way and allowing for repetition, both of which enhance learning. Darkenwald and Merriam also state that positive reinforcement is effective to facilitate learning and that retention improves with active participation.

All of these aforementioned physical and psychological factors affect learning; some are therapist-controlled while others are individually mediated. No matter what the origin of the factor, it is necessary for the therapist to arrange a setting that will optimize the learning potential of the frail elder.

CONTINUUM OF CARE

When an older person suffers from disability, considerations must be given to the care and living arrangements that will be necessary in the following days, weeks, months, and even years. Below is a description of the primary areas for receiving health care and the living arrangements associated with each type of facility.

An acute-care hospital is an inpatient care facility for an emergency or acute illness such as a stroke or hip fracture. These facilities are driven by diagnostic-related group (DRG) assessments, which means that length of stay (LOS) depends on the diagnosis. Medicare generally pays for all medications, nursing services, special care units, semiprivate room, rehabilitation, labs, x-rays, durable medical equipment, and blood transfusions while the patient is in hospital.[24] Medicare pays for all service less a $676 deduction in a 60-day benefit period; all but $169 for days 61 to 90; all but $338 for days 91 to 150; and nothing beyond 150 days. The average LOS depends on diagnosis.

Rehabilitation centers provide intensive care for rehabilitation dysfunction. The patient must be able to tolerate 3 to 5 hours of intensive rehabilitation daily. The usual LOS is 30 days. Medicare generally pays 80 percent of the costs. The usual place of discharge is home.

Skilled nursing facilities (SNF) provide care to patients who require 24-hour observation·and highly technical care of unstable medical conditions that may qualify for rehabilitation services. The patient-to-caregiver ratio is about 9:1. Staff time averages 5.7 min/hr. Average LOS is variable; it can be for a lifetime or for 1 week. Medicare Part A generally pays for all medications, nursing services, special care units, and semiprivate room, rehabilitation, labs, x-rays, durable medical equipment, and blood transfusions while the patient is in the SNF.[24] Medicare pays for 100 percent of the first 20 days; after the 21st day, there is an $87.50 (changes year) copayment. Beyond 100 days, Medicare Part A pays nothing for this care.[24] Any patient can pick up Medicare Part B for a change in function or to establish a maintenance program. After 100 days, 80 percent of rehabilitation services will be paid. Part B does pay 80 percent immediately if the patient is not covered under Part A and meets the previous criteria.[24]

Intermediate care facilities (ICF) provide care to patients who do not need round-the-clock nursing care but are still unable to function independently. An RN or LPN is on site for at least 4 hours per week. Primary care is given by nurse's aides. Patient-to-caregiver ratio is about 16:1. Staff time averages 4.25 min/h.[25] The patient must be approved for ICF. Medicare pays nothing for this type of care. The average LOS is 1 week to a lifetime. The actual facilities are rarely only SNF or ICF. There is usually a mixture of both types of patients.

Rest homes are sheltered living environments for those who need minimal assistance with activities of daily living.[25] Usually 20 or more residents live in these facilities. Staff are not required to have medical training, but home care can be ordered. Rest homes cost half of SNFs and Medicare pays for none of the charges. The average LOS is usually the rest of the person's life.

Family care homes are the same as rest homes but smaller (usually fewer than eight residents).[25] These have more of a family setting type of environment. Congregate or shared housing refers to shared living arrangements with friends and relatives or in small group homes. Medicare does not pay for this type of care.

Retirement communities are independent living arrangements with securities, emergency medical service, and some supplemental services. Some staff members are available to help with meals, laundry, recreation, and health services. Medicare does not pay for this type of care.

Home health care is skilled care consisting of rehabilitation services that can be received in the home if the person is homebound, has a doctor's referral that is updated every 60 days, needs skilled care that is intermittent in nature, is making progress, and receives rehabilitation three to five times a week. The average LOS is 6 weeks. Medicare Part A pays for five times a week and pays the full approved cost.[24] Medicare Part B pays for three times a week and pays the full approved cost.

Outpatient rehabilitation is for older patients who receive outpatient services with a doctor's prescription; they must be seen by a doctor every 30 days to continue. The patient is responsible for $100 deductible and any noncovered or unapproved amounts. If the therapist takes assignment, the patient is not responsible for the unapproved amounts. Medicare pays up to $720 (80 percent of $900 limit) for outpatient physical therapy and occupational therapy provided in a therapist-owned clinic.[24] Medicare does not pay for services by independent speech pathologists. In comprehensive outpatient rehabilitation facilities (CORFs), there is no limit on payment; however, the patient must need skilled care prescribed by the doctor.

Day care refers to daily supervised, programmed activities; lunch is provided to moderately to minimally impaired elders. Costs range from $20 to $50 per day. This arrangement allows the family caregiver to work outside the home.

Hospice care is for the terminally ill (home or inpatient). The recipient must receive care at a Medicare participating hospice or at home. Doctors must certify that the patient has fewer than 6 months to live. Hospice care is covered by Medicare and there are no deductibles. Medicare also covers nursing, doctors, drugs, rehabilitation, homemaker, social services, short-term care, respite care, and counseling.[25]

PHYSICAL RESTRAINTS

Physical restraints have been used in nursing homes and hospitals for many years in the United States. A review of the literature shows that restraints are used for several reasons.[26,27] Reasons cited include the desire to prevent the patient from falling, sliding out of the wheelchair, wandering off into unfamiliar surroundings, or getting into other patients' belongings. Restraints are used to manage incontinence and keep the patient from slipping on a wet floor and falling. In reality, the initial reasons for restraint are often lost, and there may be little or no evidence of any real danger of the patient wandering off or falling.

The adverse side effects of physical restraint use are well documented.[26–28] Restraint use has been associated with fecal and urinary incontinence, skin abrasions, pressure sores, circulatory obstructions, cardiac stress, poor appetite, dehydration, death by strangulation, loss of personal autonomy, and a cause or exacerbation of agitation. Recent literature questions the effectiveness of restraints in preventing injury.[29]

Because of the adverse effects of restraint use, its limited use in European countries, and its questionable usefulness in preventing injuries, the

Federal government has developed new regulations that govern the use of restraints:[30]

> Patients have the right to be free from physical or mental abuse, corporal punishment, involuntary seclusion, and any physical or chemical restraints imposed for purposes of discipline or convenience and not required to treat the resident's medical symptoms. Restraints may only be imposed (I) to ensure the physical safety of the resident or other residents, and (II) only upon the written order of a physician that specifies the duration and circumstances under which the restraints are to be used (except in emergency circumstances specified by the Secretary) until such an order could reasonably be obtained. (p. 188)

These regulations have been interpreted as follows

Physical restraints are any manual method or physical or mechanical device, material, or equipment attached or adjacent to the resident's body that the individual cannot remove easily and that restricts freedom of movement or normal access to one's body.[31] Leg restraints, arm restraints, hand mitts, soft ties or vests, wheelchair safety bars, and geri-chairs **are** all physical restraints.

Psychoactive drugs are drugs prescribed to control mood, mental status, or behavior. These include sedative hypnotics and antianxiety agents such as Restoril, Halcion, Ativan, Valium; antidepressants such as Elavil, Tofranil, Marplan, Nardil; antipsychotics such as Thorazine, Mellaril, Navane, Haldol.

Discipline is any action taken by the facility for the express purpose of punishing or penalizing residents.

Convenience is any action taken by the facility to control resident behavior or maintain residents with the least amount of effort by the facility and not in the residents' best interest. All of the original reasons stated for restraint use could be interpreted as convenience measures by the Department of Health, including restraint to manage incontinence, prevent falls or wandering, etc.

Less restrictive measures than restraints, such as pillows, pads, and removable lap trays, coupled with appropriate exercise, are often effective in achieving proper body position, balance, alignment, and preventing contractures. A facility must have evidence of consultation with appropriate health professionals, such as occupational or physical therapists in the use of less restrictive supportive devices *prior to* using physical restraints as defined in this guideline for such purposes.[31]

If, after a trial of less restrictive measures, the facility decides that a physical restraint would enable and promote greater functional independence, the use of the restraining device must first be explained to the resident, family member, or legal representative. If the resident, family member, or legal representative agrees to this treatment alternative, the restraining device may be used for the specific periods for which it has been determined to be an enabler.

If there are medical symptoms that are life-threatening (such as dehydration, electrolyte imbalance, urinary blockage), a restraint may be used temporarily to provide necessary life-saving treatment. Physical restraints may be used for *brief periods* to allow medical treatment to proceed, if there is documented evidence of resident or legal representative approval of the treatment.

Since the inception of OBRA 87,[30] many nursing homes are striving to achieve restraint-free or restraint-appropriate environments. Alternatives to restraint use are becoming more common. For instance, instead of side rails, vests, or body holders in bed to manage nighttime incontinence, a weight-sensitive sensor mat can be placed under the mattress. There are several commercially available units that can be hooked into the call-bell system. A less technical attempt would be to initiate frequent or anticipatory toileting for problem cases; for example, toilet residents every 2 hours. Keeping the environment as safe as possible involves keeping the side rails down, having the bed at the lowest position, keeping a night light on, having the resident's socks off, providing frequent observations, having a commode near the bed, and maintaining an obstacle-free path in the room.

If the problem is poor wheelchair positioning in which the resident continually slides out of the wheelchair, various suggestions can be made. If the resident is immobile or nonambulatory, a wedge can be used if it does not prevent standing for that particular patient. A lapboard can be used for that resident if it is documented that the lapboard is used for symmetrical posturing necessary for feeding, or that the lapboard enables the resident to perform tabletop activities for diversion or for decreasing agitated states. Adding nonslip material (Dycem) under the cushion or eliminating nylon hoyer lift cradles are often effective in alleviating sliding. Some residents slide only in the late afternoon. For these frail elders, afternoon naps are often the intervention of choice. Sliding may also be due to skin irritations and wet diapers. Alleviation of the primary problem may reduce the sliding.

If sliding is exhibited by semiambulatory or mobile patients who "voluntarily" push into extension, avoiding wheelchair use and using stationary semireclining chairs is often helpful. Additionally, frequent assisted ambulation may inhibit poor wheelchair posture. For ambulatory patients who frequently fall, avoiding use of wheelchairs is recommended because wheelchair use has been associated with increased incidence of injury and with falls.[32]

THE FUTURE OF PROVIDING CARE TO THE FRAIL ELDERLY

Resource utilization groups (RUGS) is a system of patient classification that is used for Medicaid reimbursement in a growing number of states. In the RUGS-II classification system, five general categories of care are subdivided into 16 different patient types based on the resident's ADL abilities.[33] The general category and ADL score are determined after a patient review instrument (PRI) is completed by a trained screener (usually a nurse). These scores comprise a case mix index (CMI) for each individual. The CMIs of each resident are averaged, and the nursing home CMI is compared to other nursing homes' CMIs to determine their percentage of state funding.

The general categories of care in descending reimbursement order are rehabilitation, special care, clinically complex, behavioral, and physically reduced. The rehab category includes residents who receive PT or OT at least 5 days a week and have a restorative goal. "Special care" includes patients with coma, quadriplegia, multiple sclerosis, and stage 4 pressure sores and patients who require nasogastric feedings, IVs, and suctioning. The "clinically complex" group includes residents with diagnoses of cerebral palsy, hemiplegia, urinary tract infection, dehydration, internal bleeding, stasis ulcers, or terminal illness; and those who require oxygen, wound care, chemotherapy, transfusions, or at least weekly visits by an MD. The "behavioral" group includes residents who are verbally or physically aggressive or disruptive, and residents who hallucinate. The final category is termed "physically reduced" and includes residents who do not fall into any of the other categories.

A PRI is completed for every admission to a nursing home. Figure 19–1 shows the ADL section of the PRI. It is also completed biannually for every resident to redetermine the CMI. Because the general idea of RUGS is that the more care a resident requires, the higher the reimbursement, it would be financially desirable for the therapists to treat as many residents who need restorative therapy as possible during the biannual assessments. Even though there are specific qualifiers for a resident to be considered "restorative," the RUGS system provides therapists with an incentive to treat all patients who need restorative PT or OT regardless of their payment source.

The development of RUGS-III, which emphasizes rehabilitation even more strongly, appears to be very similar to parts of the MDS. It has been posited that RUGS will be incorporated into the MDS framework so that one screening device will be used for both clinical and financial reasons. This union would facilitate greater team input, which would serve to provide the highest quality care to the residents of skilled nursing facilities.

RESOURCES FOR THE AGING INDIVIDUAL

Older persons commonly present an array of problems to the health care professional. Because older adults tend to have not one health care problem but a combination of conditions, it is especially important for the rehabilitation professional in geriatrics to be able to refer patients to and for appropriate resources. The appendix is a list of a variety of resources for aging persons.

III. ACTIVITIES OF DAILY LIVING (ADLs)

Answer questions 19–22 according to how each task was completed, 60% of the time during the past four weeks or since admission whichever is shorter (regardless of cause). Read the Changed Condition Rule and definitions in the instructions

19   EATING: PROCESS OF GETTING FOOD BY ANY MEANS FROM THE RECEPTACLE INTO THE BODY (FOR EXAMPLE, PLATE, CUP, TUBE).

1=Feeds self without supervision or physical assistance. May use adaptive equipment.

2=Requires intermittent supervision (that is, verbal enc-encouragement/guidance) and/or minimal physical assistance with minor parts of eating, such as cutting food, buttering bread or opening milk carton.

3=Requires continual help (encouragement/teaching/ physical assistance) with eating or meal will not be completed.

4=Totally fed by hand; patient does not manually participate.

5=Tube or parenteral feeding for primary intake of food. (Not just for supplemental nourishments.)

20   MOBILITY: HOW THE PATIENT MOVES ABOUT.

1=Walks with no supervision or human assistance. May require mechanical device (for example, a walker), but not a wheelchair.

2=Walks with intermittent supervision (that is, verbal cueing and observation). May require human assistance for difficult parts of walking (for example, stairs, ramps).

3=Walks with constant one-to-one supervision and/or constant physical assistance.

4=Wheels with no supervision or assistance, except for difficult maneuvers (for example, elevators, ramps). May actually be able to walk but generally does not move.

5=Is wheeled, chairfast, or bedfast. Relies on someone   else to move about, if at all.

21   TRANSFER: PROCESS OF MOVING BETWEEN POSITIONS, TO/FROM BED, CHAIR, STANDING, (EXCLUDE TRANSFERS TO/FROM BATH AND TOILET).

1=Requires no supervision of physical assistance to complete necessary transfer. May use equipment,such as railings, trapeze.

2=Requires intermittent supervision (that is, verbal cueing, guidance) and/or physical assistance for difficult maneuvers only.

3=Requires one person to provide constant guidance, steadiness and/or physical assistance. Patient may participate in transfer.

4=Requires *two* people to provide constant supervision and/or physically lift. May need lifting equipment.

5=Cannot and is not gotten out of bed.

22   TOILETING: PROCESS OF GETTING TO AND FROM A TOILET (OR USE OF OTHER TOILETING EQUIPMENT, SUCH AS BEDPAN), TRANSFERRING ON AND OFF TOILET, CLEANSING SELF AFTER ELIMINATION AND ADJUSTING CLOTHES.

1=Requires no supervision or physical assistance. May require special equipment, such as a raised toilet or grab bars.

2=Requires *intermittent* supervision for safety or encouragement; or minor physical assistance (for example, clothes adjustment or washing hands.

3=Continent of bowl and bladder. Requires constant supervision and/or physical assistance with major/all parts of the task, *including* applications (i.e., colostomy, ileostomy, urinary catheter.

4=Incontinent of bowel *and/or* bladder, but is taken to a bathroom every two to four hours during the day and as needed at night.

FIGURE 19–1. The activities of daily living of the Patient Review Instrument.

SUMMARY

By implementing the various tools and techniques presented in this chapter and by using well-thought-out treatment approaches, therapists can ensure improved outcomes for frail elderly patients. Only by working toward a better understanding of the complete treatment strategy, however, will therapists be able to provide the greatest gains for their patients. It is not sufficient to concentrate in one area while ignoring the others; a truly global approach must be envisioned and then practiced.

REFERENCES

1. Kane, RL, Ouslander, JG, and Abrass, IB: Essentials of Clinical Geriatrics, ed 2. McGraw-Hill, New York, 1989.
2. O'Neil, MB, Woodard, M, Sosa, V, Hunter, L, Mulrow, CD, Gerety, MB, and Tuley, M: Physical therapy assessment and treatment protocol for nursing home residents. Phys Ther 72:596, 1992.
3. Folstein, MF, Folstein, SE, and McHugh, PR: Mini-mental state: A practical method for grading the cognitive state of patients for the clinician. J Psych Res 12:189, 1975.
4. Pfeiffer, E: A short portable mental status questionnaire for the assessment of organic brain deficit in elderly patients. J Am Geriatr Soc 23:433, 1975.
5. Kendall, FP, McCreary, EK, and Provance, P: Muscles, Testing and Function with Posture and Pain, ed 4. Williams & Wilkins, Baltimore, 1993.
6. Daniels, L and Worthingham, C: Muscle Testing. Techniques of Manual Examination. WB Saunders, Philadelphia, 1980.
7. Huskisson, EC: Measurement of pain. Lancet 2:1127, 1974.
8. Fox, TC (ed): Long-Term Care Administration: Statndards and Guidelines for Long-Term Care Facilities. National Health Publishing, Owings Mills, MD, 1989.
9. Berg, KO, Wood-Dauphinee, SL, Williams, JI, and Maki, B: Measuring balance in the elderly: Validation of an instrument. Can J of Public Health, 83 (Suppl 2):S7, 1992.
10. Duncan, PW, Weiner, DK, Chandler, J, and Studenski, S: Functional reach: A new clinical measure of balance. J Gerontol, 45:M192, 1990.
11. Tinetti, ME: Performance-oriented assessment of mobility problems in elderly patients. J Am Geriatr Soc 34:119, 1986.
12. Wolfson, L, Whipple, R, Amerman, P, and Kleinberg, A: Stressing the postural response: A quantitative method for testing balance. J Am Geriatr Soc 34:845, 1986.
13. Nelson, AJ: Functional ambulation profile. Phys Ther 54:1059, 1974.
14. Butland, RJA, Pang, J, and Gross, ER: Two-, six-, and twelve-minute walking test in respiratory disease. Br Med J 284:1607, 1982.
15. Guyatt, GH, Sullivan, MJ, Thompson PJ, Fallen, L, Pugsley, SO, Taylor, DW, and Berman, LB: The 6-minute walk: A new measure of exercise capacity in patients with chronic heart failure. Can Med Assoc J 132:919, 1985.
16. Feldman, J and Butler, C (eds): Multistate Nursing Home Case Mix and Quality Demonstration Training Manual. Eliot Press, Natick, MA, 1992.
17. Hesse, KA and Campion, EW: Motivating the geriatric patient for rehabilitation. J Am Geriatr Soc 31:586, 1983.
18. Hesse, KA, Campion, EW, and Karamouz, E: Attitudinal stumbling blocks to geriatric rehabilitation. J Am Geriatr Soc 32:747, 1984.
19. Welford, AT: Motivation, capacity, learning, and age. In Kastenbaum, R (ed): Old Age on the New Scene. Springer, New York, 1981.
20. Pryse-Phillips, W: Examination of the highest cerebral functions in the elderly.Sem Neurol 9:8, 1989.
21. Thompson, M: Education. The older learner. Paper given at APTA Combined Sections Meeting, San Antonio, TX 1993.
22. Gardener, DL, Greenwell, SC, and Costich, JF: Effective teaching of the older adult. Top Geriatr Rehabil 6(3):1, 1991.
23. Darkenwald, G and Merriam, S: Adult Education: Foundations of Practice. Harper & Row, New York, 1982.
24. U.S. Department of Health and Human Services: The Medicare 1993 Handbook. Baltimore, MD, 1993.
25. Snow, TL, Giduz, EH, McConnell, ES, Sanchez, CJ, and Wildman, DS: Handbook of Geriatric Practice Essentials, Aspen Publishers, Rockville, MD, 1988.
26. Hiatt, LG: Restraint reduction with special emphasis on wandering behavior. Top Geriat Rehabil 8(2):55, 1992.

27. Kirshbaum, L and O'Connor, SJ: The legal impact of restraining the elderly in nursing homes. Top Geriatr Rehabil 8(2);29, 1992.
28. Ebel, S: A new approach for physical therapists in the long-term care of Alzheimer pateints. American Journal of Alzheimer's Care and Related Disorders & Research, May/June, 12, 1992.
29. Tinetti, ME, Liu, W-L, and Ginter, SF: Mechanical restraint use and fall-related injuries among residents of skilled nursing facilities. Ann Int Med 116:364, 1992.
30. Omnibus Budget Reconciliation Act of Dec 22, 1987, PL No. 100–2003, 1987 U.S. Code Cong & Admin News (101 Stat.) 188.
31. U.S. Department of Health and Human Services, Health Care Financing Administration: Medicare, Medicaid, State Operations Manual: Provider Certification, Washington, DC, 1989.
32. Berry, G, Fisher, RH, and Lang, S: Detrimental incidents, including falls, in an elderly institutional population. J Am Geriatr Soc 29:322, 1981.
33. Schneider, DP, Fries, BE, Foley, WJ, Desmond, M, and Gormley, WJ: Case mix for nursing home payment: Resource utilization groups, version II. Health Care Financing Review (Ann Suppl 39), 1988.

Appendix

Resources for Aging Persons

Associations

Alzheimer's Disease and Related Disorders Association
70 E Lake Street
Suite 600
Chicago, IL 60601
(312) 853–3060

American Aging Association
42nd and Dewey Avenue
Omaha, NE 68105
(402) 559–4416

American Association of Homes for the Aging
1129 20th Street, NW
Suite 400
Washington, DC 20036–3489
(202) 296–5960

American Association of Retired Persons
1909 K Street, NW
Washington, DC 20049
(202) 872–4700

American College of Health Care Administrators
8120 Woodmont Ave
Suite 200
Bethesda, MD 20814
(301) 652–8384

American Geriatric Society
770 Lexington Avenue
Suite 400
New York, NY 10021
(212) 308–1414

American Health Care Association
1201 L Street NW
Washington, DC 20005
(202) 842–8444

Concerned Relatives of Nursing Homes Patients
3130 Mayfield Road
Cleveland Heights, OH 44118
(216) 321–0403

The Gerontological Society of America
1411 K Street NW
Suite 300
Washington, DC 20005
(202) 393-1411

Health Insurance Association of America
1025 Connecticut Avenue NW
Suite 1200
Washington, DC 20036

Help for Incontinent People
PO Box 544
Union, SC 29379
(803) 585–8789

Hospital Home Health
67 Peachtree Park Drive NE
Atlanta, GA 30309
(404) 351–4523

International Center for Social Gerontology
1411 K Street NW
Suite 300
Washington, DC 20005
(202) 393-1411

International Federation on Aging
1909 K Street NW   .
Washington, DC 20005
(202) 662–4987

Jewish Association for Services for the Aged
40 West 68th Street
New York, NY 10023
(212) 724–3200

Mid America Congress on Aging
9400 State Avenue
Room 110
Kansas City, KS 66112
(913) 788–9766

National Action Forum for Older Women
University of Maryland
Center for Aging
College Park, MD 20742
(301) 454–3311

National Alliance of Senior Citizens
2525 Wilson Boulevard
Arlington, VA 22201
(703) 528–4380

National Association of Area Agencies on Aging
600 Maryland Avenue SW
West Wing 208
Washington, DC 20024
(202) 323–4856

National Association of Mature People
1600 Ninth Street SW
2nd Floor
Sacramento, CA 95814
(916) 323–4856

National Association of Nutrition and Aging Services Program
c/o Aging Projects, Inc.
Wiley Building, 104 North Main
Hutchinson, KS 67501
(316) 669–8201

National Association of Older Americans
Volunteer Program Directors
11481 Bingham Terrace
Reston, VA 22091

National Association of Rehabilitation Facilities
5530 Wisconsin Avenue
Suite 955
Washington, DC 20015

National Association of State Units on Aging
2033 K Street NW
Suite 304
Washington, DC 20006
(202) 785–0707

National Association of Senior Companion
Project Directors
3225 Lyndale Avenue South
Minneapolis, MN 55408
(612) 827–5641

National Caucus and Center on Black Aged, Inc.
1424 K Street NW
Suite 500
Washington, DC 20005
(202) 637–8400

National Council of Senior Citizens
925 15th Street NW
Washington, DC 20005
(202) 347–8800

National Council on the Aging, Inc.
600 Maryland Avenue SW
West Wing 100
Washington, DC 20024
(202) 479–1200

National Geriatrics Society
212 West Wisconsin Avenue
3rd Floor
Milwaukee, WI 53203
(414) 272–4130

National Interfaith Coalition on Aging
PO Box 1924
Athens, GA 30603
(404) 353–1331

National Institute of Senior Citizens
c/o National Council on Aging
600 Maryland Avenue SW
West Wing 100
Washington, DC 20024

New Choice for the Best Years
(Formerly 50 Plus)
28 West 23rd Street
New York, NY 10010
(202) 633–4600

New England Gerontological Association
81 Cutts Road
Durham, NH 03824
(617) 374–0707

Older Women's League
730 11th Street NW
Suite 300
Washington, DC 20001
(202) 783–6686

Robert Wood Johnson Foundation, Inc.
PO Box 2316
Princeton, NJ 08540
(609) 452–8701

Rehabilitation
American Congress of Rehabilitation Medicine
130 South Michigan Avenue
Suite 1310
Chicago, IL 60603

American Occupational Therapy Association, Inc.
PO Box 1725
1383 Piccard Drive, Suite 300
Rockville, MD 20850–4375
(301) 948–9626

National Pacific/Asian Resource Center on Aging
1341 G Street NW
Suite 311
Washington, DC 20005

American Occupational Therapy Association
PO Box 1725
111 North Fairfax Street
Alexandria, VA 22314
(703) 684–2782

American Physical Therapy Association
111 North Fairfax Street
Alexandria, VA 22314
(703) 684–2782

Canadian Rehabilitation Council for the Disabled
1 Yonge Street
Suite 2110
Toronto, Ontario M5E 1E5
(416) 863–0340

Dizziness and Balance Disorders Association
Resource Center
Room 300
1015 Northwest 22nd Avenue
Portland, OR 97210
(503) 229–7348

National Parkinson Foundation, Inc.
1501 Ninth Avenue, NW
Miami, FL 33136
(305) 547–6666

National Rehabilitation Association
633 S Washington Street
Alexandria, VA 22314–4193
(703) 836–0850

National Stroke Association
1420 Odgen Street
Denver, CO 80218
(303) 839-1992

United Parkinson Foundation
360 W Superior Street
Chicago, IL 60610
(312) 664–2344

General Information
Modern Maturity
4201 Long Beach Boulevard

National Health Information Center
PO Box 1133
Washington, DC 20013
(800) 336–4797 or (703) 522–2590

Hot Lines
AIDS Hotlines
(800) 432–AIDS

National Health Information Clearinghouse
PO Box 1133
Washington, DC 20013
(800) 336–4797 or (703) 522–2590

Y-ME National Organization for Breast Cancer
(800) 221–2141 or (708) 799–8228

Support Groups
The American Self-Help Clearinghouse
St Clares Riverside Medical Center
Denville, NJ 07834
(201) 625–7101

National Self-Help Clearinghouse
25 West 43rd Street
New York, NY 10036
(212) 840–7606

Patient and Professional Education
Department of Health and Human Services
Public Health Services
Agency for Health Care Policy and Research
Executive Office Center
2101 East Jefferson Street
Suite 501
Rockville, MD 20910
(301) 594–1360

Robert Wood Foundation
Consumer Information Center
Pueblo, CO 81009

Women's Health Issues
The American College of Obstetrics and Gynecologists
600 Maryland Avenue SW
Suite 300 E
Washington, DC 20024
(202) 638–4680

Center for Climacteric Studies
University of Florida
901 NW 8th Avenue
Suite B1
Gainesville, FL 32601
(904) 392–3184

Hysterectomy Education Resources
422 Bryn Mawr Avenue
Bala Cynwyd, PA 19004
(215) 667–7757

National Women's Health Network
224 7th Street SE
Washington, DC 20024
(202) 223–6886

NIA Information Center
2209 Distribution Circle
Silver Spring, MD 20910

Nutrition and Physical Fitness
The American Dietetic Association
430 N Michigan Avenue
Chicago, IL 607611
(312) 280–5000

President's Council on Physical Fitness and Sports
450 5th Street NW
Suite 7103
Washington, DC 20001
(202) 272–3421

Medications
The AARP Pharmacy Service
PO Box NUIA
1 Prince Street
Alexandria, VA 22314
(703) 684–9244

American Pharmaceutical Association
2215 Constitution Avenue NW
Washington, DC 20037
(202) 628–4410

Food and Drug Administration
Division of Regulatory Affairs
Center for Drugs and Biologics
5600 Fisher Lane
Rockville, MD 20857
(301) 295–8012

Accident Prevention
American Association of Retired Persons
55 Alive/Mature Driving Program
Traffic and Driver Safety Program
601 E Street NW
Washington, DC 20004
(202) 434–2277 or 1 (800) 434–2277

National Safety Council
44 N Michigan Avenue
Chicago, IL 60611
(312) 527–4800

Osteoporosis
American Academy of Orthopedic Surgeons
222 S Prosperity Avenue
Park Ridge Avenue, IL 60068
(312) 823–7186

National Institute of Arthritis and Musculoskeletal and Skin Diseases
Public Information Office
Building 31, Room B2B15
Bethesda, MD 20892
(301) 496–9818

National Institute on Aging
Public Information Office
Building 31, Room 5C35
Bethesda, MD 20892
(301) 496–2947

National Osteoporosis Foundation
1625 Eye Street NW
Suite 1011
Washington, DC 20006
(202) 223–2226

Osteoarthritis
American Rheumatism Association
17 Executive Park Drive NE
Suite 280480
Atlanta, GA 30329
(404) 633–2377

Arthritis Foundation
1314 Spring Street
Atlanta, GA 30309
(404) 872–7100

Urinary Incontinence
Continence Restored
785 Park Avenue
New York, NY 10021
(212) 879–3131
or
407 Strawberry Hill Avenue
Stamford, CT 06902
(203) 348–0601

Help for Incontinent People Organization
PO Box 544
Union, SC 29379
(803) 579–7900

Simon Foundation
PO Box 835X
Wilmette, IL 60091
(800) 237–4666

Cognitive Changes
The Alzheimer's Disease Education and Referral Center
PO Box 8250
Silver Spring, MD 20907–8250
(301) 495–3311

National Mental Health Association, Inc.
1021 Prince Street
Alexandria, VA 22314–2971
(703) 684–7722

National Institute of Neurological and Communicative Disorders and
    Stroke
Public Information Office
Building 31, Room 8A06
Bethesda, MD 20892
(301) 496–5751

Cancer
American Cancer Society
District of Columbia Division
1825 Connecticut Avenue NW
Washington, DC 10009
(202) 483–2600

Canadian Cancer Society
77 Bloor Street W
Suite 1702
Toronto, Ontario M5S 3A1
(416) 961–7223

National Cancer Institute
9000 Rockville Pike
Building 31, Room 10A18
Bethesda, MD 20892
(800) 4–CANCER

Diabetes
American Diabetes Association
Two Park Avenue
New York, NY 10016
(212) 683–7444

Heart Disease
American Heart Association
7320 Greenville Avenue
Dallas, TX 75231
(214) 373–6300

National Heart, Lung and Blood Institute
900 Rockville Pike
Bethesda, MD 20892
(301) 496–4236

High Blood Pressure
High Blood Pressure Information Center
120/80 National Institute of Health
Bethesda, MD 20892
(301) 496–4000

Alcoholism
National Council on Alcoholism
12 W 21st Street
New York, NY 10010
(212) 206–6770

Database Resources
Compuserve
(800) 848–8199

Directory of Online Healthcare Databases
(503) 471–1627

Health Resources, Inc.
(501) 329–5272

Long-Term Housing Options
American Association of Homes for the Aging
1129 20th Street NW ˙
Washington, DC 20036
(202) 296–5960

National Association of Home Care
519 C Street NE
Stanton Park
Washington, DC 20002
(202) 547–7424

National Citizens' Coalition for Nursing Home Reform
1424 16th Street NW
Room L2
Washington, DC 20036
(202) 797–0657

Nursing Home Information Center
National Council of Senior Citizens
National Senior Citizens Education and Research Center
925 15th Street NW
Washington, DC 20005

Financial Planning
Social Security Administration
Office of Public Inquiries
6401 Security Boulevard
Baltimore, MD 21235
(410) 594–1234

Women's Equity Action League
1250 Eye Street NW
Suite 305
Washington, DC 20005
(202) 898–1588

Caregiving
Administration on Aging
Office of Human Development DHHS
330 Independence Avenue SW
Washington, DC 20201
(202) 245–0724

Children of Aging Parents
2761 Trenton Road
Levittown, PA 19056
(215) 945–6900

National Council for Homemaker-Home Health Aide Service, Inc.
235 Park Avenue South
New York, NY 10003

National Hospice Organization
1901 N Fort Myer Drive
Suite 307
Arlington, VA 22209
(703) 243–5900

National Institute on Adult Day Care
600 Maryland Avenue SW
West Wing 100
Washington, DC 20024
(202) 479–1200

Widowhood
ACTION
806 Connecticut Avenue NW
Washington, DC 20525
(800) 424–8580

Displaced Homemaker Network
1411 K Street NW
Washington, DC 20005
(202) 628–6767

Political Issues
The Grey Panthers
3635 Chestnut Street
Philadelphia, PA 19104
(215) 382–3300

Legal Issues
Commission on Legal Problems of the Elderly
1800 M Street NW
Washington, DC 20036
(202) 331–2297

National Senior Citizens Law Center
2025 M Street NW
Suite 400
Washington, DC 20036
(202) 887–5280

Index

An "f" indicates a figure. A "t" indicates a table.